T0323037

ACADEMY OF REHABILITATION PSYCHOLOGY SERIES

Series Editors

Bruce Caplan, Editor-in-Chief
Timothy Elliott
Janet Farmer
Robert Frank
Barry Nierenberg
George Prigatano
Daniel Rohe
Stephen Wegener

Volumes in the Series

Ethics Field Guide: Applications in Rehabilitation Psychology
Thomas R. Kerkhoff and Stephanie L. Hanson

The Social Psychology of Disability
Dana S. Dunn

Disability-Affirmative Therapy: A Case Formulation Template for Clients with Disabilities
Rhoda Olkin

Validity Assessment in Rehabilitation Psychology and Settings
Dominic A. Carone and Shane S. Bush

Suicide Prevention after Neurodisability: An Evidence-Informed Approach
Grahame K. Simpson and Lisa A. Brenner

Understanding the Experience of Disability: Perspectives from Social and Rehabilitation Psychology
Dana S. Dunn

Disability as Diversity: Developing Cultural Competence
Erin E. Andrews

Teaching Disability: Practical Activities for In Class and Homework
Rhoda Olkin

Critical Care Psychology and Rehabilitation: Principles and Practice
Kirk J. Stucky and Jennifer E. Jutte

Critical Care Psychology and Rehabilitation

PRINCIPLES AND PRACTICE

Edited by Kirk J. Stucky, PsyD, ABPP-CN, RP and
Jennifer E. Jutte, PhD, MPH

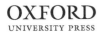
OXFORD
UNIVERSITY PRESS

OXFORD
UNIVERSITY PRESS

Oxford University Press is a department of the University of Oxford. It furthers
the University's objective of excellence in research, scholarship, and education
by publishing worldwide. Oxford is a registered trade mark of Oxford University
Press in the UK and certain other countries.

Published in the United States of America by Oxford University Press
198 Madison Avenue, New York, NY 10016, United States of America.

Library of Congress Cataloging-in-Publication Data
Names: Stucky, Kirk J., editor. | Jutte, Jennifer E., editor.
Title: Critical care psychology and rehabilitation : principles and practice /
[edited by] Kirk J. Stucky and Jennifer E. Jutte.
Description: New York, NY : Oxford University Press, [2022] |
Series: Academy of rehab psych series | Includes bibliographical references and index. |
Identifiers: LCCN 2021027772 (print) | LCCN 2021027773 (ebook) |
ISBN 9780190077013 (paperback) | ISBN 9780190077037 (epub) |
ISBN 9780197604199
Subjects: LCSH: Medicine and psychology. | Critical care medicine.
Classification: LCC R726.5 .C75 2022 (print) | LCC R726.5 (ebook) |
DDC 616.02/8—dc23
LC record available at https://lccn.loc.gov/2021027772
LC ebook record available at https://lccn.loc.gov/2021027773

DOI: 10.1093/oso/9780190077013.001.0001

For Hurley Medical Center and the patients, families, staff, and multifaceted community it serves. I have received immeasurably more than what has been given. Thank you.
Kirk J. Stucky

For mentors who provided inspiration and collaboration throughout my journey. For my husband and children who may not always understand the what or how of what I do, but who provide endless support for the why. Thank you.
Jennifer E. Jutte

Contents

List of Illustrations

TABLES

BOXES

Preface

THIS BOOK HOLDS much personal significance for me.

During the time I was completing my editorial review of the text, I was diagnosed with a relatively rare condition—constrictive pericarditis—in which abnormal growth on the outside of the pericardium interferes with normal functioning of the heart. Consequences included shortness of breath and deteriorating kidney function. The treatment of choice was surgical intervention to remove the pericardium to be followed by several days in intensive care. It was pure serendipity that I was concurrently immersed in the chapters of this book. I read them with a view to preparing myself for whatever time I would need to spend in the ICU.

The surgery went smoothly, as did my recovery. I spent 5 days in the hospital and was discharged home, intending to begin cardiac rehabilitation. However, 2 weeks later, an unrelated complication (bleeding ulcer) derailed this plan. The ulcer was cauterized in a local emergency room, and I was transferred to (a different) ICU, where I remained for 2 weeks. During that time, I was intubated/extubated and heavily sedated on two occasions and placed on a ventilator for 2 days.

It was during the second stint in ICU that I made most use of the knowledge and insights I had gleaned from this text as well as recalling relevant episodes from my career as a rehabilitation neuropsychologist. A couple of examples may suffice.

First, I was better prepared for the inevitable sleep disruption, which was the product of several factors: physical discomfort, nighttime noise on the unit, a nasogastric tube that hindered breathing, and occasional intrusions by staff needing to take vital signs or administer pills or injections. After several consecutive nights with little sustained sleep, confusion set in. I awoke convinced that I had just been in the living room at home drinking tea that I had made in the kitchen, and this misperception persisted for at least an hour. Subsequently, I was able to "normalize" that experience as a common reaction to an abnormal situation.

Having been confined to bed for over a week, I was eager to begin mobilization and to see just how physically degraded I had become. Repeated inquiries about when physical therapy would start were met with assurances that it would start "soon." However, it was not until 3 days before discharge that any therapy was provided, and this consisted of three sessions lasting a total of about 30 minutes. In the meantime, my frustration and demoralization spiked, as I imagined (incorrectly, as it turned out) that it would be several weeks before I could walk, even with the use of a walker.

While I found most staff to be cordial and responsive to my many questions, I share the view of Eileen Rubin (Chapter 2) that the nurses were the kindest and most encouraging of all, dealing with me as an adult rather than a "patient" and willing to converse and encourage me to see beyond my time in the ICU. While frustration and discouragement about my current limitations were unavoidable during my time in ICU, with the help of certain nurses I was able to remind myself of a point I had frequently made during my work life to rehabilitation patients who were demoralized at their slow pace of improvement—specifically, a reminder that while it might be impossible to avoid comparing their current condition to their pre-illness or pre-injury state, an alternate (and less distressing) perspective was to contrast the current level with that at the time of entry into the ICU, thereby encouraging recognition of some degree of progress.

Several authors in this book address the importance of keeping family members informed and involved. I would add a related point: the inestimable value of having an articulate and forceful advocate to solicit (and convey) information to staff about a patient's status, needs, concerns, and so forth and to question staff about the purpose(s) of various treatments as well as goals and plans for discharge. One's status as an ICU patient is often accompanied by depletion of energy and critical thinking ability that can incline one to simply "go along" without raising a fuss. An advocate can raise those necessary fusses on behalf of loved ones who may not have the energy or capacity to do so. In my own case, a far-too-premature discharge was avoided with the help of vigorous intervention by my wife.

While these anecdotes may provide readers with some idea of the value of the well-established principles and practices of rehabilitation psychology in the ICU, the current text will more adequately equip rehabilitation psychologists who elect to meet the challenges of working in this heretofore-overlooked venue. ICU staff can certainly benefit from the observations, perspectives, and interpretations provided by rehabilitation psychologists. In orchestrating this volume, Drs. Stucky and Jutte have done a great service to the specialty and the patients we serve.

Bruce Caplan, PhD, ABPP (RP, CN)

May 2021

Acknowledgments

The idea for this book was born in 2014 during a lively collegial conversation at the American Psychological Association's 16th annual Division 22 (Rehabilitation Psychology) midwinter conference in San Antonio, Texas. The group was enjoying dinner together after completing a well-received symposium that highlighted the work of rehabilitation psychologists in critical care settings across the United States. Among those present, Drs. Ann Marie Warren, James Jackson, Joseph Bienvenu, Lester Butt, and Nancy Merbitz stand out in memory as strong advocates, each one interested in promoting the insertion of behavioral health principles into critical care settings. Not long after, Dr. Bruce Caplan approached the first editor about writing a book on the subject for the Oxford series in rehabilitation psychology. After discussion, we agreed that more peer-reviewed literature was needed before a book would make sense. The momentum of these symposia and conversations inspired the second editor to approach Dr. Stephen Wegener about a special section in the *Journal of Rehabilitation Psychology*, which ultimately came to be and was entitled "The Role of Rehabilitation Psychology in Critical Care and Acute Medical Settings" (Jackson & Jutte, 2016). During the same time, multiple publications emerged, revealing a growing interest and enough scientific literature to justify an opus on the subject.

In the process of writing this volume we have learned a great deal and become increasingly dedicated to the goal of integrating psychological and rehabilitation principles into critical care across and outside of the United States. First and foremost we would like to thank our patients, families, and critical care staff who have inspired and taught us so much. We are humbled and honored to have been a part of so many unique lives and to work side by side with such dedicated professionals. Second, gratitude to the authors, many of whom are widely recognized experts in critical care and very busy professionals. We greatly appreciate their willingness to share valuable time, knowledge, expertise, and insights.

A very special thanks to Dr. Caplan, who diligently and meticulously reviewed every chapter, each time providing invaluable feedback and editorial suggestions. We profited immensely from his efforts and desire to make the book the very best it could be. We also want to recognize Dr. Barry Nierenberg, who was the first President of the Academy of Rehabilitation Psychology and, along with Joan Bossert, developed the Oxford series concept. Appreciation to Dr. Wegener as well, who gave all of us the opportunity to expand the number of peer-reviewed articles in this emerging field, groundbreaking work that was necessary before a book like this could be justified. We would also like to recognize Jennifer Godlesky, MLIS, library manager at Hurley Medical Center, who relentlessly searched for and diligently verified innumerable citations used throughout the text. Finally, gratitude to our loved ones, who have graciously accepted our time away from other responsibilities and provided so much support in the process.

Reference

Jackson, J. C. & Jutte, J. E. (2016). Rehabilitating a missed opportunity: Integration of rehabilitation psychology into the care of critically ill patients, survivors, and caregivers. *Rehabilitation Psychology, 61,* 115–119. http://dx.doi.org/10.1037/rep0000091

About the Editors

Kirk J. Stucky obtained his PsyD from Florida Tech in 1995. He completed his internship at Union Memorial Hospital in Baltimore, Maryland, and his residency at Hurley Medical Center in Flint, Michigan. He is currently chair of the Department of Behavioral Health at Hurley Medical Center and an assistant professor for the Michigan State University College of Human Medicine, Department of Medicine. As a program director, he has had the privilege of teaching and supervising trainees for 25 years and mentoring a talented cadre of professionals who have moved on to productive and meaning-filled careers. Being board certified in rehabilitation psychology and clinical neuropsychology, he has been dedicated to advancing the interests of both specialties, including the development of integrated training standards and exploring new opportunities for advanced hospital practice. He is a long-term member of the level 1 trauma and inpatient rehabilitation teams at Hurley Medical Center. All of these roles and experiences, especially the latter, inspired a growing interest in promoting the practice of integrated critical care.

Jennifer E. Jutte earned her MPH from the Rollins School of Public Health at Emory University in Atlanta, Georgia. In between her MPH and PhD, she worked as an infectious disease epidemiologist and program coordinator at the Centers for Disease Control and Prevention in Atlanta, Georgia. She then went on to earn her PhD in clinical psychology from Washington State University in Pullman, Washington. After completing a residency and postdoctoral fellowship in rehabilitation psychology and neuropsychology at the University of Washington in Seattle, she began her critical care psychology career in the Department of Physical Medicine and Rehabilitation at the Johns Hopkins University. While she was at Hopkins, she achieved an early career grant from the National Institutes of Health to develop an anxiety management intervention with critically ill patients in the intensive care unit. She then returned to the Pacific Northwest and was on faculty at the University of Washington/Harborview Medical Center (level 1 trauma center). In each of these positions, she taught, supervised, and mentored rehabilitation psychology interns, postdoctoral fellows, medical students, and early career faculty. Dr. Jutte also has been involved in advocacy and leadership roles within the American Psychological Association (APA) and APA's Division 22 (Rehabilitation Psychology). Currently, she is in independent practice in the greater Seattle area providing health and behavior interventions, psychotherapy, coaching, and consultation services to individuals who have experienced a critical illness or catastrophic injury as well as frontline providers. All of these experiences have helped to shape and broaden her passion for critical care psychology and inspired continued engagement in academic pursuits—such as this book.

Contributors

O. Joseph Bienvenu, MD, PhD
Associate Professor
Psychiatry and Behavioral Sciences
Johns Hopkins University School of
  Medicine
Baltimore, MD, USA

Jonathan Brigham, MD
Clinical Instructor
Department of Psychiatry and
  Behavioral Sciences
University of Washington
Seattle, WA, USA

Valerie Canary, MSN, RN, CPNP
Pediatric Trauma Program Manager
Organ Donation Liaison
Hurley Medical Center
Flint, MI, USA

Crystal L. Cederna-Meko, PsyD
Pediatric Psychologist
Hurley Children's Hospital
Associate Professor, Department of
  Pediatrics and Human Development
Michigan State University College of
  Human Medicine
Flint, MI, USA

Nancy Ciccolella, PsyD
Temple University Hospital
Philadelphia, PA, USA

**Judy E. Davidson, DNP, RN,
MCCM, FAAN**
Nurse Scientist, University of
  California San Diego Health
Research Scientist, University of
  California San Diego School of
  Medicine
Department of Psychiatry
San Diego, CA, USA

Scott Davidson, MD
Trauma Surgery Services
Bronson Methodist Hospital
Kalamazoo, MI, USA

Shannon L. Dennis, PhD
Pediatric Neuropsychologist
Hurley Children's Hospital
Adjunct Assistant Professor,
    Department of Psychiatry and
    Behavioral Sciences
Michigan State University College of
    Human Medicine
Flint, MI, USA

Maria C. Duggan, MD, MPH
Geriatric Research Education and
    Clinical Center, Department of
    Veteran Affairs, Tennessee Valley
    Healthcare System
Division of Geriatric Medicine,
    Vanderbilt University School of
    Medicine
Nashville, TN, USA

Rebecca E. H. Ellens, PsyD
Pediatric Psychologist
Hurley Children's Hospital
Assistant Professor, Department of
    Pediatrics and Human Development
Michigan State University College of
    Human Medicine
Hurley Medical Center
Flint, MI, USA

E. Wesley Ely, MD, MPH
Geriatric Research Education and
    Clinical Center, Department of
    Veteran Affairs, Tennessee Valley
    Healthcare System
Center for Health Services
    Research, Vanderbilt University
    Medical Center
Division of Allergy, Pulmonary, and
    Critical Care Medicine, Vanderbilt
    University School of Medicine
Nashville, TN, USA

Joan Fleishman, PsyD
Oregon Health & Science University
Portland, OR, USA

Brighid Fronapfel, PhD
Nevada Center for Excellence in
    Disabilities
University of Nevada
Reno, NV, USA

Macarena Gálvez Herrer, PDH
Psychologist
Project HU-CI
Scientist, Personality, Stress and
    Health Research Team, Faculty of
    Psychology
Universidad Autónoma
Madrid, Spain

Ted Avi Gerstenblith, MD
Assistant Professor
Department of Psychiatry and
    Behavioral Sciences
Johns Hopkins University School of
    Medicine
Baltimore, MA, USA

Christina J. Hayhurst, MD
Assistant Professor of Anesthesiology
    and Critical Care
Vanderbilt University School of
    Medicine
Nashville, TN, USA

Julie Highfield, BSc, ClinPsyD
Consultant Clinical Psychologist
Cardiff Critical Care
Cardiff, UK

Ramona O. Hopkins, PhD
Psychology Department
Brigham Young University
Provo, UT, USA

Megan M. Hosey, PhD
Assistant Professor
Physical Medicine and Rehabilitation
Johns Hopkins University School of
    Medicine
Baltimore, MA, USA

**David C. J. Howell, PhD,
FFICM, FRCP**
Divisional Clinical Director
Critical Care, University College
    London Hospitals
London, UK

James C. Jackson, PsyD
Critical Illness, Brain Dysfunction,
    and Survivorship Center, Vanderbilt
    University Medical Center
Geriatric Research Education and
    Clinical Center, VA Tennessee Valley
    Healthcare System
Department of Medicine, Division of
    Allergy, Pulmonary and Critical Care
    Medicine, Vanderbilt University
    School of Medicine
ICU Recovery Center at Vanderbilt,
    Vanderbilt University School of
    Medicine
Nashville, TN, USA

Hannah Kamsky, BSN, RN, CCCTM
Oregon Health & Science University
Portland, OR, USA

Jennifer E. Jutte, PhD, MPH
Independent Practice
Seattle, WA, USA

Gabriel Heras La Calle, MD
Intensive Care Unit, Hospital Comarcal
    de Santa Ana
Motril, Granada, Spain
Project HU-CI, Ph.D. (cand.), School
    of Medicine, Universidad Francisco
    de Vitoria
Madrid, Spain

Caroline L. Lassen-Greene, PhD
Critical Illness, Brain Dysfunction,
    and Survivorship Center, Vanderbilt
    University Medical Center
Geriatric Research Education and
    Clinical Center, VA Tennessee Valley
    Healthcare System
Nashville, TN, USA

Alan Lewandowski, PhD
Department of Psychiatry
Western Michigan University School of
    Medicine
Kalamazoo, MI, USA

Michelle Maxson, MSN, RN,
ACCNS-AG
Senior Manager of Trauma Operations
Hurley Medical Center
Flint, MI, USA

Nancy Merbitz, PhD
VA Northeast Ohio Healthcare System
Cleveland, OH, USA

Leo C. Mercer, MD, FACS
Chair, Trauma & Acute Care Surgery
Trauma Medical Director
Director, Surgical Services Clinical
    Operations
Hurley Medical Center
Flint, MI, USA

Matt Morgan, PhD, MBBCh, BSc,
FICM, FRCA
Consultant in Intensive Care Medicine
Cardiff Critical Care
Cardiff, UK

Sandeep Nayak, MD
Postdoctoral Research Fellow
Department of Psychiatry and
    Behavioral Sciences
Johns Hopkins University School of
    Medicine
Baltimore, MA, USA

Mina Nordness, MD
PGY4 Resident
Department of Surgery
Vanderbilt University Medical Center
Nashville, TN, USA

Elizabeth Prince, DO
Instructor
Department of Psychiatry and
    Behavioral Sciences
Johns Hopkins University School of
    Medicine
Baltimore, MA, USA

Eileen Rubin, JD
President, ARDS Foundation
Northbrook, IL, USA

Carla M. Sevin, MD
Critical Illness, Brain Dysfunction,
    and Survivorship Center, Vanderbilt
    University Medical Center
Department of Medicine, Division of
    Allergy, Pulmonary and Critical Care
    Medicine, Vanderbilt University
    School of Medicine
ICU Recovery Center at Vanderbilt,
    Vanderbilt University School of
    Medicine
Nashville, TN, USA

Deborah Smyth, BSc
Senior Nurse
Research and Development
Critical Care and Anaesthetics
University College London Hospitals
London, UK

Jack Spector, PhD
Independent Practice
Baltimore, MA, USA

Kirk J. Stucky, PsyD, ABPP-CN, RP
Chairman, Department of
    Behavioral Health
Director of Rehabilitation Psychology
    and Neuropsychology
Program Director, Postdoctoral
    Fellowship Program, Rehabilitation
    Psychology
Hurley Medical Center
Flint, MI, USA

Stephanie Sundborg, PhD
Portland State University
Portland, OR, USA

Kirk Szczepkowski, MA
Clinical Psychology Program
Midwestern University
Glendale, AZ, USA

Jamie Lynne Tingey, MS
Seattle Pacific University
Seattle, WA, USA

Paul Twose, MSc
Physiotherapist
Cardiff Critical Care
Cardiff, UK

Julie Van, BA
Geriatric Research Education and
    Clinical Center, Department of
    Veteran Affairs, Tennessee Valley
    Healthcare System
Division of Allergy, Pulmonary, and
    Critical Care Medicine, Vanderbilt
    University School of Medicine
Nashville, TN, USA

Dorothy Wade, PhD
Consultant Psychologist
North East London Foundation Trust
    and UCL
London, UK

Ann Marie Warren, PhD, ABPP
Baylor Scott & White Research
    Institute
Dallas, TX, USA

1 Introduction to Critical Care Psychology and Rehabilitation

Kirk J. Stucky and Jennifer E. Jutte

WHEN CONTEMPLATING THE broad field of critical care and all of its complexities, rehabilitation and psychology practice is not likely among the top 10 services that clinicians, patients, or the public think of, and rightly so. The vast majority of patients who require intensive care arrive at death's door, and many linger in a limbo-like space somewhere between life and the afterlife. The primary focus at this juncture is often on pressing matters such as reestablishing and stabilizing basic bodily functions, optimizing lifesaving machine settings, and deciding who does and does not need additional, urgent interventions. Still, just beneath the surface of this fascinating, multilayered environment, the need for psychologists and rehabilitation-oriented clinicians is everywhere, in large part because intensive care stands among the most emotionally intense and physically taxing hospital-based settings for everyone involved—patients, families, caregivers, and staff alike. Despite this, recognition that psychologists and rehabilitation-oriented professionals could and should be more integrated within the critical care team is uncommon. In fact, it can be argued that some European countries are ahead of the United States in this regard (Agarwala et al., 2011; Andreoli et al., 2001; Jackson & Jutte, 2016; Peris et al., 2011; Sukantarat et al., 2007; Tan et al., 2009; Van den Born–van Zanten et al., 2016). Fortunately, there are growing integrative trends in the United States. In 2010, a conference was convened by the Society of Critical Care Medicine with broad goals to

Kirk J. Stucky and Jennifer E. Jutte, *Introduction to Critical Care Psychology and Rehabilitation* In: *Critical Care Psychology and Rehabilitation*. Edited by: Kirk J. Stucky and Jennifer E. Jutte, Oxford University Press. © Oxford University Press 2022. DOI: 10.1093/oso/9780190077013.003.0001 inform stakeholders about the multiple long-term consequences of critical illness (e.g., postintensive care syndrome [PICS]) and initiate improvements across the continuum of care for critical illness survivors. In addition to critical care specialists, this meeting included professionals from rehabilitation, outpatient, and community care settings. Among the many insights and recommendations made, Needham and colleagues (2012) indicated that one of the largest barriers to integration was the existence of "silos" in clinician groups, creating gaps in the continuity of care when patients transfer from the intensive care unit (ICU) to other settings. They also stated that "[a]n ideal setting for survivors would be comprehensive multidisciplinary outpatient ICU follow-up clinics that provide assessments from all relevant clinician groups and that coordinate a plan for rehabilitation care" (p. 506). Barriers to this aspirational standard beyond clinical silos included underutilization of rehabilitation, limited awareness of critical illness outcomes (unlike traumatic brain injury [TBI] and stroke), insurance and financial issues, and regulatory requirements.

It is well known that the core critical care team has a great deal to keep track of when in the midst of saving a life, and it is not surprising that they may not have the time, expertise, or inclination to think about nuanced "downstream" psychological risks and responses or long-term treatment planning. In modern medicine there is simply too much to do and too much to know, making it impossible for any single physician leader or small team of clinicians to manage it all. A potential solution to this dilemma is to link and integrate critical care and rehabilitation teams in an interdisciplinary fashion across the continuum. This philosophy of care brings a variety of professionals to the patient's bedside in the ICU, although the frequency and intensity of their interventions will most certainly vary and evolve over time. For example, in the early stages of acute respiratory distress syndrome (ARDS), the intensivist, nurse, and respiratory therapist play primary roles in ensuring the patient's survival and preventing complications. However, as the patient becomes more stable and ventilator weaning trials begin, the physiatrist, speech-language pathologist, and physical therapist become more involved, while others turn their focus to the more critically ill and new arrivals. Finally, once the patient is off the ventilator, the psychologist, social worker, and occupational therapist lead efforts to address cognitive, emotional, and functional residuals while working collaboratively with the rest of the team.

Although, in an integrated model, all of these professionals are aware of the patient from the day of admission, the intensity of their involvement in care waxes and wanes as the patient's condition evolves and their needs change. Along with the other authors in this volume, we have witnessed firsthand the power and potential of this advanced model and mindset, which in turn fueled a desire to write more about it. We kept in mind three primary goals while writing this book:

1. Provide an introduction to critical care for psychologists and rehabilitation-oriented professionals who are interested in, or who are already providing services, in intensive care environments.

2. Expand on the growing literature that emphasizes the benefits of integrating rehabilitative and psychological principles into the continuum of critical care practice.

3. Present summative reviews of the literature, treatment techniques, and innovative developments in various intensive care settings geared toward helping professionals appreciate how integrated critical care practice can benefit all stakeholders—patients, families, caregivers, staff, institutions, and society at large.

In the midst of preparing this volume, we were faced with a "novel" critical illness, the magnitude of which had not been experienced by critical care or rehabilitation psychologists in the United States—the SARS-CoV-2 virus (i.e., COVID-19). This virus has changed psychology practice in several important ways, beginning with how we interact with patients, their family supports, and the care team, and the ways in which we assess, treat, and conduct research. Many of these practices have transitioned from personalized in-person care to virtual telemedicine options, which have had both positive (e.g., better access to care for some) and negative (e.g., transition away from "interdisciplinary" to "siloed" care) effects on patient care and psychologist engagement with the care team. We have included an important chapter on the intersection of infectious diseases and critical illnesses (see Chapter 8) and we also have included COVID-19–related information in relevant chapters (see Chapters 3, 4, 6, 9, 17). At the time of the writing of this volume, there are limited data on long-term outcomes for survivors of COVID-19 and related ICU hospitalization. We are able to surmise, however, that the outcomes are likely to mirror those associated with other critical illnesses (i.e., the physical, cognitive, and mental health phenotypes associated with PICS and postintensive care syndrome—family [PICS-F]).

Although the published literature on PICS and PICS-F has been steadily growing, few books have been devoted to the topic of critical care psychology and rehabilitative practice across the continuum of critical care settings. In 2017 Bienvenu, Jones, and Hopkins edited a groundbreaking book entitled *Psychological and Cognitive Impact of Critical Illness*, which highlighted emotional, psychosocial, and cognitive outcomes of critical illness. We hope that this volume will further those efforts. Chapters cover a wide range of psychological and rehabilitative topics relevant to various critical care settings. They have been intentionally written to pique the interest of psychologists who work in hospital settings as well as other critical care professionals from diverse disciplines (physicians; allied health professionals;

nurses; chaplains; speech-language pathologists, physical and occupational therapists). Considerations across the lifespan are covered from pediatrics to geriatrics (see Chapters 9 and 10). Furthermore, although critical care issues are discussed broadly, there is a primary focus on rehabilitative and behavioral health science interventions and assessment techniques; we recognize that many of our colleagues in critical care are intuitively employing these, although they may not always be aware of their scientific underpinnings. This is intended to elucidate, emphasize, and reinforce the point that all critical care providers should be trained in, and mindful of, nonpharmacologic rehabilitative and behavioral health tools and techniques that can help those in their charge. In doing so, we hope that the book will contribute to the existing literature, inspire innovations, and serve as a practical resource for clinicians in critical care settings.

It is also important to recognize the broad diversity of practice models and patterns in critical care medicine. While working on this project we acquired an increasing appreciation that, with regard to rehabilitation and psychology integration, there is tremendous variability in critical care practice throughout North America and the world. Some hospitals offer little to no psychology or rehabilitation services in critical care, while others have developed sophisticated and inclusive interdisciplinary systems. Furthermore, in the United States there is already an established rehabilitation pathway for individuals who have sustained TBI, stroke, and polytrauma, but this is not yet true for survivors of critical illness. With that in mind we have, throughout this opus, discussed both critical illness and critical injury, appreciating that current practices in fields like neurorehabilitation can help inform the treatment of critical illness survivors as well. We also strove to provide practical, basic information for clinicians entertaining the possibility of adopting aspects of a more integrated model while also outlining how sophisticated systems function in various critical care settings. In line with the view of the critical care team as a diverse, integrated body of clinicians, the chapters offer perspectives from a variety of professionals who work in intensive care settings and many who have published and/or presented at national conferences regarding advanced critical care practice (in particular see Chapters 3, 4, and 7). When appropriate, authors discuss staff support and training, future directions, areas that require more study, and how to navigate barriers to establishing more integrative care models (in particular see Chapters 12, 13, and 17).

As a final note, none of the chapters in this volume are intended to provide in-depth coverage of all things relevant to the main subject, as comprehensive reviews of the literature would far exceed space limitations. Instead, we asked authors to provide a brief, yet broad, overview of psychology and rehabilitative practice in critical care settings and their relevance to contemporary research and practice. The ideas and cited references, therefore, are also intended to point interested readers to more directed and in-depth study. In the following sections, we provide an introduction to central concepts in this volume, including critical care settings and essential terminology; the intensity of intensive care; survivorship; staff support, education, and training; and trends in critical care–focused psychology practice and rehabilitation.

Critical care settings and essential terminology

In this volume, *critical care* is defined as the direct delivery of care to a critically ill or critically injured patient. Critical illness and/or injury acutely impairs one or more vital organ system(s), resulting in a high probability of imminent death or life-threatening deterioration if effective medical care is not administered promptly. It should also be noted that the terms *critical care* and *intensive care* are often used interchangeably. For example, critical care units, intensive therapy units, or intensive treatment units all refer to areas in the hospital where seriously ill or injured patients receive specialized care such as advanced life support. However, for our purposes, *critical care* primarily refers to the practice of critical care medicine while *intensive care* refers to the venues in which that care is delivered (i.e., hospital units/wards). Table 1.1 lists the various types of ICUs.

Throughout this volume, various medical and psychological terms are used that may not be familiar to readers from a variety of professional backgrounds, including psychologists. As one of our primary goals was to make this book an easy-to-read introduction to rehabilitation and psychological practices and principles in critical care, a glossary of terms with summary explanations is provided, as well as three appendices (A: Trauma-Informed Care Practices in the ICU; B: Links to Resources; C: Anxiety Management and Ventilator Liberation Strategies).

The intensity of intensive care

In the ICU there is no end to tragic tales, heroic efforts, unexpected joys sometimes called "miracles," and inevitable loss. Consider what is required of an intensivist who has to tell an overwhelmed family that their loved one developed new, unexpected complications and is not likely to survive the night. What is the long-term psychological impact on critical care staff who regularly interact with patients who are delirious, combative, depressed, and/or terrified by the nature of their situation? What should a team member do when they discover that one of their colleagues is dealing with acute stress disorder related to the unexpected death of a child with asthma, and the clinician's symptoms may be affecting patient care? How about the experience of a parent who receives an unexpected phone call and that of the trauma surgeon who has to explain that their adolescent daughter was caught in a crossfire

TABLE I.I.

Types of ICUs*

Unit name	Abbreviation	Patient population
Burn injury care unit	BICU	Patients who have sustained burn and/or inhalation injuries
Coronary care unit**	CCU	Patients who have coronary/cardiac conditions (e.g., heart attack, congestive heart failure)
Cardiothoracic units**	CTU	Patients who have undergone cardiac and thoracic surgery
Long-term intensive care units	LICU	Patients with prolonged critical care needs (e.g., mechanical ventilation, dialysis)
Medical intensive care unit	MICU	Patients with medical conditions who do not require surgery
Neuro intensive care unit	Neuro-ICU	Patients with acute neurologic injury or events (e.g., TBI, stroke)
Neonatal intensive care unit	NICU	Newborn infants with serious medical problems
Pediatric intensive care unit	PICU	Children with a variety of serious medical conditions
Surgical intensive care unit	SICU	Surgical patients
Trauma intensive care unit	TICU	Patients typically with serious polytrauma (e.g., multiple fractures, internal injuries)

* During the SARS-CoV-2 pandemic, patients who were critically ill with COVID-19 infection were treated in a variety of ICUs as well as acute care wards, depending on the number of beds needed.

** In some hospitals similar units might be combined into one. For example, a cardiac and thoracic critical care unit (CTCCU) is a specialist unit that cares for patients with a range of cardiac, thoracic, and vascular problems, both surgical and medical.

and now may not survive emergency surgery? How can the critical care psychologist best support patients and team members within a critical care team fragmented in the midst of a pandemic crisis? These delicate situations can be handled in ways that vary from the clumsy, blunt, and unprofessional to the empathic, effective, and sophisticated. Furthermore, critical care situations inevitably raise ethical, moral, and clinical dilemmas with no clear solutions but profound implications for individuals, clinicians, communities, and society at large. The way in which clinicians assess, process, and deal with these issues can strongly influence not only patient outcomes but also staff wellness and the health care system itself (see Chapters 14 and 15 for more detailed discussion).

After nearly three decades working in various critical care environments, we have come to know that skilled clinicians often employ techniques such as reflective listening, crisis management, environmental control, and other strategies that are firmly grounded in behavioral and rehabilitative science. Although clinicians in the trenches may not align their approach with, or be aware that they are employing, such techniques, this does not lessen their importance. Because of this and growing supportive literature (Jackson & Jutte, 2016; Needham et al., 2012), we believe that the practice of critical care medicine is on the brink of an evolution in which it will move away from a traditional multidisciplinary (i.e., clinical silo type) approach toward more inclusive interdisciplinary team models that fully integrate rehabilitation and behavioral health professionals. We also anticipate that this change in philosophy will help stimulate new ideas with regard to evolving roles, activities, opportunities, and treatment guidelines in the practice of critical care.

Survivorship—the patient

Thanks to advances in critical care, more people are surviving critical illnesses, catastrophic injuries, and medical complications that were previously associated with high mortality rates. This success is directly related to the growing sophistication of medical technologies, research, and clinical practice guidelines (Barr et al., 2013; Devlin et al., 2018). More than 6 million people in North America are admitted to ICUs annually with life-threatening conditions such as sepsis, ARDS, and multisystem organ failure (Deutschman et al., 2012; Halpern & Pastores, 2010; Society of Critical Care Medicine, 2011). In addition, in the United States, over 1 million people are hospitalized at level 1 or level 2 trauma centers annually with varying levels of downstream disability (Hall et al., 2010; National Center for Injury Prevention and Control, 2011; Prin & Guohua, 2016). A large percentage of these patients experience delirium, and many experience their critical illnesses and/or ICU hospitalization as traumatic, as do their families. During the COVID-19 pandemic the stressful nature of this experience has been magnified for patients and families due to the physical distancing requirements and inability to be near their loved ones while they are hospitalized regardless of diagnosis. Indeed, the collective toll of critical illness and injury is difficult to overestimate. For example, about one in three ICU survivors have newly acquired or exacerbated clinically debilitating cognitive impairment that can last for years (Ely et al., 2001; Girard et al., 2010; Ouimet et al., 2007; Pandharipande et al., 2013), and between one quarter and one third of survivors report symptoms of posttraumatic stress disorder (PTSD), anxiety, and/or depressive symptoms (Bienvenu et al., 2012; Davydow, Desai et al., 2008; Davydow,

Gifford et al., 2008; Davydow et al., 2009; Jackson et al., 2016; Kapfhammer et al., 2004; Parker et al., 2015; Schelling et al., 1998) (see Chapters 5 and 11 for more in-depth discussion). Considering the losses, stressors, and other unexpected challenges loved ones often endure, this number may be even higher among their family members (Azoulay et al., 2005).

PICS phenotypes and the costs of survivorship, as well as PICS-F phenotypes, are associated with diverse difficulties and poor quality of life (Bienvenu et al., 2012; Davidson et al., 2017; Davydow, Desai et al., 2008; Davydow et al., 2009; Desai et al., 2011; Dowdy et al., 2006; Hopkins et al., 2010; Stevenson et al., 2013; Van der Schaaf et al., 2009). Classifying and better understanding these phenotypes can help inform clinicians working with patients and family members with regard to key areas of assessment and treatment that may be helpful for both short- and long-term recovery. Moreover, growing awareness of PICS has been a prime factor in justifying the need for early rehabilitation to promote wellness among survivors, their families, and caregivers to better support them in the long process of recovery (Eakin et al., 2015; Needham et al., 2012). In addition, considering the presence of significant psychological and cognitive morbidity, it is not surprising that the investigation of psychological issues has been identified as a top research priority by the Multisociety Strategic Planning Task Force for Critical Care Research (Deutschman et al., 2012).

Because these survivors are at high risk for recurrent rehospitalization, debility, and premature death, there is an emerging understanding of the need for ongoing treatment with a variety of skilled professionals versed in the art and science of collaborative care (Davydow, Desai et al., 2008; Desai et al., 2011). Thus, the concern among critical care providers has shifted from a narrow focus on preventing mortality to a broader focus on issues of quality of life and survivorship (Iwashyna et al., 2010).

Fortunately, the value of progressive mobility, the ICU liberation bundle (aka ABCDEF bundle), and other rehabilitative techniques, during and after critical care, has strong support in the literature (Ely, 2017; Harrison & Kirkpatrick, 2011; Hoenig et al., 2015; Jutte et al., 2015, 2017; Merbitz et al., 2012, 2016; Musicco et al., 2003; Pun et al., 2019). In addition, an expanding body of evidence indicates that psychologists can assist in early identification and/or interventions for those at risk in critical care, with potentially desirable influences on outcomes and quality of life (Andreoli et al., 2001; Archer et al., 2012; Davidson et al., 2012; Jackson et al., 2016; Merbitz et al., 2016; Van der Schaaf et al., 2009).

Unfortunately, despite an increased understanding of and attention to the problems of survivors, many patients are still lost to follow-up after discharge from intensive care (Dowdy et al., 2005; Griffiths et al., 2006). To address this issue, some hospital systems in the United Kingdom, Europe, and the United States have established outpatient treatment centers specifically designed to address survivor needs (Jackson & Jutte, 2016; Van den Born–van Zanten et al., 2016) (also see Chapter 13). In some of these settings, psychologists and other rehabilitation-oriented clinicians are at the forefront of identification, treatment, and prevention of psychological, physical, and cognitive complications frequently seen during or following critical illness (see Chapter 4).

Survivorship—the family

In the early stages of ICU admission while patients are typically nonverbal, minimally responsive, or intentionally sedated, loved ones face significant emotional and practical challenges including, but not limited to, the initial shock of ICU admission and prospect of loss, making difficult and often unanticipated decisions regarding care (e.g., surgical pros and cons, advance directives), and handling the person's affairs in and outside of the hospital (McAdam et al., 2010; Warren et al., 2016). Simultaneously, family members (often with no or very limited medical knowledge) are expected to consolidate information provided by a variety of hospital staff and specialists who deliver important bits of information pertaining to the patient's situation. It is not surprising that many family members feel overwhelmed or confused, often because they are striving to keep up with, understand, or organize the complex information delivered. At times this can also be related to the way in which the information is being conveyed or received, especially given that family members are typically experiencing heightened stress and some may be in shock. During a pandemic, when communication with families is made all the more challenging by physical distancing, personal protective equipment (PPE), and telemedicine constraints, family members can become even more confused, distanced, and disengaged. The situation and the stress of it all can compromise the family's ability to make important decisions on behalf of their loved ones.

The chronic issues that survivors live with, sometimes years beyond the original hospitalization, affect not only them but family members and caregivers as well. Following ICU discharge family members may act as primary caregivers, sometimes reducing their work hours or leaving the workforce altogether, often with real financial consequences that only add to the overall stress (Finkelstein et al., 2006). Therefore, it is not surprising that multiple studies have shown that family members, caregivers, and loved ones are at increased risk for developing depression, anxiety, and PTSD during or following the critical care experience (Davidson & Zisook, 2017; Paul & Rattray, 2008; Pochard et al., 2001; Schmidt & Azoulay, 2012). Unfortunately, the psychological impact on the patient's support system is too often overlooked (Azoulay et al., 2005; Kross et al., 2011; Van den Born–van Zanten et al., 2016). This phenomenon has been referred to in various ways, such as "the burden of survivorship" (Iwashyna & Netzer, 2012), caregiver burden, and caregiver strain (Thornton & Travis, 2003).[1] In line with this, experts in the field proposed criteria for PICS-F, which refers to the physical, cognitive, and social strains faced by the caregiver (Davidson et al., 2017; Davidson & Zisook, 2017; Needham et al., 2012). Terms like PICS-F and PICS provide a common language for clinicians in various specialties and a pathway to developing comprehensive care plans that include the patient's support system (Jackson & Jutte, 2016). It should also be noted that some limited research has been done pertaining to interventions that alleviate family stress, and this is explored further in Chapter 12 (Garrouste-Orgeas et al., 2012; Jones et al., 2010, 2012).

Staff support, education, and training

The whole is greater than its collective parts, and everyone has something they can learn from others. Ideally, critical care teams should be interdisciplinary, and to some degree transdisciplinary, in that each member understands the others' primary role(s) and how they optimally interface with and complement one another. In turn, this knowledge and philosophical approach allows the team to more fully take advantage of their strengths while minimizing weaknesses or gaps in service delivery. When teams work and learn together, the synergy can lead to unique contributions to the program that extend far beyond patient care. Some of those potential benefits and value-added services are briefly discussed next.

STAFF SUPPORT

Staff who care for the critically ill or injured, day in and day out, are taking an emotional risk every time they enter the ICU. Repeated exposure to trauma, critical illness, death and dying, and other such highly charged emotional situations inevitably tests the resilience and psychological health of professionals, no matter how experienced or well trained they are. Unfortunately, in the culture of critical care, staff members often do not readily recognize or share the need to address emotional issues. Instead, practitioners may engage in or even encourage their colleagues to minimize or "swallow" psychological reactions due to fear that it might negatively affect patient care or how they are perceived by colleagues. Furthermore, the clinical pace and ICU culture typically do not allow time for the team to discuss or process difficult experiences. Unfortunately, denying, avoiding, or ignoring mounting stress and chronic issues can ultimately diminish performance, relationships, team dynamics, and patient care. Moreover, mounting emotional residuals can result in burnout, secondary traumatic stress, and compassion fatigue (Figley, 1995; Moss et al., 2016). In several publications, the first author and others proposed that, although psychologists cannot act as the team's therapist, they can provide services such as acute crisis management, advising staff about self-care and stress management, or directing staff members to appropriate services when needed (Stucky & Warren, 2019; Warren et al., 2013).

EDUCATION

Large hospitals with advanced ICUs are also often teaching hospitals in which everyone shares a commitment to lifelong learning. In the healthiest team environment, everyone has an opportunity to teach and learn from one another. During formal rounds, case conferences, and other educative activities, team members should take turns teaching and listening to one another. In our opinion, when executed ideally, this parallel process ultimately leads to higher-quality and more comprehensive patient care and staff wellness. Most psychologists do not typically receive formal training in intensive care settings. It has been our experience that, once established, competent and appropriately trained psychologists can teach hospital staff, medical students, residents, and other trainees about behavioral health concepts such as the complexities of psychiatric conditions, their treatment, and the role of psychological factors in adjustment to illness or injury. Psychologists also can assist team members with effective communication strategies, ways to prevent or ameliorate burnout, and how to best establish boundaries with patients, caregivers, and coworkers. Finally, as integrated members of the critical care team, psychologists can also uniquely contribute to research endeavors (see Chapter 16).

TRAINING

Rehabilitation professionals, including physical and occupational therapists and speech–language pathologists, often have limited exposure to critical care during and after training. Furthermore, the field of health service psychology has yet to establish specific training guidelines or competencies for psychologists who work in critical care settings. Thus, most psychologists involved in critical care today did not complete a formal internship or residency specifically focused on the delivery of psychological services in intensive care settings. Instead, health service psychologists have translated and applied evidence-based treatments from other hospital environments in an effort to determine which interventions and assessment techniques work best with the ICU population. We foresee the eventual development of guidelines and/or suggestions regarding how rehabilitation professionals (including psychologists) can be properly prepared to work in these unique and challenging settings. We also believe that critical care psychology may become a specialty area within rehabilitation psychology. If this comes to be, training requirements should include internship and postdoctoral experiences and exposure to working in an intensive care environment. In addition, the critical care psychologist should have broad background (during graduate school at the minimum) experiences that provide a strong base for the development of foundational competencies. The authors of various chapters throughout this volume offer additional insights regarding current training and educational pathways as well as what the future may hold. Considering that the model and ideas proposed in this book are relatively new, we anticipate that training programs, attending providers, and trainees might be interested in those insights as well. Moreover, related critical care professionals—such as intensivists, trauma surgeons, case managers, nurses, unit administrators, social workers, psychiatric nurse practitioners, physician assistants, and psychiatrists—might also find the information relevant to their program and staff development initiatives.

Trends in critical care-focused psychology practice and rehabilitation

Some authors have argued that rehabilitation psychologists have a unique set of skills and specific competencies that make them especially well suited for practice in critical care environments such as level 1 trauma centers (Jackson & Jutte, 2016; Stucky et al., 2016; Stucky & Warren, 2019; Warren et al., 2013). In the United Kingdom and other European countries, psychologists are routinely members of the critical care team (Agarwala et al., 2011; Sukantarat et al., 2007; Tan et al., 2009). In the United States, this practice model is not as common but appears to be growing in some regions. For example, in 2016, a U.S.-based survey confirmed the hypothesis that psychologists from various specialties in health care psychology are involved in critical care settings such as level 1 trauma centers (Stucky et al., 2016). Furthermore, there have been several well-received symposia on this subject at national conferences, including the 2015 and 2016 American Psychological Association (APA) Division 22 midwinter conferences. These events inspired the creation of a special section in the *Rehabilitation Psychology* journal ("The Role of Rehabilitation Psychology in Critical Care and Acute Medical Settings;" Jackson & Jutte, 2016). That journal contained articles addressing issues such as caregiver strain, PTSD, and the integration of rehabilitation psychology principles into the care of patients and families in intensive care settings; those familiar with that publication will recognize that we have relied on it heavily in writing this book.

Some authors have suggested that, at a minimum, interaction with a supportive provider such as a rehabilitation psychologist can be helpful in not only addressing psychological distress but also reducing stigma associated with mental health concerns (Warren et al., 2013). Although evidence suggests that psychological interventions are used in many ICUs, the effectiveness of these interventions and their impact on long-term outcomes remains largely unknown (Peris et al., 2011). Chapter 4 provides a more detailed summary of this fascinating field of research, including studies on nonpharmacologic interventions in the ICU, family and caregiver emotional adjustment, cognitive rehabilitation, and the psychological impact on critical care staff.

Conclusion

Critical care practice has steadily evolved thanks to the ingenuity, perseverance, and quality care provided by countless pioneering clinicians. As a consequence, it is increasingly understood that there are costs associated with survivorship, including persistent psychological, cognitive, and physical issues that affect survivors and families alike. We believe that properly trained clinicians with a rehabilitative and psychologically minded approach have something unique to offer in the critical care environment, not only to patients and families but also to the treatment team, institution, and society at large. This book was designed to provide a broad overview of rehabilitation and psychology practice across the continuum of critical care settings. Although most chapters emphasize contemporary psychology practice, the book is written to appeal to an interdisciplinary audience. It is our hope that in the future, high-quality and sophisticated intensive care and postintensive care will be characterized by more integrated involvement of rehabilitation-oriented professionals, including psychologists.

Note

1. It should be noted that some in the disability community take issue with the term "burden" because it assumes and makes a judgement regarding the family and patient's experience. It is well known that persons with disability often live full, productive lives and are not thought of as a "burden" by their support network. Thus, individual differences in patient outcomes, family resources and other relevant variables should be considered in assessing existence and degree of "burden."

References

Agarwala, R., Ahmed, N., & Patil, K. (2011). An audit of adult critical care rehabilitation processes in a UK district general hospital based on NICE guidelines. *Critical Care, 15*(Suppl 1), P532.

Andreoli, P., Novaes, M., Karam, C., & Knobel, E. (2001). The ICU humanization program: Contributions from the psychologist team. *Critical Care, 5*(Suppl 3), Article P80.

Archer, K. R., Castillo, R. C., Wegener, S. T., Abraham, C. M., & Obremskey, W. T. (2012). Pain and satisfaction in hospitalized trauma patients: The importance of self-efficacy and psychological distress. *Journal of Trauma and Acute Care Surgery, 72*(4), 1068–1077.

Azoulay, E., Pochard, F., Kentish-Barnes, N., Chevret, S., Aboab, J., Adrie, C., . . . FAMIREA Study Group. (2005). Risk of post-traumatic stress symptoms in family members of intensive care unit patients. *American Journal of Respiratory and Critical Care Medicine, 171*(9), 987–994.

Barr, J., Fraser, G. L., Puntillo, K., Ely, E. W., Gélinas, C. Dasta, J. F., . . . Jaeschke, R. (2013). Clinical practice guidelines for the management of pain, agitation, and delirium in adult patients in the intensive care unit. *Critical Care Medicine, 41*(1), 263–306.

Bienvenu, O. J., Colantuoni, E., Mendez-Tellez, P. A., Dinglas, V. D., Shanholtz, C., Husain, N., . . . Needham, D. M. (2012). Depressive symptoms and impaired physical function after acute lung injury: A 2-year longitudinal study. *American Journal of Respiratory and Critical Care Medicine, 185*(5), 517–524.

Bienvenu, O. J., Jones, C., & Hopkins, R. O. (2017). *Psychological and cognitive impact of critical illness*. Oxford University Press.

Davidson, J. E., Jones, C., & Bienvenu, O. J. (2012). Family response to critical illness: Postintensive care syndrome-family. *Critical Care Medicine, 40*(2), 618–624. http://dx.doi.org/10.1097/CCM.0b013e318236ebf9

Davidson, J., McDuffie, M., & Campbell, K. (2017). Family centered care. In S. Goldsworthy, R. Kleinpell, & G. E. Speed (Eds.), *International best practices in critical care* (pp. 311–368). World Federation of Critical Care Nursing.

Davidson, J. E., & Zisook, S. (2017). Implementing family-centered care through facilitated sensemaking. *AACN Advanced Critical Care, 28*(2), 200–209.

Davydow, D. S., Desai, S. V., Needham, D. M., & Bienvenu, O. J. (2008). Psychiatric morbidity in survivors of the acute respiratory distress syndrome: A systematic review. *Psychosomatic Medicine, 70*(4), 512–519.

Davydow, D. S., Gifford, J. M., Desai, S. V., Needham, D. M., & Bienvenu, O. J. (2008). Posttraumatic stress disorder in general intensive care unit survivors: A systematic review. *General Hospital Psychiatry, 30*(5), 421–434.

Davydow, D. S., Gifford, J. M., Desai, S. V., Bienvenu, O. J., & Needham, D. M. (2009). Depression in general intensive care unit survivors: A systematic review. *Intensive Care Medicine, 35*(5), 796–809.

Desai, S. V., Law, T. J., & Needham, D. M. (2011). Long-term complications of critical care. *Critical Care Medicine, 39*(2), 371–379.

Deutschman, C. S., Ahrens, T., Cairns, C. B., Sessler, C. N., & Parsons, P. E. (2012). Multisociety task force for critical care research. *Chest, 141*(1), 201–209.

Devlin, J. W., Skrobik, Y., Gélinas, C., Needham, D. M., Slooter, A. J. C., Pandharipande, P., . . . Alhazzani, W. (2018). Clinical practice guidelines for the prevention and management of pain, agitation/sedation, delirium, immobility, and sleep disruption in adult patients in the ICU. *Critical Care Medicine, 46*(9), e825–e873.

Dowdy, D. W., Eid, M. P., Dennison, C. R., Mendez-Tellez, P. A., Herridge, M. S., Guallar, E., . . . Needham, D. M. (2006). Quality of life after acute respiratory distress syndrome: A meta-analysis. *Intensive Care Medicine, 32*(8), 1115–1124.

Dowdy, D. W., Eid, M. P., Sedrakyan, A., Mendez-Tellez, P. A., Pronovost, P. J., Herridge, M. S., & Needham, D. M. (2005). Quality of life in adult survivors of critical illness: A systematic review of the literature. *Intensive Care Medicine, 31*(5), 611–620.

Eakin, M. N., Ugbah, L., Arnautovic, T., Parker, A. M., & Needham, D. M. (2015). Implementing and sustaining an early rehabilitation program in a medical intensive care unit: A qualitative analysis. *Journal of Critical Care, 30*(4), 698–704.

Ely, E. W. (2017). The ABCDEF bundle: Science and philosophy of how ICU liberation serves patients and families. *Critical Care Medicine, 45*(2), 321–330.

Ely, E. W., Inouye, S. K., Bernard, G. R., Gordon, S., Francis, J., May, L., . . . Margolin, R. (2001). Delirium in mechanically ventilated patients: Validity and reliability of the confusion assessment method for the intensive care unit (CAM-ICU). *Journal of the American Medical Association, 286*(21), 2703–2710.

Figley, C. R. (1995). Compassion fatigue: Toward a new understanding of the costs of caring. In B. H. Stamm (Ed.), *Secondary traumatic stress: Self care issues for clinicians, researchers, and educators* (pp. 3–28). Sidran Press.

Finkelstein, E. A., Corso, P. S., & Miller, T. R. (2006). *Incidence and economic burden of injuries in the United States.* Oxford University Press.

Garrouste-Orgeas, M., Coquet, I., Périer, A., Timsit, J. F., Pochard, F., Lancrin, F., . . . Angeli, S. (2012). Impact of an intensive care unit diary on psychological distress in patients and relatives. *Critical Care Medicine, 40*(7), 2033–2040.

Girard, T. D., Jackson, J. C., Pandharipande, P. P., Pun, B. T., Thompson, J. L., Shintani, A. K., . . . Ely, E. W. (2010). Delirium as a predictor of long-term cognitive impairment in survivors of critical illness. *Critical Care Medicine, 38*(7), 1513–1520.

Griffiths, J. A., Barber, V. S., Cuthbertson, B. H., & Young, J. D. (2006). A national survey of intensive care follow-up clinics. *Anaesthesia, 61*(10), 950–955. http://dx. doi.org/10.1111/j.1365-2044.2006.04792.x

Hall, M. J., DeFrances, C. J., Williams, S. N., Golosinskiy, A., & Schwartzman, A. (2010). *National hospital discharge survey: 2007 summary.* US Department of Health and Human Services, Centers for Disease Control and Prevention, National Center for Health Statistics.

Halpern, N. A., & Pastores, S. M. (2010). Critical care medicine in the United States 2000–2005: An analysis of bed numbers, occupancy rates, payer mix, and costs. *Critical Care Medicine, 38*(1), 65–71.

Harrison, J. P., & Kirkpatrick, N. (2011). The improving efficiency frontier of inpatient rehabilitation hospitals. *Health Care Manager, 30*(4), 313–321.

Hoenig, H., Lee, J., & Stineman, M. (2015). Conceptual overview of frameworks for measuring quality in rehabilitation. *Topics in Stroke Rehabilitation, 17*(4), 239–251. https://doi.org/10.1310/tsr1704-239

Hopkins, R. O., Key, C. W., Suchyta, M. R., Weaver, L. K., & Orme, J. F. (2010). Risk factors for depression and anxiety in survivors of acute respiratory distress syndrome. *General Hospital Psychiatry, 32*(2), 147–155.

Iwashyna, T. J., Ely, E. W., Smith, D. M., & Langa, K. M. (2010). Long-term cognitive impairment and functional disability among survivors of severe sepsis. *Journal of the American Medical Association, 304*(16), 1787–1794.

Iwashyna, T. J., & Netzer, G. (2012). The burdens of survivorship: An approach to thinking about long-term outcomes after critical illness. *Seminars in Respiratory and Critical Care Medicine, 33*(4), 327–338. http://dx.doi.org/10.1055/s-0032-1321982

Jackson, J. C., & Jutte, J. E. (2016). Rehabilitating a missed opportunity: Integration of rehabilitation psychology into the care of critically ill patients, survivors, and caregivers. *Rehabilitation Psychology, 61*(2), 115–119.

Jackson, J. C., Jutte, J. E., Hunter, C. H., Ciccolella, N., Warrington, H., Sevin, C., & Bienvenu, O. J. (2016). Posttraumatic stress disorder (PTSD) after critical illness: A conceptual review of distinct clinical issues and their implications. *Rehabilitation Psychology, 61*(2), 132–140. http://dx.doi.org/10.1037/rep0000085

Jones, C., Backman, C., Capuzzo, M., Egerod, I., Flaatten, H., Granja, C., . . . Griffiths, R. D. (2010). Intensive care diaries reduce new-onset posttraumatic stress disorder following critical illness: A randomised, controlled trial. *Critical Care, 14*(5), R168.

Jones, C., Backman, C., & Griffiths, R. D. (2012). Intensive care diaries and relatives' symptoms of posttraumatic stress disorder after critical illness: A pilot study. *American Journal of Critical Care, 21*(3), 172–176.

Jutte, J. E., Erb, C., & Jackson, J. C. (2015). Physical, cognitive and psychological disability following critical illness: What is the risk? *Seminars in Respiratory Critical Care, 36*, 1–16.

Jutte, J. E., Jackson, J. C., & Hopkins, R. (2017). Rehabilitation psychology insights for treatment of critical illness. In O. J. Bienvenu, C. Jones, & R. O. Hopkins (Eds.), *Psychological and cognitive impact of critical illness* (pp. 105–139). Oxford University Press.

Kapfhammer, H-P., Rothenhäusler, H-B., Krauseneck, T., Stoll, C., & Schelling, G. (2004). Posttraumatic stress disorder and health-related quality of life in long-term survivors of acute respiratory distress syndrome. *American Journal of Psychiatry, 161*(1), 45–52.

Kross, E. K., Engelberg, R. A., Gries, C. J., Nielsen, E. L., Zatzick, D., & Curtis, J. R. (2011). ICU care associated with symptoms of depression and posttraumatic stress disorder among family members of patients who die in the ICU. *Chest, 139*(4), 795–801.

McAdam, J. L., Dracup, K. A., White, D. B., Fontaine, D. K., & Puntillo, K. A. (2010). Symptom experiences of family members of intensive care unit patients at high risk for dying. *Critical Care Medicine, 38*(4), 1078–1085.

Merbitz, N. H., Merbitz, C. T., & Ripsch, J. P. (2012). Rehabilitation outcomes and assessment: Toward complex adaptive rehabilitation. In P. Kennedy (Ed.), *Oxford handbook of rehabilitation psychology* (pp. 96–127). Oxford University Press.

Merbitz, N. H., Westie, K., Dammeyer, J. A., Butt, L., & Schneider, J. (2016). After critical care: Challenges in the transition to inpatient rehabilitation. *Rehabilitation Psychology, 61*, 186–200. http://dx.doi.org/10.1037/rep0000072

Moss, M., Good, V. S., Gozal, D., Kleinpell, R., & Sessler, C. N. (2016). A critical care societies collaborative statement: Burnout syndrome in critical care health-care professionals. A call to action. *American Journal of Respiratory and Critical Care Medicine, 194*(1), 106–113. https://doi.org/10.1164/rccm.201604-0708ST

Musicco, M., Emberti, L., Nappi, G., & Caltagirone, C. (2003). Italian multicenter study on outcomes of rehabilitation of neurological patients. Early and long-term outcome of rehabilitation in stroke patients: The role of patient characteristics, time of initiation, and duration of interventions. *Archives of Physical Medicine and Rehabilitation, 84*(4), 551–558.

National Center for Injury Prevention and Control. (2011). Web-based Injury Statistics Query and Reporting System (WIQARS). Centers for Disease Control and Prevention. http://www.cdc.gov/injury/wisqars

Needham, D. M., Davidson, J., Cohen, H., Hopkins, R. O., Weinert, C., Wunsch, H., . . . Harvey, R. N. (2012). Improving long-term outcomes after discharge from intensive care unit: Report from a stakeholders' conference. *Critical Care Medicine, 40*(2), 502–509. http://dx.doi.org/10.1097/CCM.0b013e318232da75

Ouimet, S., Kavanagh, B. P., Gottfried, S. B., & Skrobik, Y. (2007). Incidence, risk factors and consequences of ICU delirium. *Intensive Care Medicine, 33*, 66–73.

Pandharipande, P. P., Girard, T. D., Jackson, J. C., Morandi, A., Thompson, J. L., Pun, B. T., . . . Ely, E. W. (2013). Long-term cognitive impairment after critical illness. *New England Journal of Medicine, 369*(14), 1306–1316.

Parker, A. M., Sricharoenchai, T., Raparla, S., Schneck, K. W., Bienvenu, O. J., & Needham, D. M. (2015). Posttraumatic stress disorder in critical illness survivors: A metaanalysis. *Critical Care Medicine, 43*(5), 1121–1129.

Paul, F., & Rattray, J. (2008). Short-and-long-term impact of critical illness on relatives: Literature review. *Journal of Advanced Nursing, 62*(3), 276–292.

Peris, A., Bonizzoli, M., Iozzelli, D., Migliaccio, M. L., Zagli, G., Bacchereti, A., . . . Belloni, L. (2011). Early intra-intensive care unit psychological intervention promotes recovery from posttraumatic stress disorders, anxiety and depression symptoms in critically ill patients. *Critical Care, 15*, R41. doi:10.1186/cc10003

Pochard, F., Azoulay, E., Chevret, S., Lemaire, F., Hubert, P., Canoui, P., . . . Dhainaut, J. F. (2001). Symptoms of anxiety and depression in family members of intensive care unit patients: Ethical hypothesis regarding decision-making capacity. *Critical Care Medicine, 29*(10), 1893–1897.

Prin, M., & Guohua, L. (2016). Complications and in-hospital mortality in trauma patients treated in intensive care units in the United States, 2013. *Injury Epidemiology, 3*(1), 18. doi:10.1186/s40621-016-0084-5

Pun, B. T., Balas, M. C., Barnes-Daly, M. A., Thompson, J. L., Aldrich, J. M., Barr, J., . . . Ely, E. W. (2019). Caring for critically ill patients with the ABCDEF bundle: Results of the ICU liberation collaborative in over 15,000 adults. *Critical Care Medicine, 47*(1), 3–14.

Schelling, G., Stoll, C., Haller, M., Briegel, J., Manert, W., Hummel, T., . . . Klaus, P. (1998). Health-related quality of life and posttraumatic stress disorder in survivors of the acute respiratory distress syndrome. *Critical Care Medicine, 26*(4), 651–659.

Schmidt, M., & Azoulay, E. (2012). Having a loved one in the ICU: The forgotten family. *Current Opinion in Critical Care, 18*(5), 540–547. http://dx.doi.org/10.1097/MCC.0b013e328357fl41

Society of Critical Care Medicine. (2011). *Critical care units: A descriptive analysis* (2nd ed.). Society of Critical Care Medicine.

Stevenson, J. E., Colantuoni, E., Bienvenu, O. J., Sricharoenchai, T., Wozniak, A., Shanholtz, C., . . . Needham, D. M. (2013). General anxiety symptoms after acute lung injury: Predictors and correlates. *Journal of Psychosomatic Research, 75*(3), 287–293.

Stucky, K., Jutte, J. E., Warren, A. M., Jackson, J. C., & Merbitz, N. (2016). A survey of psychology practice in critical care settings. *Rehabilitation Psychology, 61*(2), 201–209.

Stucky, K. J., & Warren, A. M. (2019). Rehabilitation psychologists in critical care settings. In L. A. Brenner, S. Reid-Arndt, T. R. Elliott, R. G. Frank, & B. Caplan (Eds.), *The rehabilitation psychology handbook* (3rd ed., pp. 483–496). American Psychological Association.

Sukantarat, K., Greer, S., Brett, S., & Williamson, R. (2007). Physical and psychological sequelae of critical illness. *British Journal of Health Psychology*, *12*(1), 65–74.

Tan, T., Brett, S. J., & Stokes, T. (2009). Rehabilitation after critical illness: Summary of NICE guidance. *British Medical Journal, 338*, b822.

Thornton, M., & Travis, S. S. (2003). Analysis of the reliability of the modified caregiver strain index. *Journals of Gerontology: Series B: Psychological Sciences and Social Sciences*, *58*(2), S127–S132. http://dx.doi.org/10.1093/geronb/58.2.S127

Van den Born–van Zanten, S. A., Dongelmans, D. A., Dettling-Ihnenfeldt, D., Vink, R., & Van der Schaaf, M. (2016). Caregiver strain and posttraumatic stress symptoms of informal caregivers of intensive care unit survivors. *Rehabilitation Psychology*, *61*(2), 179–185. http://dx.doi.org/10.1037/rep0000080

Van der Schaaf, M., Beelen, A., Dongelmans, D. A., Vroom, M. B., & Nollet, F. (2009). Functional status after intensive care: A challenge for rehabilitation professionals to improve outcome. *Journal of Rehabilitation Medicine, 41*, 360–366.

Warren, A. M., Rainey, E., Weddle, R. J., Bennett, M., Roden-Foreman, K., & Foreman, M. L. (2016). The ICU experience: Psychological impact on family members of patients with and without traumatic brain injury. *Rehabilitation Psychology*, *61*(2), 179–185.

Warren, A. M., Stucky, K., & Sherman, J. J. (2013). Rehabilitation psychology's role in the level I trauma center. *Journal of Trauma and Acute Care Surgery, 74*, 1357–1362.

2 In a Split Second

ONE PATIENT'S PERSPECTIVE OF A LIFE CHANGED BY CRITICAL ILLNESS

Eileen Rubin

EDITORIAL INTRODUCTION: we believe that clinicians, as a rule, aspire to provide quality care to those in their charge. Sometimes clinicians are unaware of undesirable outcomes because patients don't tell them, and without that feedback clinicians don't have the opportunity to change practice patterns. We asked Eileen Rubin to share her story from her point of view without making substantial changes or additions. It is our hope that after reading this, clinicians will be even more convinced regarding the value of psychologically informed critical care, sophisticated rehabilitation, and follow-up care after discharge, all of which may have resulted in more favorable long-term outcomes for Eileen.

My world changed forever when I was 33 years old. I had been working as a criminal prosecutor for 7 years and had just gone into business as a sole practitioner doing criminal defense work. As I was developing my new practice, I began to experience excruciating low back pain. Initially, I did not allow this pain to interfere with my work, but eventually I could no longer tolerate it. After examining me, my internist told me that I must have pulled a muscle. I protested, because I knew I had not hurt myself. Nonetheless, I was sent home with two muscle relaxants. About 6 days later,

Eileen Rubin, *In a Split Second* In: *Critical Care Psychology and Rehabilitation*. Edited by: Kirk J. Stucky and Jennifer E. Jutte, Oxford University Press. © Oxford University Press 2022. DOI: 10.1093/oso/9780190077013.003.0002

I saw the internist's associate because my pain was now in my chest and back. At that time, I had deteriorated so much that I could not drive. I looked terrible. An exam was repeated, but no tests were ordered; the associate appeared to follow the notes from my original doctor, repeating that I had pulled a muscle. I was again sent home with the same medications.

The following day, I woke in such extreme pain that I had to crawl out of bed. I called the doctor's office at 5 a.m. and spoke to the associate; he told me to call back at 10 a.m. to speak to my own doctor. When I did so, much to my utter shock, she told me that she would not see me because they had seen me yesterday.

As I hung up the phone, I was in tears. I panicked but then called another doctor who agreed to see me later that afternoon. By the time of that appointment, I needed assistance to walk, my blood pressure was 70/50, and I had blood in my urine. I was shaky and struggling mentally. The doctor took blood and ordered a chest x-ray. However, he stated that if I went to the hospital for the chest x-ray, the hospital would likely admit me, and he did not urge me to go there. He gave me a choice, but I was incapable of making an informed decision about what would be best for me. I had my outpatient chest x-ray and returned home.

The next morning, the doctor called me early and said that I needed to go to the emergency department (ED) immediately. I became extremely emotional and started crying. When I arrived in the ED I was diagnosed with septic shock. No etiology was determined. I was admitted directly to the intensive care unit (ICU). That night, my kidneys failed. The next day, I felt slightly better, but my chest x-rays were getting worse. The following morning, 2 days into my admission to the ICU, I said to my mother, "I can't breathe; I think I'm dying."

My mother found my internist, who told her that I was fine and that I was "just anxious." Nonetheless, he (reluctantly) returned to my room. At that point, my family was removed from the room, a code was called, and chaos ensued. My family stayed in the waiting room for over 2 hours. When they came back to see me, I was sedated and on a ventilator, fighting for my life. Shortly after that, I was diagnosed with acute respiratory distress syndrome (ARDS).

After those initial 2 days, I was sedated quite heavily. Because I was very agitated, additional paralytics were administered to the point that I was completely deconditioned. My oxygen level was at 100% and my positive end-expiratory pressure (PEEP), though it changed, was high. At some point, both lungs collapsed, and I needed two chest tubes. During these weeks, I also suffered fluid overload, causing my body to balloon up in weight, and my eyes were taped closed. I was also restrained at my wrists. When the fluid overload subsided, my body weight had dropped from 104 pounds to only 82 pounds. I had a main line placed, and a tracheostomy was performed sometime around 10 to 14 days into my hospitalization.

After only 2 weeks, my physicians suggested "pulling the plug" because they said that they had done all they could do medically. They told my family that I would never breathe without supplemental oxygen and, worse, that I would never be weaned from mechanical ventilation. They stressed that I likely had suffered brain damage, and it had become a "quality of life" issue. My family declined and directed medical professionals to do everything they could to save my life.

Doctors told my family that my spleen had deteriorated by 90%, requiring surgery; however, as I was too sick to endure the procedure, it was cancelled. I also received four units of blood, a spinal tap, and many other tests to try to determine the precipitating cause of the ARDS that I was fighting. Throughout my hospitalization, I was intermittently delirious, and I nearly died several times.

After about 4 weeks in the ICU, the sedation was lifted and I began to awaken. I remained on the ventilator with my oxygen at 100% and my PEEP at a high level. Although I do not recall anything specific while in the medically induced coma, I know that I was taking in some information. For example, once I regained consciousness, each provider introduced themselves and told me their specialty area. Despite never having met any of them prior to hospitalization, I already knew who each doctor was and their specialty and, most of all, I knew who I liked and who I did not like.

I was so physically deconditioned that I could not even lift a finger. I was unable to communicate in any way, even by mouthing words to medical staff and family. There were no communications boards, and there was no attempt to establish eye blinking as a method of communication. This was terribly frustrating. One day, a doctor came into my room, told me that I was watching too much television and simply switched to the hospital music channel. I was outraged. I wanted the channel switched back, but as much as I willed my finger to move, nothing happened. I was unable to press the call button for the nurses. I became so anxious that I was literally screaming inside my head. I finally collapsed asleep, and when I awoke, I was relieved to find that the television was back on a regular channel.

A few days after emerging from my medically induced coma, I was told that I was being moved to the ventilator floor. This alarmed me, as the transfer was taking place late at night and I did not know why. It would also take me away from all of the hospital staff that I had come to know and trust. I immediately became highly anxious. How would visitors find me? I was not thinking clearly. I recall my family telling me that this meant I was getting better, but I was convinced that I was not. I eventually learned that a single room had become available on the vent floor, and they did not want to pass up the opportunity for me to have my own room.

When I got to the vent floor, they told my family that visiting hours were over and they had to leave. Suddenly, my only support was gone. Shortly after that, I fell into a terrible delirium and narcotic withdrawal. I had strange and vivid dreams, my hands were shaking uncontrollably, and my mouth hung open. Some visitors were so alarmed at my condition that two of them never came back, it so troubled them. An uncle who saw me during this time called my cousins and said, "Eileen is going to die."

Finally, after a few days, a neurological consult was ordered. I recall being angry that they were adding yet another doctor to my case. I felt I had no control over my health and decisions that were being made on my behalf. Although I am not certain what my reasoning was, I decided not to cooperate with this new doctor. Clearly, I was disoriented, and I was reacting in a defiant manner without even knowing why. I recall that I refused to follow any of his requests. He read the notes, spoke to my family and staff, and examined me. He raised my right arm over my head and dropped it, then my left arm and dropped it. He then explained to me and my family that he believed that my transfer to another floor in the hospital and the discontinuation of my sedating medications had produced a "hospital psychosis." Because he spoke to both my family and to me, it was the first time I had felt like part of the "team." After four tests, including another spinal tap, my morphine was reintroduced and then tapered slowly. I gradually emerged from my delirium and narcotic withdrawal.

During the next 4 weeks, I remained on the ventilator. One day, my temperature spiked to 105 degrees. Doctors told me that a *Pseudomonas aeruginosa* infection had developed in my tracheostomy. During my weeks on the vent floor, both lungs collapsed a second time, requiring three more chest tubes. At that point, I was considered to be vent-dependent. I was not progressing with weaning from the ventilator. When, without letting me know, the staff tried another method of breathing that forced me to take breaths on my own, almost immediately I panicked, and this had to be discontinued. I experienced persistent anxiety, several panic attacks, and a depressed mood. I was still struggling with mobility. Just trying to move from lying down to sitting up caused my blood pressure to drop quickly and resulted in my body reacting with fear, panic, and shaking. Any time therapists or nurses moved me in such a way, I would physically react like that. I had physical therapy (PT) and occupational therapy (OT), but I was progressing very slowly. I was also provided with speech therapy, but I dismissed the therapist, writing on my notes, "If I can't talk and I can't walk, I don't care if I can think."

One day, one of my pulmonologists came to update me regarding my condition. I began writing notes on my pad of paper, but when I looked up, the doctor had turned his back and was walking out of the room. I tried to throw my pad of paper at him to get his attention but missed. I was too weak, but I was infuriated.

Eventually, I began to wean from the ventilator, about 5% a day. I was able to do more with my physical and occupational therapists. During my seventh week in the hospital, my physical therapist told me we were going to walk from my chair out into the hallway. A physical therapist walked on one side of me, and a nurse walked on the other side, both assisting me. A respiratory therapist was at my side "bagging" me as I walked, since I was still on the ventilator. When I finally sat down, the staff at the nurse's station gave me a standing ovation. I was like a baby who had just taken her first steps. I felt wonderful when I realized how these nurses were so invested in my progress.

After 8 weeks on the ventilator, I finally weaned successfully. I spent 1 more week in the hospital, during which I passed my swallow test. My chest tubes and nasogastric (NG) tube were removed, and I continued PT and OT. After all of this was accomplished, I was finally discharged to my home.

To say this was the fight of my life would be an understatement. However, this momentous hospitalization was not just about me. It was also about my devoted and dedicated family, who were at my bedside each of the 63 days I was in the hospital. My parents spent every day there, and my brothers, their wives, and my sister were there every day as well, asking questions, doing research, and letting people know that I had a family that cared about me that they needed to answer to.

This story is also about those nurses, who held my hand, comforted me, calmed me, cared for me. I cannot overestimate how much the connection with my nurses lifted me, both physically and metaphorically when I could not lift myself. It is also about my devoted doctors who were always there or on call during my worst crisis . . . and I was in crisis so often. Nonetheless, those doctors did more than their "jobs" because in me, I believe they saw their wives, sisters, or children, and they would not let me die on their watch. And thankfully, they did not. It is also about the physical and occupational therapists, who made sure I kept moving and thinking and remained motivated, and certainly my respiratory therapists, who were overall very kind and gentle, especially when suctioning secretions from my throat and mouth.

After surviving ARDS against the odds, my doctors advised me that recovery would be difficult but after about a year, I would be fine and back to "normal." This was not completely accurate.

I did struggle during the year following my hospital discharge. I was completely dependent on others for almost everything. I needed help bathing. I needed someone to stand outside of my bathroom door to make sure I did not fall. Someone had to create and serve my meals. I spent the next several months in outpatient physical therapy. When I walked and exercised at home, someone needed to accompany me to make sure I did not fall. I could not drive for almost 4 months.

I was very isolated, and I was feeling depressed. My days were long, and I was alone too often. When I fell asleep at night, I would wake up about an hour or two later, and then I could not fall back to sleep. I was reliving my hospitalization over and over. Even now, decades later, I still have difficulty sleeping. Further, I still suffer long-term effects of my hospitalization that result in anxiety or incidents of post-traumatic stress disorder relating to surviving ARDS.

On the other hand, after about 4 months, I went to work part time, doing filing and light computer work. This was so beneficial, as it enabled me to begin to reorient myself and experience the responsibility of a schedule and work environment. Four months later, I went back to work as an attorney part time. I also got pregnant about 6 months after my discharge from the hospital. I had my first child 15 months after my hospital discharge and my second child 22 months after that.

I realize that my life did not return to "normal." That is not to say that I did not achieve a life worth living, but this process was very slow and very arduous. As a patient, being in the hospital, especially in the ICU, is a frightening, anxiety-filled time. It is likely the worst time one can experience. From my experience, I believe that greater effort to include patients and families as part of the care team would likely contribute to a reduction of anxiety, stress, and terror. It would increase a cooperative environment for everyone involved in the care of that patient, and everyone would benefit. Also, as a survivor, while it is difficult to feel exactly like I felt before getting ARDS, I have found a different sense of "normal" and, definitely, I live a life worth living.

I always thought that I would do something to "give back" after my hospitalization, but I was not sure how it would manifest itself. Five years after my discharge, I co-founded the nonprofit organization ARDS Foundation in December 2000. Initially, the goal was merely to create a brochure in plain language that could be understood by patients and families with ARDS. With the assistance of medical professionals, the brochure was created and the ARDS Foundation's website went online. Almost immediately, we were contacted by people all over the world, and we realized that people were hungry for an organization that offered support, education, information, and awareness of ARDS.

In the years that have followed, the ARDS Foundation has connected with thousands of patients and families affected by ARDS and related medical complications. As president and CEO of the ARDS Foundation, I have had the opportunity to offer the patient and family perspective to many medical professionals at meetings or conferences. Aside from speaking, I have worked with professional medical societies and sat on a number of committees with the goal of offering the patient perspective on critical care issues. I have been co-author on a number of publications that have appeared in a variety of medical journals, and I have gone to Capitol Hill for a Congressional briefing addressing ARDS. In the past, the ARDS Foundation has offered partnership medical grants for new research and also graduate-level nursing scholarships for candidates continuing their master's degrees in critical care medicine. Finally, I have been personally engaged in research, being principal investigator for a 2017–2018 Patient-Centered Outcomes Research Institute (PCORI) Pipeline to Proposal Tier A Award for Humanizing Critical Care for Patients and Families.

The ARDS Foundation continues to work with those devoted medical professionals who have dedicated themselves to their work with ARDS and its aftermath. But most important is the work that we do for patients and families who face the devastating diagnosis of ARDS. I knew that if I survived ARDS and had done nothing for others with that diagnosis who followed me, I would not be able to live with myself. The ARDS Foundation, and helping others after a diagnosis of ARDS, is now my passion.

Editorial comment: We thank the author for being so candid in sharing her story and remaining dedicated to helping other critical illness survivors. Some of the details provided are likely difficult for clinicians to read, but they are necessary in order to more clearly understand the patient experience and to inspire us to continually work toward a more integrated standard of care. Eileen's anger and frustration toward her initial providers is palpable throughout her narrative. Would she feel less angry if she perceived that her providers had listened better? Her challenging critical care admission was punctuated by delirium, which likely impacted her overall perception and memory regarding what actually occurred. Would that have been positively impacted if a psychologist had worked with her regularly? Communication issues, isolation, and anxiety were also major concerns. If ICU humanization initiatives had been in place, is it reasonable to assume that she would have been more satisfied with her overall experience. Finally, some of her most positive experiences were with therapists, nurses, and physicians during the initial stages of rehabilitation and recovery. Would this have been even more effective and memorable if rehabilitation principles were integrated throughout the continuum of care? The chapters that follow in this book unpack and discuss each of these relevant issues in more depth.

3 Critical Care, Psychology, and Rehabilitation

INTEGRATIVE ASPIRATIONS

Kirk J. Stucky

Introduction

A central argument throughout this book is that the integration of early psycho-logical and rehabilitative interventions into critical care can have a positive and pro-found impact on desired outcomes, both short and long term. In 2010 the Society of Critical Care Medicine (SCCM) convened a stakeholders' conference to encourage improvements across the continuum of care for critical illness survivors, especially those dealing with postintensive care syndrome (PICS) (Needham et al., 2012). The conference participants indicated that ideally these survivors would have ongoing access to sophisticated rehabilitation services, including outpatient follow-up clin-ics. Barriers to realizing this vision included the existence of what they referred to as "silos" in clinician groups and a host of other factors that interfere with the coordi-nation of care. Today, there is tremendous variability worldwide in practice. Some hospitals have little to no psychology or rehabilitation involvement across the criti-cal care continuum while others have developed sophisticated systems (Jackson & Jutte, 2016). In this chapter, various integrative concepts are outlined along with a summary of the literature supporting the efficacy of rehabilitation during and after the intensive care unit (ICU) stay. To set a foundation that supports this philosophy

Kirk J. Stucky, *Critical Care, Psychology, and Rehabilitation* In: *Critical Care Psychology and Rehabilitation*. Edited by: Kirk J. Stucky and Jennifer E. Jutte, Oxford University Press. © Oxford University Press 2022. DOI: 10.1093/oso/9780190077013.003.0003 of care, it is first important to define alternative models to make clear how they can or might be applied within and throughout the continuum.

Health care team models

The depth and breadth of health care knowledge is far too complex and expansive for any one clinician to master. This reality, especially in the era of modern medicine, has made clear the need for many types of professionals, hospitals, and clinics and flexible approaches to service delivery. In the health care system, in general, there are three types of teams: multidisciplinary, interdisciplinary, and transdisciplinary. Each model has a different approach to treatment, leadership, and team coordination. Although there are similarities and differences with regard to how these models are defined and described, for the purposes of this chapter they generally align with Karol's description of team models in neurorehabilitation (2014). An in-depth discussion regarding the pros and cons of these approaches is beyond the scope of this chapter, but the reader is referred to the article by Karol (2014) for a more detailed exploration. For present purposes the models are generally defined as outlined in Table 3.1.

Karol put forth the idea that in neurorehabilitation the transdisciplinary model is the most sophisticated and patient-centered. However, as will be illustrated, in critical care settings a transdisciplinary model is not necessarily ideal for a variety of reasons.

Toward a more sophisticated team model in critical care

Due to the complexity of issues and shifting needs of the patient, family, and staff over time, none of the models will ideally meet all situational demands. Instead, a hybrid approach that primarily combines interdisciplinary and transdisciplinary team philosophies is required. For example, when a new patient is admitted to the ICU, the intensivist leads a small interdisciplinary team and directs all of the acute interventions. Each clinician has very specific duties and responsibilities that they "own" and know well (e.g., setting up intravenous lines, performing intubation, monitoring vital signs, administering medications, performing surgical interventions). Similar to the multidisciplinary approach, during this acute phase, the attending physician might call for consultations from various specialists but will not expect or even want that specialist to take over aspects of care without explicit permission. If the patient survives but remains at risk for an undesirable outcome

TABLE 3.1.

Comparison between team models in health care

	Multidisciplinary	Interdisciplinary	Transdisciplinary
Orientation	Profession-centered: Care is provided within specific boundaries and clinicians are not routinely required to coordinate their efforts with other professionals.	Mixed professional- and patient-centered: Care is provided by multiple professionals with acknowledgment of overlapping boundaries and that aspects of care can be shared.	Patient/family-centered: Care is designed to be optimally patient- and family-centered. The team focuses on the needs of the patient and family as a whole, identifying their unique assets and issues in order to tailor goals to specific needs. Team members share responsibilities and embrace overlapping roles and responsibilities.
Team composition, coordination, and coverage	Variable: Clinicians may come and go during the course of care depending on the attending physician's requests. Team members may change frequently or intermittently and team cohesion may not be a priority.	Semi-stable: A core team of professionals is involved but they may rotate on and off frequently during the course of care.	Relatively stable: The team is one cohesive and consistent unit that is closed to outside "float" staff or the "pool." The same clinicians remain involved throughout the course of care, although there is necessary rotation when staff have days off. New providers may be added if the patient's needs change.
Team communication	Disciplines report to the physician, who then makes decisions about how to proceed with treatment. If rounds or meetings are held, they are typically run by the physician.	Team meetings are held regularly, typically run by the physician. Core team members talk with one another formally and informally to coordinate care and discuss shared goals.	Coordination and mutual understanding of the goals and roles of team members is crucial to success. This requires that clinicians talk with one another often and freely. Team meetings are held often. Leadership may change or rotate depending on the patient's specific needs.

Patient/family communication	Individual practitioners talk to the patient about their specific area of focus. Alternatively, the physician gathers information from the team and relays that to the patient and family. The patient and family are often not considered members of the team and are not typically invited to team conferences, rounds, or other collaborative discussions.	Patient and family are typically considered part of the team. Conferences for the patient and family are held in which they can ask questions of team members, provide feedback, and make requests.	The patient and family are considered to be part of the team and fully integrated whenever possible. When appropriate, rounds are held at the bedside so that the patient and family can participate.
Treatment and treatment planning	Each individual professional owns and is solely responsible for their piece of the treatment plan. The physician remains aware of these various activities and modifies the overall plan as needed. Although team members may talk with or read one another's notes, they do not typically create or own a joint treatment plan.	Disciplines may share some aspects of the treatment plan but not all. Clinicians work together and establish shared, as well as discipline-specific, goals. Meetings are held in which broad goals are discussed (e.g., barriers to functional recovery, increased quality of life).	All disciplines are equally responsible for executing the treatment plan and work synergistically to accomplish broad goals. Treatment plans are holistic with tailored goals to address the patient's specific needs.
Workload demands	Standard; professionals are only responsible for specific tasks and a restricted range of duties according to their areas of expertise. Coordinated co-treatment does not occur or occurs very rarely.	Medium; professionals have shared responsibilities, meetings, and other requirements. Their scopes of practice may overlap. Co-treatment may also occur.	High; all disciplines are equally responsible and work synergistically to accomplish broad goals. Co-treatment is common and sometimes results in "role release" in which clinicians are not required to practice outside of their scope but function within a team philosophy that allows them to safely use skillsets that might otherwise be discouraged in other models.

(e.g., delirium, debility, psychological complications), the core critical care team follows protocols that call in other professionals, recognizing that they will not be able to manage all of the patient and family needs without assistance. At this point the team model shifts toward an interdisciplinary and transdisciplinary mindset because of the need for more coordination, family integration, and co-treatment (e.g., early mobility for a ventilated patient; nurse, respiratory therapist, and physical therapist coordinate care with a psychologist who can assist in addressing motivational issues and avoidance behaviors). During this stage on the ICU, there may be two or more interdisciplinary teams working in tandem while interfacing periodically to address specific issues (see Figure 3.1 for an example). After ICU discharge, the patient may enter an inpatient rehabilitation program where an interdisciplinary team addresses the survivor's physical, cognitive, and psychological issues. The focus at this stage will likely be on improving strength and endurance, learning adaptive strategies, and managing basic activities of daily living (ADLs) (e.g., hygiene, transfers). Finally, when the patient can be discharged

OT = Occupational Therapy; PA = Physicians Assistant; PT = Physical Therapy; NP = Nurse Practitioner; SLP = Speech and Language Pathology; RT = Respiratory Therapy; SW = Social Work

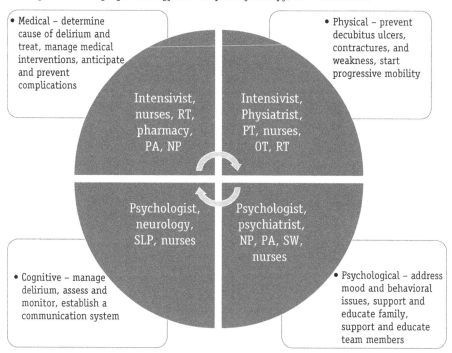

FIGURE 3.1 Overlapping interdisciplinary teams with a ventilated, delirious patient.

home, the team's attention turns to community reentry, higher-level ADLs, and advanced functional goals (e.g., shopping, driving, independent living). At this stage of recovery, an outpatient rehabilitation program that employs both interdisciplinary and transdisciplinary approaches becomes necessary.

Although a fully integrated model that spans the continuum of care is considered to be optimal, there may be organizational, financial, and even practical reasons why this may not be possible in some settings. Ultimately, the institution has to decide which approach to care will best meet the needs of the patients in their charge. Considering the wide range of ICU settings and practice locations, it is not possible to provide specific standards or directives regarding ideal team models in specific settings, circumstances, or phases of care. Consequently, I will not attempt to provide a detailed review of all potential permutations and combinations of team approaches. However, a few broad organizational considerations should be touched upon before moving on to a more detailed discussion regarding rehabilitation and its application to critical care practice.

First, the traditional medical model calls upon the critical care team to save the patient's life. Once the patient is stable, they yield care to a separate team, often with no or very limited expectation for the critical care professionals to follow up. In some hospitals, rehabilitation teams may not have the access, or the workforce necessary, to address the difficulties experienced by patients and their families on the ICU. In fact, in some settings, the rehabilitation system is intentionally excluded until the critical care team consults them, often when the patient is almost ready for ICU discharge. These traditional, although arguably outdated, models did not develop accidentally. There is practicality built into them in that most health care teams are already stretched for coverage, and often the culture, business model, and accrediting bodies do not require or incentivize a more holistic approach. Thus, considering the differences in philosophy, staff availability, and external pressures, it is not surprising that integrating these two teams can be very challenging and in many settings is not easily accomplished.

Second, in teaching hospitals, the team and educational models should be synchronized. As trainees advance, they tend to mirror what they learned from their supervisors—or do the opposite if their experience was negative. If professionals in training do not obtain positive experiences in coordinated care delivery, they are not likely to value or think to join such models when they become independent practitioners. Thus, in addition to acquiring specific competencies, trainees need to learn why a specific team approach is being used and how that relates to protocols, coordination, and the overall plan of care. Making these systemic features explicit can help trainees understand the "big picture" and experience firsthand the efficacy and efficiencies realized through coordinated care. In addition, the level of "buy-in" from the faculty, core clinical staff, and trainees regarding the model's value can have a profound impact on patient care, the quality of training, and the institution as a whole.

Third, if the hospital has an ICU but does not have a rehabilitation unit, the interface between critical care and rehabilitation teams may not be possible unless there is administrative commitment to hiring those clinicians to work on the ICU. This may be especially challenging for smaller hospitals and settings in which more complicated patients are typically transferred to level 1 trauma centers or other large specialty hospitals.

Fourth, if the hospital has an ICU and some rehabilitation staff but no psychologist, it will likely be difficult to establish more sophisticated systems of care that address the cognitive and psychological complications often encountered by survivors and families dealing with PICS or postintensive care syndrome–family (PICS-F). Although social workers, psychiatric nurse practitioners, and psychiatrists have valuable skillsets, the rehabilitation-oriented psychologist is uniquely trained to provide a wide range of services and can act as a bridge between critical care and rehabilitation (Stucky & Warren, 2019; Warren et al., 2013). For example, psychologists in critical care settings commonly provide cognitive assessment and capacity evaluations. A recent survey found that rehabilitation-oriented psychologists, relative to other psychologists, were also much more likely to provide family support and education, behavioral management, and help in determining the appropriateness for rehabilitation admission (Stucky et al., 2016). Those same authors also suggested that rehabilitation psychologists can be instrumental in facilitating transfer to rehabilitation by

(a) asking open-ended questions for patients/family members to describe their thoughts pertaining to transfer; (b) ascertain what type of information might be helpful to them; (c) providing imaginal exposure to the acute care medical floor; (d) introducing one of their providers prior to transition; (e) and meeting with . . . them immediately following the transition (and beyond if necessary). (Stucky et al., 2016, p. 202)

Finally, psychologists on the critical care team are in a unique position to provide staff support through didactic sessions, provision of educational materials and resources, and active and consistent guidance on working with complicated patients.

Rehabilitation in critical care: the case for integration

In the United States there are already established pathways from the ICU to rehabilitation for individuals who have sustained traumatic brain injury (TBI), spinal cord injury (SCI), stroke, burn injury, and polytrauma. Unfortunately, this is not yet true for survivors of critical illness (Needham et al., 2012), but current best practices in fields like neurorehabilitation can help inform the development of new systems of care. A number of centers have described their efforts to integrate rehabilitation into the continuum of critical care (Brummel et al., 2012; Dammeyer et al., 2013; Eakin et al., 2015; Needham & Korupolu, 2010). Some of those articles list a variety of barriers to this aspirational standard beyond clinical "silos," including underutilization of rehabilitation, limited awareness of critical illness outcomes, insurance restrictions, financial issues, and regulatory requirements (Hall et al., 2010; Needham et al., 2012). However, a growing body of literature makes clear that patients can benefit from rehabilitation throughout the continuum of care (Agarwala et al., 2011; Bailey et al., 2007; Berney et al., 2015). Although an integrated approach is also holistic, in the sections that follow we elaborate on the benefits of rehabilitation in addressing physical health due to the fact that other chapters in this text are dedicated to psychological and cognitive issues (please also see Chapters 4, 6, 11, and 13).

Intensive care

At a very basic level patients on the ICU can be separated into two broad categories: those with critical illness or injury who are not cognitively impaired (e.g., acute respiratory distress syndrome, patient in sickle cell crisis, SCI survivor) and those who are (e.g., delirium, sepsis, TBI, stroke). Tables 3.2 and 3.3 outline some examples of interventions that might be provided for patients on the ICU and the primary disciplines involved. As can be seen, rehabilitative approaches and treatment strategies with cognitively impaired and cognitively intact patients can be either quite different or nearly identical depending on the needs and circumstances. For example, patients with cognitive impairment typically require a structured routine that includes a low-stimulation protocol, frequent cognitive assessment with instruments like the Confusion Assessment Measure for the Intensive Care Unit (CAM-ICU), and interventions aimed at managing or reducing the length of confusion (Ely et al., 2001). On the other hand, a cognitively intact patient on the ICU who is still on the ventilator but cannot write may require a structured routine that includes protected time for adaptive communication with staff in order to promote careful

TABLE 3.2.

Team intervention examples with a cognitively impaired patient on the ICU

Intervention/Assessment	Purpose	Primary team (lead listed first)
Physical		
Basic range of motion (ROM)	Prevent contractures, skin breakdown, and muscle wasting	PT, OT, nursing, family/caregivers
Progressive mobility	• Improve strength, endurance, and cardiovascular health • Reduce ventilator days, ICU length of stay, and length of delirium • Enhance patient motivation and participation despite pain or emotional distress	PT, OT, nursing, respiratory therapy* Psychologists and family/caregivers for support and encouragement
Cognitive		
Sedation/coma assessment	• Monitor time to follow commands for those in coma or minimally conscious state • Optimize/minimize sedation	Physicians, nursing, psychology, SLP
Cognitive assessment (e.g., CAM-ICU)	• Monitor orientation and reorientation • Track delirium and assess change to inform treatment	Nursing, psychology, SLP
Low-stimulation/controlled stimulation	• Avoid over- and under-stimulation • Maintain structured environment and predictable schedule for therapy interventions	Nursing, psychology, all other providers and family/caregivers
Behavioral/Psychological		
Delirium management	• Identify likely causes of delirium • Sleep/wake cycle stabilization • Family education and support • Monitor protocols and plans for behavioral and environmental management	Physicians, psychologist, nursing

TABLE 3.2. Continued

Intervention/Assessment	Purpose	Primary team (lead listed first)
Behavioral management	• Address agitation • Reduce risk of harm to self and others • Family education and support • Interventions and plans for behavioral and environmental management	Psychologist, nursing, physicians, OT, SLP, PT, family/caregivers
Depression/anxiety	• Address and treat symptoms • Crisis management • Reduce risk of persistent acute stress/PTSD • Support for family/caregivers	Psychologist, nursing, social work, physicians (i.e., psychiatrist, intensivist, neurologist)
Functional		
Basic ADLs (e.g., toileting, hygiene)	• Determine level of care requirements and establish short- and long-term functional goals • Evaluate potential for rehab after ICU discharge • Improve self-efficacy • Determine readiness for discharge home or to an alternate setting	OT, nursing, PT, family/caregivers
Capacity assessment	Determine patient's ability to perform/manage higher-level ADLs and functional tasks (e.g., financial management, medical decision-making)	Psychologist, nursing, OT, SLP

*Especially if the patient is on a ventilator

CAM-ICU = Confusion Assessment Method for the Intensive Care Unit, OT = occupational therapy, PT = physical therapy, RT = respiratory therapy, SLP = speech and language pathology, ADLs = activities of daily living

TABLE 3.3.

Team intervention examples with a cognitively intact, ventilated patient on the ICU

Intervention/Assessment	Purpose	Primary team (lead listed first)
Physical		
Basic range of motion (ROM)/manual stretching	Prevent contractures, skin breakdown, and muscle wasting.	PT, OT, nursing, family/caregivers
Bed exercises	• Improve ROM, prevent stiffness, build strength • Prepare for more difficult exercises • Assess tolerance for increased activity	PT, OT, nursing, family/caregivers
Out-of-bed schedule	Build hemodynamic tolerance to sitting and out-of-bed activities	PT, OT, nursing, respiratory therapy, family/caregivers, psychology*
Progressive mobility	• Improve strength, endurance, and cardiovascular health • Reduce ventilator days and ICU length of stay • Enhance motivation and participation despite pain and emotional distress	PT, OT, nursing, respiratory therapy, family/caregivers, psychology*
Momentum schedules	Start with easy tasks and slowly increase difficulty based on patient performance/tolerance • Provide encouragement and reinforcement of desirable behaviors; emphasize progress	PT, OT, nursing, respiratory therapy, family/caregivers, psychology
Cognitive		
Establish communication	• Enhance patient's ability to communicate wants and needs and ask questions • Introduce adaptive tools (e.g., writing, letter or picture board, iPad)	SLP, psychology, nursing

TABLE 3.3.   Continued

Intervention/Assessment	Purpose	Primary team (lead listed first)
Determine patient's concerns/questions	• Use communication system to ensure that patient has information necessary to make informed choices • Increase patient's sense of control/autonomy	SLP, psychology, nursing, family/caregivers
Behavioral/Psychological		
Address depression/low motivation	• Determine if cause is psychological, physiologic, or both • Psychotherapy, activities (e.g., cards, music) to reduce isolation, address negative thoughts, and promote resilience	Psychology, psychiatry, social work, nursing
Address anxiety, refusal, and avoidance	• Use techniques to address patient anxiety about specific procedures or goals (e.g., blood draws, vent weaning) • Educate patient on purpose of monitors/treatment, psychotherapeutic techniques (e.g., systematic desensitization, distraction, music) • Recruit family members to assist	Psychology, psychiatry, social work, nursing
Ventilator weaning	Look at the ventilator and attempt to initiate larger tidal volume breaths on a pressure support setting	Nursing, RT, physicians, allied health
Functional		
Basic ADLs (e.g., toileting, hygiene)	• Determine level of care requirements and establish short- and long-term functional goals • Evaluate potential for rehab after ICU discharge • Improve self-efficacy.	OT, nursing, PT, family/caregivers

*Especially if anxiety, behavioral, and motivational issues are present

OT = occupational therapy, PT = physical therapy, RT = respiratory therapy, SLP = speech and language pathology, ADLs = activities of daily living explanation of the treatment plan and a clear understanding of the patient's concerns and informed choices.

In what follows, interventions for ICU-acquired weakness and other physical issues, mechanical ventilation (MV), pain management, cognitive/communication issues, and psychological issues are explored through an interdisciplinary lens. Detailed discussion of these areas falls beyond the scope of this chapter, but the references provided offer a solid foundation for more in-depth exploration if desired.

ICU-ACQUIRED WEAKNESS AND OTHER PHYSICAL CHALLENGES

It is not surprising that survivors of critical illness and injury, especially after long ICU admissions, frequently develop debility marked by weakness and low endurance (Fletcher et al., 2003; Stevens et al., 2007, 2009). For patients who require MV and have prolonged immobility, muscle catabolism often occurs, ultimately leading to declines in strength, anaerobic capacity, and diaphragmatic strength (Athari et al., 2019; Babb et al., 2012; Batt et al., 2017). In the most extreme cases, critical illness myopathy can result in profound declines in neuromuscular integrity and functional quadriparesis (Desai et al., 2011; Hermans & Van den Berghe, 2015; Latronico et al., 2017). In a review of 24 studies involving patients with sepsis, prolonged MV, and multiorgan failure, Needham (2008) found that neuromuscular dysfunction occurred in 46% of patients. Other individuals experience persistent joint stiffness, contractures, and pain that can linger long after the critical illness or injuries have primarily resolved.

Fortunately, studies have shown that early rehabilitation intervention and mobilization on the ICU is both safe and feasible (Brummel et al., 2014; Dubb et al., 2016; Jackson et al., 2012). When combined with sound medical practice, rehabilitative interventions can improve muscle strength (Connolly et al., 2016; Doiron et al., 2018), physical functioning (Geense et al., 2019; SCCM, 2011, Tan et al., 2009), pain (Archer et al., 2012; Barr et al., 2013), sleep (Devlin et al., 2018; Kamdar et al., 2011), and delirium (Schweickert et al., 2009) and also reduce the frequency of certain complications such as decubitus ulcers (Dickinson et al., 2013; Haesler, 2014; Shahin et al., 2009), joint stiffness (Laurent et al., 2016; Nydahl et al., 2014), contractures (Reid et al., 2018), and ICU-acquired weakness (De Jonghe et al., 2002; Dos Santos et al., 2016; Elliott et al., 2011; Kress & Hall, 2014). Reduced ventilator days and ICU length of stay have also been demonstrated (Girard et al., 2016; Pun et al., 2018). Occupational therapists (OTs) and physical therapists (PTs) can assist with mobility goals while also introducing other interventions unique to their discipline (e.g., progressive splinting for contractures, assisting with basic ADLs) (Dinglas et al., 2013; Miller et al., 2015; Prohaska et al., 2019; Weinreich et al., 2017). OTs and PTs can assist nurses in ensuring that timely turning, passive range of motion, and pressure relief are performed regularly to preserve joints, avoid skin breakdown, improve strength, and potentially decrease time on MV.

These same team members can teach family members to safely perform certain techniques (e.g., massage, passive range of motion), which gives the patient's loved ones a greater understanding and a productive role in executing the treatment plan. Loved ones are often overwhelmed, feel helpless, and are looking for ways to help (Paul & Rattray, 2008; van den Born–van Zanten et al., 2016; Warren et al., 2016). Being welcomed as part of the team and given new knowledge or specific tasks can empower them and direct emotional energy in a much more fruitful fashion (Davidson & Zisook, 2017).

MECHANICAL VENTILATION

Not surprisingly, the sensation of being unable to breathe or being short on air causes a great deal of distress and has been referred to as "air hunger" (see Chapter 11 for more detailed discussion). Individuals who remember being on MV often describe the awkward sensation of having air forced into their lungs and the peculiar experience of having to learn to breathe both with and without the machine on various settings. In addition, the process of weaning from MV can be anxiety-provoking and potentially traumatic, especially if weaning protocols are initiated but do not include proper education, preparation, reassurance, and emotional support. When anxious, breathing can become quick and shallow, which further contributes to the individual's perception that they are not able to breathe. While anxiety can be addressed by modifications in medications, as well as ventilator settings, these strategies are sometimes not enough. Along with other members of the team, psychologists can coach the family and patient through the process, perhaps teaching relaxation strategies in an effort to reduce anxiety and improve the odds of successful ventilator weaning.

PAIN MANAGEMENT

Pain is a common issue on the ICU. It can hamper response to rehabilitative efforts and also contribute to increased confusion and psychological distress (Archer et al., 2012). The optimization of pain control and reducing sedation before therapy sessions requires considerable coordination between the critical care and rehabilitation team. For example, to foster participation and tolerance of exercises and stretching, PTs and OTs will likely prefer to coordinate the administration of pain medication, typically 30 to 45 minutes prior to treatment. Psychologists, nurses, and other providers can teach cognitively intact patients nonpharmacologic strategies for pain management such as distraction, calm breathing, visualization and the like (Boutron et al., 2008; Gélinas et al., 2013). While a confused patient is not likely to benefit from nonpharmacologic techniques like mindfulness or distraction, the team can make other recommendations. For example, due to the difficulty in properly gauging their needs at any specific point in time, a delirious patient may respond better to scheduled pain medication dosing rather than an "as needed" format. Finally, recruiting trusted loved ones to encourage patients through, or to be present during, uncomfortable procedures and activities can be particularly effective in curbing anxiety, resistance, paranoia, and other counterproductive psychological reactions (for more in-depth discussion of pain management see Chapter 7).

COGNITIVE AND COMMUNICATION ISSUES

Patients on the ICU are often in, or vacillating between, various stages of cognitive compromise (e.g., coma, minimally conscious, confused, emerging from delirium) and can benefit from various nonpharmacologic techniques that are also frequently used in neurorehabilitation. Fortunately, these approaches with the confused patient are quite similar whether the diagnosis is TBI, stroke, or delirium. Psychologists, working in concert with the rehabilitation and critical care teams, can help establish and maintain low-stimulation and environmental management protocols, behavioral management plans, and delirium management initiatives such as those in the ICU liberation bundle (Ely, 2017; Gelinas et al., 2013; Girard et al., 2018) (also see Chapter 6). Numerous authors have written about various speech and swallowing complications during and after extubation and have also described adaptive communication interventions in the hospital setting (Heffner, 2010; Husain et al., 2001; Macht et al., 2014; Mirzakhani et al., 2013; Skoretz et al., 2010).

Cognitive and communication interventions are not limited to use with cognitively impaired patients. Psychologists, psychiatrists, and neurologists have unique assessment skills that can be used to determine an individual's decision-making capacity and also identify patients who are cognitively intact but simply do not have the means to communicate effectively. Patients in this situation frequently report high levels of distress and frustration (Pennock et al., 1994; Rotondi et al., 2002). When identified, specific interventions can be implemented with far-reaching impacts on the patient, family, and quality of care. For example, consider a cognitively intact patient who is on the ventilator but cannot write. Staff from speech–language pathology (SLP) and psychology introduce an adaptive communication system that initially consists of letter and picture boards, later advancing to use of an iPad. Medical staff and the family are then able to use this system to learn the patient's concerns and informed choices as care progresses. Unfortunately, on most ICUs, staff primarily rely on unaided strategies such as silent articulation (mouthing words), gestures, and body language, although evidence suggests that they are insufficient and frequently frustrating for all parties (Broyles et al., 2012; Happ et al., 2011). Mobasheri and colleagues (2016) make useful recommendations on the use of augmentative and alternative communication aids for patients with transient loss of speech, including pen and paper, picture boards, computer-based devices with synthesized speech, and tablet-based platforms. Furthermore, for nonverbal patients with tetraplegia or locked-in syndrome, eye-tracking computer systems are available and it is critical to establish use as early as possible. More detailed discussion is beyond the scope of this chapter, but suffice it to say that early involvement of staff from SLP and psychology can go a long way in implementing sophisticated adaptive and augmentative communication that will have a meaningful impact on patient care, potentially reducing the risk of undesirable psychological outcomes (Mobasheri et al., 2016).

PSYCHOLOGICAL ISSUES

It is well known that patients and family members on the ICU are at increased risk for anxiety (Hopkins et al., 2010; Sukantarat et al., 2007), depression (Bienvenu et al., 2012; Davydow et al., 2009; Pochard et al., 2001), and posttraumatic stress disorder (Jackson et al., 2016; Kapfhammer et al., 2004; Peris et al., 2011). When psychological and behavioral issues are present, psychologists are uniquely trained to diagnose, treat, and direct comprehensive treatment plans, potentially calling in psychiatrists for specific pharmacologic interventions (Azoulay et al., 2005; Bienvenu et al., 2017) (also see Chapter 11). Psychologists, along with other staff, can introduce ICU diaries, coping skills training, and psychoeducation for families in need of support, empathy, and understanding (Garrouste-Orgeas et al., 2012; Jones et al., 2010, 2012; Nielsen et al., 2019). Also, psychologists can offer assistance in crisis management for the patient and family, something that other team members typically do not have the time, training, or comfort to provide (Davidson et al., 2012; Jackson & Jutte, 2016; Warren et al., 2013).

Staff on the critical care and rehabilitation teams are often called on to provide emotional support, education, and reassurance. Coupled with their many other duties, this can be psychologically taxing and time-consuming for critical care clinicians (Moss et al., 2016). An embedded psychologist or behavioral health professional can serve to offload some of this work, resulting in numerous downstream benefits for the patient, family, and staff (e.g., reduce risk of compassion fatigue, better resource allocation, improved family support). Previous publications have argued that rehabilitation psychologists have specific competencies in these and the aforementioned areas that make them uniquely well suited for practice in the ICU environment (Stucky et al., 2016; Stucky & Warren, 2019; Warren et al., 2013).

Keys to ICU implementation

Some studies have shown that with critically ill patients, PTs working with nursing staff can achieve greater levels of mobilization than nursing staff alone (Garzon-Serrano et al., 2011). Despite this, rehabilitation professionals are not usually consulted until after extubation or near the end of the ICU admission. For example, Hodgin and colleagues (2009) found that PTs automatically evaluated ICU patients at only 1% of hospitals in the United States. One of the primary reasons for late consultation of rehabilitation professionals is thought to be related to concern that too much or overly aggressive therapy can harm vulnerable patients and lead to more complications (e.g., accidentally pulling out lines, threats to physiologic stability). To address this, in more recent years, the SCCM and others (e.g., Dammeyer et al., 2013) have started to establish guidelines for early mobilization along with specific exclusion criteria and safety measures that are employed before, during, and after mobility sessions (Table 3.4). Notably, although a medical intensivist participated in and supported the project, the implementation was driven by nurses at the bedside, and therapy consults were entered automatically. In addition, a comprehensive orientation was developed for staff, with lectures and written manuals outlining techniques for airway clearance, managing lines, and physical handling and positioning techniques.

The value of progressive mobility and the ICU liberation bundle (aka ABCDEF bundle) has mounting support in the literature (Ely, 2017; Harrison & Kirkpatrick, 2011; Hoenig et al., 2015; Jutte et al., 2015, 2017; Musicco et al., 2003; Pun et al., 2018), but implementation is not easy. For example, early mobility for ventilated patients is not possible without, at minimum, approval by physicians and close collaboration among staff from respiratory therapy, nursing, and physical therapy. Also, the process itself is quite labor-intensive, requiring multiple staff to simultaneously provide physical assistance, manage equipment, and monitor physiologic status. Initially these efforts increase the workload for everyone, and true cultural change does not occur until the staff recognize the interventions as effective, safe, and best for the patient. Providing staff with evidence-based literature supporting reduced ventilator days, reduced length of stay, lower restraint use, and better functional outcomes can help providers consider a change in practice (Dammeyer et al., 2013). Researchers have also indicated that establishing an early mobility program requires recognition

TABLE 3.4.

Exclusion criteria and contraindications for mobility

Exclusion criteria	Contraindications for initiating PT session	Contraindications for continuing active PT session
Ventilatory settings	Vital signs	Vital signs
FIO$_2$ > 60%	MAP < 60	MAP < 60
PEEP > 12	SBP > 180	SBP > 200 sustained for 5 min (not resolving with rest break)
	Heart rate > 140	Heart rate > 165 sustained for 5 min (sinus tach only, not resolving with rest)
	Respiratory rate > 40	Respiratory rate > 40 sustained for 5 min (not resolving with rest)
	Pulse oximetry < 88%	Pulse oximetry < 85% sustained for 5 min
		or
		Symptomatic shortness of breath (not resolving with rest)
Other	Other	Other
*CRRT, if tenuous access with frequent alarms	*Agitation requiring increased sedative administration in last 30 min	*Patient distress as evidenced by nonverbal cues, gestures, agitation
*Arteriovenous fistula access	*New arrhythmia	*New arrhythmia
*Two vasopressors	*Concern for myocardial ischemia	*Concern for myocardial ischemia
*Active delirium tremens	*Concern for airway device integrity	*Concern for airway device integrity
*Gastrointestinal bleed/variceal hemorrhage with hypotension		
*Acute coronary syndrome		
*Increased intracranial pressure		
*Unstable tachyarrhythmias		
*Pulmonary artery catheter		

CRRT, continuous renal replacement therapy; FIO$_2$, fraction of inspired oxygen; MAP, mean arterial pressure; PEEP, positive end-expiratory pressure; PT, physical therapy; SBP, systolic blood pressure; SOB. Reproduced with permission from Dammeyer, J. A., Baldwin, N., Packard, D., Harrington, S., Christofferson, B., Christopher, J., Strachan, C. L., & Iwashyna, J. (2013). Mobilizing outcomes: Implementation of a nurse-led multidisciplinary mobility program. *Critical Care Nursing Quarterly, 36*(1), 109–119.

that this was connected to other related goals such as better sedation management, delirium recognition, and improving sleep/wake cycles. At Johns Hopkins, Eakin and colleagues (2015) reported on their efforts to implement and sustain an early rehabilitation program on an ICU. Similar to others, they identified multiple factors necessary for success. An integrated summary of suggestions made by various authors (Dammeyer et al., 2013; Eakin et al., 2015; Needham et al., 2012) has been provided to assist programs that are considering transition to interdisciplinary models that include critical care and rehabilitation team coordination:

Leadership: If new team models are imposed on a group by an outside authority without some "believers" on the team, the effort is likely to fail. Thus, specific members of the critical care and rehabilitation team (preferably in multiple disciplines) need to be passionate about, and invested in, the process of implementation. The team needs a "champion" who can jumpstart the integration of rehabilitation practices into the team. This requires a clear vision of what the new model will look like as well as an understanding of the preexisting team culture and anticipating barriers to implementation. Ideally these champions will present a well-thought-out proposal to administration and also be integral to preventing relapse into the older model once implementation begins.

Administrative support: Hospital leadership will be more likely to consider and tolerate increased costs if there is a likelihood of cost savings through reduced length of stay, lower complication rates, and other value-added outcomes. Therefore, clinical leaders need to present compelling and supportive evidence along with a specific plan for implementation. Extra resources (e.g., staff, equipment, training) have to be available and guaranteed long term to support such programs with a recognition that cost savings and improved patient satisfaction and outcomes may not be immediately apparent.

Addressing safety concerns: Concerns about inadvertent removal of medical devices and physiologic instability are understandable from staff who are skeptical about, or have not observed, early intervention. Literature on implementation suggests that staff had to believe that early rehabilitation was safe and beneficial prior to implementation. Case conferences to review outcomes, reassure staff, and finetune processes can be helpful. Some have noted that staff resistance to culture change and safety concerns often faded only after staff experienced firsthand the benefits of early intervention (Hodgson et al., 2014, 2016).

Staff training and buy-in: Because the integrated model increases the complexity and workload for everyone, varying degrees of resistance to change should be anticipated, especially if staff are unaware of the advantages. Ways to circumvent this potential barrier include didactics on evidence-based research supporting efficacy and venues in which staff can discuss patients and new protocols openly (e.g., team rounds, morbidity and mortality conferences). Ideally, staff should also be involved in the process of revamping procedures and reorganizing workflows.

Communication and cooperation: To function as an interdisciplinary team, rounds or huddles must occur regularly. Protocols and workflows have to be established that require and encourage coordination and cotreatment. During team meetings leaders should review clinical data while providing examples of how individuals worked as a team, complementing clinicians publicly for successful integration efforts. Reinforcing that the treatment plan and outcomes are owned by the team as a whole can help solidify commitment to the model and possibly improve job satisfaction. Some studies have reported improved patient outcomes and increased job satisfaction once an early mobility program was fully implemented (Dammeyer et al., 2013; Eakin et al., 2015).

Sedation practice and delirium management : Early mobility and rehabilitation can only be accomplished if combined with sophisticated sedation practices as outlined in the ICU liberation protocol (e.g., limited use of benzodiazepines, timing medications to complement rehabilitative initiatives) (Ely, 2017; Ely et al., 2001).

INPATIENT REHABILITATION

People who survive critical illness or injury almost always require some level of rehabilitation after discharge from the ICU. From the first contact, practitioners with a rehabilitative mindset are thinking about short- and long-term functional goals, barriers to independence, and interventions that will maximize the person's quality of life. However, Van der Schaaf and colleagues (2009) indicated that, as a result of changes in health care and health care financing, a higher proportion of patients are being discharged from the acute medical setting with little to no exposure to rehabilitative interventions. In fact, in the United States, patients who qualified for and received intensive inpatient rehabilitation in the past are no longer admitted due to more stringent admission criteria and numerous restrictions created by new Medicare guidelines, private insurance limitations, discharge planning requirements, reduced length of stay, and the prioritization of cost savings or cost cutting (Ottenbacher et al., 2004). Unfortunately, despite clear need, some survivors are determined to be ineligible for inpatient rehabilitation—for example, a patient who is ambulatory and can perform basic ADLs, but still has severe cognitive impairments. Although the patient clearly needs 24-hour supervision due to impulsivity, poor judgment, and memory impairment, the insurance company may not approve admission because they are deemed "too high functioning." Unfortunately, suitable placement options and rehabilitation programs for these patients are often limited, especially if there are behavioral issues or inadequate resources to pay for necessary care. Rehabilitation professionals who are familiar with the patient can sometimes anticipate and advocate in advance. As noted by various authors and in the preceding sections, there are likely multiple downstream benefits with regard to continuity of care when the patient and family continue to receive services from familiar professionals after discharge from the ICU (Merbitz et al., 2012). This becomes possible if rehabilitation professionals work on both the ICU and inpatient rehabilitation unit (Merbitz et al., 2016; Stucky & Warren, 2019). However, in larger medical centers where teams work on only one unit, this can be facilitated if the ICU team communicates with, and ensures a smooth transition to, the next team.

Successful rehabilitation is often measured by determining the degree and significance of functional recovery over time. During inpatient rehabilitation the focus is not typically on cure but rather on maximizing function and reducing the overall level of care required for that individual. If the patient will require long-term assistance, the emphasis may be on teaching patients how to direct their own care and advocate for themselves while also training caregivers in specific functions. Ideally, after a patient has survived critical illness or injury, successful inpatient rehabilitation prepares the patient and family for return home or transition to the least restrictive environment where quality of life is maximized, additional functional goals can be pursued, and the patient can resume engaging in important pursuits such as employment and social connection (Dowdy et al., 2005, 2006; Schelling et al., 1998).

OUTPATIENT FOLLOW-UP CLINICS

In the past two decades there has been increasing interest in the development of outpatient treatment centers to address the long-term needs of critical illness survivors (Cuthbertson et al., 2009; Griffiths et al., 2006; Jackson & Jutte, 2016; Walsh et al., 2012). Programs at Vanderbilt University, University of Indiana, University of San Diego, and Massachusetts General Hospital are examples of health care systems that are conducting research regarding the effectiveness of these programs and how to make them better. Some of these were modeled after cancer survivorship programs but with a focus on challenges specifically associated with PICS. They are based on the observation that patients sometimes lose gains made due to poor follow-through on home exercise, reverting to undesirable behavioral/health patterns, and/or inadequate education about what they are or are not supposed to do. These programs can also assist in these and other areas such as continued psychological/emotional support, cognitive rehabilitation, and physical interventions. Unfortunately, in systems that do not have ICU follow-up clinics, after discharge some patients are lost to follow-up and do not receive this type of ongoing rehabilitative care (also see Chapter 13). We hope that someday these holistic programs will be much more common and will function in a fashion similar to those designed for individuals with cancer, TBI, SCI, and burn injury.

REHABILITATION IN THOSE WITH INFECTIOUS DISEASE RESTRICTIONS

It is not unusual for patients with critical illness or injury to contract serious infections that mandate isolation and other aggressive precautions, such as methicillin-resistant *Staphylococcus aureus* (MRSA), severe acute respiratory syndrome (SARS), tuberculosis, and Middle East respiratory syndrome (MERS). This has become a more prominent reality during the novel coronavirus disease (COVID-19) pandemic and has created significant challenges beyond those already mentioned in this chapter, in part due to high patient volumes and logistical challenges. Notably, personal protective equipment (PPE) such as N95 masks, face shields, and gowns must be worn by anyone in contact with the patient (Ceravolo et al., 2020). In the early stages of the pandemic, there was considerable concern about the availability of these supplies that led to rationing. Furthermore, certain units or rooms must be set aside to house these infected patients, and strict procedures designed to minimize spread of the disease must be adhered to, which in turn stretches or divides limited resources for other patients (Simpson & Robinson, 2020).

Like others, individuals with highly infectious conditions also require progressive mobility, periodic evaluation of cognitive status due to high risk of delirium, and monitoring of emotional adjustment due to critical illness factors, coupled with the effects of increased isolation. In the delivery of these rehabilitation services, it is critical to consider whether they must be provided "hands on" or if they can be administered remotely. Considerations gleaned from Ceravolo and colleagues (2020), Sakai and colleagues (2020), and Simpson and Robinson (2020) are briefly discussed next.

Hands-on care

Standard nursing care and progressive mobility clearly fit into this category. Strategies to ensure implementation have to be built into the treatment plan proactively; otherwise, significant debility and complications might occur that could have been prevented or minimized. After ICU discharge these patients often require inpatient rehabilitation and/or outpatient care, which may be difficult to access during surges in case numbers or environments that are unprepared to manage patients adequately. The need to educate and protect health care staff has become a major focus for health care systems in order to (1) maintain the commitment and availability of specialty staff who are often in limited supply and high demand; (2) prevent infection spread; and (3) ensure that patients receive the same standard of care delivered to other patients.

Remote options

When hospitals establish reliable and ready telehealth platforms, it creates a number of apparent benefits. For example, using an iPad and Google Meets platform, the author of this chapter and his team have been able to conduct cognitive screens and interviews to assess emotional adjustment and intellectual functioning. These assessments, in turn, have allowed for more sophisticated monitoring and treatment planning. Without access to these tools, patients and families may not see one another for weeks or months, which can result in considerable emotional strain on them as well as the staff, who are often especially sensitive to the patient's angst, most particularly in those patients who are dying.

Some studies of intensive care patients that have investigated combined in-person rehabilitation and telerehabilitation interventions found this approach to be safe and feasible and to improve cognitive function at 3-month follow-up (Brummel et al., 2014; Jackson et al., 2012). However, telerehabilitation has clear limitations, including limited availability of equipment, restrictions on the physical examination, and reduced personnel to implement activities and ensure safety (Simpson & Robinson, 2020). As the COVID-19 pandemic evolves, it is anticipated that additional research will illuminate these issues and lead to advances in care delivery, staff support, and changes in the health care system.

Summary

People now survive critical illness and injury at higher rates thanks to advances in critical care, but those survivors and their families are often left to deal with a host of physical, cognitive, and psychological consequences (Herridge et al., 2011; Iwashyna, 2010; Iwashyna et al., 2010; Iwashyna & Netzer, 2012). Unfortunately, rehabilitation service lines are not as available to critical illness survivors as they are for individuals who have sustained stroke, TBI, burn injury, or SCI. A growing body of literature and programs across the world forecasts an expanding evolution in the continuum of critical care toward the integration of rehabilitation and psychological principles. Ideally, the interface between critical care and rehabilitation teams should be a hybrid model—interdisciplinary and to some degree transdisciplinary—in that each member understands the others' primary role(s) and how they optimally work with and complement one another. This conceptual approach allows the teams to take greatest advantage of their strengths while minimizing gaps in service delivery. When teams work and learn together, the synergy can also lead to unique contributions to the program, training, and institution as a whole. In the future it is hoped that holistic, patient- and family-centered models will be increasingly incorporated to address the needs of critical illness survivors and their families. This mindset, along with growing research, will likely promote the development of new ideas, innovations, and techniques that will further improve outcomes and positively affect society in a manner that extends far beyond patient care alone.

References

Agarwala, R., Ahmed, N., & Patil, K. (2011). An audit of adult critical care rehabilitation processes in a UK district general hospital based on NICE guidelines. *Critical Care, 15*(1), 1–190.

Archer, K. R., Castillo, R. C., Wegener, S. T., Abraham, C. M., & Obremskey, W. T. (2012). Pain and satisfaction in hospitalized trauma patients: The importance of self-efficacy and psychological distress. *Journal of Trauma and Acute Care Surgery, 72*(4), 1068–1077.

Athari, F., Hillman, K. M., & Frost, S. A. (2019). The concept of frailty in intensive care. *Australian Critical Care, 32*(2), 175–178.

Azoulay, E., Pochard, F., Kentish-Barnes, N., Chevret, S., Aboab, J., Adrie, C., . . . FAMIREA Study Group. (2005). Risk of post-traumatic stress symptoms in family members of intensive care unit patients. *American Journal of Respiratory and Critical Care Medicine, 171*(9), 987–994.

Babb, T., Levine, B., & Philley, J. (2012). ICU-acquired weakness: An extension of the effects of bed rest. *American Journal of Respiratory and Critical Care, 185*(2), 230–231.

Bailey, P., Thomsen, G. E., Spuhler, V. J., Blair, R., Jewkes, J., Bezdjian, L., . . . Hopkins, R. O. (2007). Early activity is feasible and safe in respiratory failure patients. *Critical Care Medicine, 35*(1), 139–145.

Barr, J., Fraser, G. L., Puntillo, K., Ely, E. W., Gélinas, C., Dasta, J. F., . . . Jaeschke, R. (2013). Clinical practice guidelines for the management of pain, agitation, and delirium in adult patients in the intensive care unit. *Critical Care Medicine, 41*(1), 263–306.

Batt, J., Herridge, M., & Dos Santos, C. (2017). Mechanism of ICU-acquired weakness: Skeletal muscle loss in critical illness. *Intensive Care Medicine, 43*(12), 1844–1846.

Berney, S. C., Rose, J. W., Bernhardt, J., & Denehy, L. (2015). Prospective observation of physical activity in critically ill patients who were intubated for more than 48 hours. *Journal of Critical Care, 30*(4), 658–663.

Bienvenu, O. J., Colantuoni, E., Mendez-Tellez, P. A., Dinglas, V. D., Shanholtz, C., Husain, N., . . . Needham, D. M. (2012). Depressive symptoms and impaired physical function after acute lung injury: A 2-year longitudinal study. *American Journal of Respiratory and Critical Care Medicine, 185*(5), 517–524.

Bienvenu, O. J., Jones, C., & Hopkins, R. O. (2017). *Psychological and cognitive impact of critical illness.* Oxford University Press.

Boutron, I., Moher, D., Altman, D. G., Schultz, K., Ravaud, P., & CONSORT Group (2008). Extending the CONSORT Statement to randomized trials of nonpharmacologic treatment: Explanation and elaboration. *Annals of Internal Medicine, 148*(4), 295–309.

Broyles, L. M., Tate, J. A., & Happ, M. B. (2012). Use of augmentative and alternative communication strategies by family members in the intensive care unit. *American Journal of Critical Care, 21*, E21–E32.

Brummel, N. E., Girard, T. D., Ely, E. W., Pandharipande, P. P., Morandi, A., Hughes, C. G., . . . Jackson, J. C. (2014). Feasibility and safety of early combined cognitive and physical therapy for critically ill medical and surgical patients: The Activity and Cognitive Therapy in ICU (ACT-ICU) trial. *Intensive Care Medicine, 40*(3), 370–379.

Brummel, N. E., Jackson, J. C., Girard, T. D., Pandharipande, P. P., Schiro, E., Work, B., . . . Ely, E. W. (2012). A combined early cognitive and physical rehabilitation program for people who are critically ill: The Activity and Cognitive Therapy in the Intensive Care Unit (ACT-ICU) trial. *Physical Therapy, 92*(12), 1580–1592.

Ceravolo, M. G., de Sire, A., Andrenelli, E., Negrini, F., & Negrini, S. (2020). Systematic rapid "living" review on rehabilitation needs due to COVID-19: Update to March 31st, 2020. *European Journal of Physical Rehabilitation Medicine, 56*(3), 347–353. doi:10.23736/S1973-9087.20.06329-7

Connolly, B., O'Neill, B., Salisbury, L., & Blackwood, B. (2016). Physical rehabilitation interventions for adult patients during critical illness: An overview of systematic reviews. *Thorax, 71*(10), 881–890.

Cuthbertson, B. H., Rattray, J., Campbell, M., Gager, M., Roughton, S., Smith, A., . . . Waldmann, C. (2009). The PRaCTICaL study of nurse-led, intensive care follow-up programmes for improving long term outcomes from critical illness: A pragmatic randomized controlled trial, *BMJ, 339*, b3723. doi:10.1136/bmj.b3723

Dammeyer, J. A., Baldwin, N., Packard, D., Harrington, S., Christofferson, B., Christopher, J., . . . Iwashyna, J. (2013). Mobilizing outcomes: Implementation of a nurse-led multidisciplinary mobility program. *Critical Care Nursing Quarterly, 36*(1), 109–119. doi:10.1097/CNQ.0b013e31827535db

Davidson, J. E., Jones, C., & Bienvenu, O. J. (2012). Family response to critical illness: Postintensive care syndrome—family. *Critical Care Medicine, 40*(2), 618–624. http://dx.doi.org/10.1097/CCM.0b013e318236ebf9

Davidson, J. E., & Zisook, S. (2017). Implementing family-centered care through facilitated sensemaking. *AACN Advanced Critical Care, 28*(2), 200–209.

Davydow, D. S., Gifford, J. M., Desai, S. V., Bienvenu, O. J., & Needham, D. M. (2009). Depression in general intensive care unit survivors: A systematic review. *Intensive Care Medicine, 35*(5), 796–809.

De Jonghe, B., Sharshar, T., Lefaucheur, J. P., Authier, F. J., Durand-Zaleski, I., Boussarasar, M., ... Bastuji-Garin, S. (2002). Paresis acquired in the intensive care unit: A prospective multicenter study. *Journal of the American Medical Association, 288*(22), 2859–2867.

Desai, S. V., Law, T. J., & Needham, D. M. (2011). Long-term complications of critical care. *Critical Care Medicine, 39*(2), 371–379.

Devlin, J. W., Skrobik, Y., Gelinas, C., Needham, D. M., Slooter, A. J. C, Pandharipande P. P., ... Alhazzani, W. (2018). Clinical practice guidelines for the prevention and management of pain, agitation/sedation, delirium, immobility, and sleep disruption in adult patients in the ICU. *Critical Care Medicine, 46*(9), e825–e873.

Dickinson, S., Tschannen, D., & Shever, L. L. (2013). Can the use of an early mobility program reduce the incidence of pressure ulcers in a surgical critical care unit? *Critical Care Nursing Quarterly, 36*(1), 127–140.

Dinglas, V. D., Colantuoni, E., Ciesla, N., Mendez-Tellez, P. A., Shanholtz, C., & Needham, D. M. (2013). Occupational therapy for patients with acute lung injury: Factors associated with time to first intervention in the intensive care unit. *American Journal of Occupational Therapy, 67*(3), 355–362.

Doiron, K. A., Hoffmann, T. C., & Beller, E. M. (2018). Early intervention (mobilization or active exercise) for critically ill adults in the intensive care unit. *Cochrane Database Systematic Review, 3*, CD010754.

Dos Santos, C., Hussain, S. N., Mathur, S., Picard, M., Herridge, M., Correa, J., ... Batt, J. (2016). Mechanisms of chronic muscle wasting and dysfunction after an intensive care unit stay: A pilot study. *American Journal of Respiratory and Critical Care Medicine, 194*(7), 821–830.

Dowdy, D. W., Eid, M. P., Dennison, C. R., Mendez-Tellez, P. A., Herridge, M. S., Guallar, E., ... Needham, D. M. (2006). Quality of life after acute respiratory distress syndrome: A meta-analysis. *Intensive Care Medicine, 32*(8), 1115–1124.

Dowdy, D. W., Eid, M. P., Sedrakyan, A., Mendez-Tellez, P. A., Pronovost, P. J., Herridge, M. S., & Needham, D. M. (2005). Quality of life in adult survivors of critical illness: A systematic review of the literature. *Intensive Care Medicine, 31*(5), 611–620.

Dubb, R., Nydahl, P., Hermes, C., Schwabbauer, N., Toonstra, A., Parker, A. M., ... Needham, D. M. (2016). Barriers and strategies for early mobilization of patients in intensive care units. *Annals of the American Thoracic Society, 13*(5), 724–730.

Eakin, M. N., Ugbah, L., Arnautovic, T., Parker, A. M., & Needham, D. M. (2015). Implementing and sustaining an early rehabilitation program in a medical intensive care unit: A qualitative analysis. *Journal of Critical Care, 30*(4), 698–704.

Elliott, D., McKinley, S., Alison, J., Aitken, L. M., King, M., Leslie, G. D., ... Burmeister, E. (2011). Health-related quality of life and physical recovery after a critical illness: A multi-centered randomised controlled trial of a home-based physical rehabilitation program. *Critical Care, 15*(3), R142.

Ely, W. (2017). The ABCDEF bundle: Science and philosophy of how ICU liberation serves patients and families. *Critical Care Medicine, 45*(2), 321–330.

Ely, E. W., Inouye, S. K., Bernard, G. R., Gordon, S., Francis, J., May, L., ... Margolin, R. (2001). Delirium in mechanically ventilated patients: Validity and reliability of the confusion assessment method for the intensive care unit (CAM-ICU). *Journal of the American Medical Association, 286*(21), 2703–2710.

Fletcher, S. N., Kennedy, D. D., Ghosh, I. R., Misra, V. P., Kiff, K., Coakley, J. H., & Hinds, C. J. (2003). Persistent neuromuscular and neurophysiologic abnormalities in long-term survivors of prolonged critical illness. *Critical Care Medicine, 31*(4), 1012–1016.

Garrouste-Orgeas, M., Coquet, I., Périer, A., Timsit, J. F., Pochard, F., Lancrin, F., . . . Angeli, S. (2012). Impact of an intensive care unit diary on psychological distress in patients and relatives. *Critical Care Medicine, 40*(7), 2033–2040.

Garzon-Serrano, J., Ryan, C., Waak, K., Hirschberg, R., Tully, S., Bittner, E. A., . . . Eikermann, M. (2011). Early mobilization in critically ill patients: Patients' mobilization level depends on health care provider's profession. *PM&R Journal, 3*(4), 307–313. doi:10.1016/j.pmrj.2010.12.022

Geense, W. W., van den Boogaard, M., van der Hoeven, J. G., Vermeulen, H., Hannink, G., & Zegers, M. (2019). Nonpharmacologic interventions to prevent or mitigate adverse long-term outcomes among ICU survivors: A systematic review and meta-analysis. *Critical Care Medicine, 47*(11), 1607–1618.

Gélinas, C., Klein, K., Naidech, A., & Skrobik, Y. (2013) Pain, sedation, and delirium management in the neurocritically ill: Lessons learned from recent research. *Seminars in Respiratory Critical Care Medicine, 34*(02), 236–243.

Girard, T.D., Alhazzani, W., Kress, J. P., Ouellette, D. R., Schmidt, G. A., Truwit, J. D., . . . Morris, P. E. (2016). An official American Thoracic Society/American College of Chest Physicians clinical practice guideline: Liberation from mechanical ventilation in critically ill adults. Rehabilitation protocols, ventilator liberation protocols, and cuff leak tests. *American Journal of Respiratory and Critical Care Medicine, 195*(1), 120–133.

Girard, T. D., Thompson, J. L., Pandharipande, P. P., Brummel, N. E., Jackson, J. C., Patel, M. B., . . . Ely, E. W. (2018). Clinical phenotypes of delirium during critical illness and severity of subsequent long-term cognitive impairment: A prospective cohort study. *Lancet Respiratory Medicine, 6*(3), 213–222.

Griffiths, J. A., Barber, V. S., Cuthbertson, B. H., & Young, J. D. (2006). A national survey of intensive care follow-up clinics. *Anaesthesia, 61*(10), 950–955.

Haesler, E. (2014). *Prevention and treatment of pressure ulcers: Critical practice guideline.* Cambridge Media.

Hall, M. J., DeFrances, C. J., Williams, S. N., Golosinskiy, A., & Schwartzman, A. (2010). National hospital discharge survey: 2007 summary. *National Health Statistics Report, 29*, 1–20.

Happ, M. B., Garrett, K., Thomas, D. D., Tate, J., George, E., Houze, M., . . . Sereika, S. (2011). Nurse–patient communication interactions in the intensive care unit. *American Journal of Critical Care, 20*, e28–340.

Harrison, J. P., & Kirkpatrick, N. (2011). The improving efficiency frontier of inpatient rehabilitation hospitals. *Health Care Manager, 30*(4), 313–321.

Heffner, J. E. (2010) Swallowing complications after endotracheal extubation: Moving from "whether" to "how." *Chest, 137*(3), 509–510.

Hermans, G., & Van den Berghe, G. (2015) Clinical review: Intensive care unit acquired weakness. *Critical Care, 19*, 274.

Herridge, M. S., Tansey, C. M., Matte, A., Tomlinson, G., Diaz-Granados, N., Cooper, A., . . . Cheung, A. M. (2011). Functional disability 5 years after acute respiratory distress syndrome. *New England Journal of Medicine, 364*(14), 1293–1304.

Hodgin, K. E., Nordon-Craft, A., McFann, K. K., Mealer, M. L., & Moss, M. (2009). Physical therapy utilization in intensive care units: Results from a national survey. *Critical Care Medicine, 37*(2), 561–568.

Hodgson, C. L., Bailey, M., Bellomo, R., Berney, S., Buhr, H., Denehy, L., . . . Webb, S. (2016). A binational multicenter pilot feasibility randomized controlled trial of early goal-directed mobilization in the ICU. *Critical Care Medicine, 44*(6), 1145–1152.

Hodgson, C. L., Stiller, K., Needham, D. M., Tipping, C. J., Harrold, M., Baldwin, C. E., . . . Webb, S. A. (2014). Expert consensus and recommendations on safety criteria for active mobilization of mechanically ventilated critically ill adults. *Critical Care, 18*(6), 658.

Hoenig, H., Lee, J., & Stineman, M. (2015). Conceptual overview of frameworks for measuring quality in rehabilitation. *Topics in Stroke Rehabilitation, 17*(4), 239–251. https://doi.org/10.1310/tsr1704-239

Hopkins, R. O., Key, C. W., Suchyta, M. R., Weaver, L. K., & Orme, J. F. (2010). Risk factors for depression and anxiety in survivors of acute respiratory distress syndrome. *General Hospital Psychiatry, 32*(2), 147–155.

Husain, T., Gatward, J. J., & Harris, R. D. (2001). Use of subglottic suction port to enable verbal communication in ventilator-dependent patients. *American Journal of Respiratory and Critical Care Medicine, 184*(3), 384.

Iwashyna, T. J. (2010) Survivorship will be the defining challenge of critical care in the 21st century. *Annals of Internal Medicine, 153*(3), 204–205.

Iwashyna, T. J., Ely, E. W., Smith, D. M., & Langa, K. M. (2010). Long-term cognitive impairment and functional disability among survivors of severe sepsis. *Journal of the American Medical Association, 304*(16), 1787–1794.

Iwashyna, T. J. & Netzer, G. (2012). The burdens of survivorship: An approach to thinking about long-term outcomes after critical illness. *Seminars in Respiratory and Critical Care Medicine, 33*(4), 327–338. http://dx.doi.org/10.1055/s-0032-1321982

Jackson, J. C., Ely, E. W., Morey, M. C., Anderson, V. M., Denne, L. B., Clune, J., . . . Hoenig, H. (2012). Cognitive and physical rehabilitation of intensive care unit survivors: Results of the RETURN randomized controlled pilot investigation. *Critical Care Medicine, 40*(4), 1088–1097.

Jackson, J. C., & Jutte, J.E. (2016). Rehabilitating a missed opportunity: Integration of rehabilitation psychology into the care of critically ill patients, survivors, and caregivers, *Rehabilitation Psychology, 61*(2), 115–119.

Jackson, J. C., Jutte, J. E., Hunter, C. H., Ciccolella, N., Warrington, H., Sevin, C., & Bienvenu, O. J. (2016). Posttraumatic stress disorder (PTSD) after critical illness: A conceptual review of distinct clinical issues and their implications. *Rehabilitation Psychology, 61*(2), 132–140. http://dx.doi.org/10.1037/rep0000085

Jones, C., Backman, C., Capuzzo, M., Egerod, I., Flaatten, H., Granja, C., . . . Griffiths, R. D. (2010). Intensive care diaries reduce new-onset posttraumatic stress disorder following critical illness: A randomised, controlled trial. *Critical Care, 14*(5), R168.

Jones, C., Backman, C., & Griffiths, R. D. (2012). Intensive care diaries and relatives' symptoms of posttraumatic stress disorder after critical illness: A pilot study. *American Journal of Critical Care, 21*(3), 172–176.

Jutte, J. E., Erb C., & Jackson J. C. (2015). Physical, cognitive and psychological disability following critical illness. What is the risk? *Seminars in Respiratory and Critical Care, 36*, 1–16.

Jutte, J. E., Jackson, J. C., & Hopkins, R. (2017). Rehabilitation psychology insights for treatment of critical illness. In O. J. Bienvenu, C. Jones, & R. O. Hopkins (Eds.), *Psychological and cognitive impact of critical illness* (pp. 105–139). Oxford University Press.

Kamdar, B. B., Needham, D. M., & Collop, N. A. (2011). Sleep deprivation in critical illness: Its role in physical and psychological recovery. *Journal of Intensive Care Medicine, 27*(2), 97–111.

Kapfhammer, H. P., Rothenhäusler, H. B., Krauseneck, T., Stoll, C., & Schelling, G. (2004). Posttraumatic stress disorder and health-related quality of life in long-term survivors of acute respiratory distress syndrome, *American Journal of Psychiatry, 161*(1), 45–52.

Karol, R. L. (2014). Team models in neurorehabilitation: Structure, function, and culture change. *NeuroRehabilitation, 34*(4), 655–669.

Kress, J. P., & Hall, J. B. (2014). ICU-acquired weakness and recovery from critical illness. *New England Journal of Medicine, 370*(17), 1626–1635.

Latronico, N., Herridge, M., Hopkins, R.O., Angus, D., Hart, N., Hermans, G., Iwashyna, T., . . . Needham, D. M. (2017). The ICM research agenda on intensive care unit-acquired weakness. *Intensive Care Medicine, 43*(9), 1270–1281.

Laurent, H., Aubreton, S., Richard, R., Gorce, Y., Caron, E., Vallat, A., . . . Coudeyre, E. (2016). Systematic review of early exercise in intensive care: A qualitative approach. *Anaesthesia, Critical Care & Pain Medicine, 35*(2), 133–149.

Macht, M., White, S. D, & Moss, M. (2014). Swallowing dysfunction after critical illness. *Chest, 146*(6), 1681–1689.

Merbitz, N. H., Merbitz, C. T., & Ripsch, J. P. (2012). Rehabilitation outcomes and assessment: Toward complex adaptive rehabilitation. In P. Kennedy (Ed.), *Oxford handbook of rehabilitation psychology* (pp. 96–127). Oxford University Press.

Merbitz, N. H., Westie, K., Dammeyer, J. A., Butt, L., & Schneider, J. (2016). After critical care: Challenges in the transition to inpatient rehabilitation. *Rehabilitation Psychology, 61*, 186–200. http://dx.doi.org/10.1037/rep0000072

Miller, M. A., Govindan, S., Watson, S. R., Hyzy, R. C., & Iwashyna, T. J. (2015). ABCDE, but in that order? A cross-sectional survey of Michigan intensive care unit sedation, delirium and early mobility practices. *Annals of the American Thoracic Society, 12*(7), 1066–1071.

Mirzakhani, H., Williams, J. N., Mello, J., Joseph, S., Meyer, M. J., Waak, K., . . . Eikermann, M. (2013). Muscle weakness predicts pharyngeal dysfunction and symptomatic aspiration in long-term ventilated patients. *Anesthesia, 119*(2), 389–397.

Mobasheri, M. H., King, D., Judge, S., Arshad, F., Larsen, M., Safarfashandi, Z., Shah, H., . . . Darzi, A. (2016). Communication aid requirements of intensive care unit patients with transient speech loss. *Augmentative & Alternative Communication, 32*(4), 261–271.

Moss, M., Good, V. S., Gozal, D., Kleinpell, R., & Sessler, C. N. (2016). A critical care societies collaborative statement: Burnout syndrome in critical care health-care professionals. A call to action. *American Journal of Respiratory and Critical Care Medicine, 194*(1), 106–113.https://doi.org/10.1164/rccm.201604-0708ST

Musicco, M., Emberti, L., Nappi, G., & Caltagirone, C. (2003). Italian multicenter study on outcomes of rehabilitation of neurological patients. Early and long-term outcome of rehabilitation in stroke patients: The role of patient characteristics, time of initiation, and duration of interventions. *Archives of Physical Medicine and Rehabilitation, 84*(4), 551–558.

Needham, D. M. (2008). Mobilizing patients in the intensive care unit: Improving neuromuscular weakness and physical function. *Journal of the American Medical Association, 300*(14), 1685–1690.

Needham, D. M., Davidson, J., Cohen, H., Hopkins, R. O., Weinert, C., Wunsch, H., . . . Harvey, R. N. (2012). Improving long-term outcomes after discharge from intensive care unit: Report from a stakeholders' conference. *Critical Care Medicine, 40*(2), 502–509. http://dx.doi.org/10.1097/CCM.0b013e318232da75

Needham, D. M., & Korupolu, R. (2010). Rehabilitation quality improvement in an intensive care unit setting: Implementation of a quality improvement model. *Topics in Stroke Rehabilitation, 17*(4), 271–281.

Nielsen, A. H., Egerod, I., Hansen, T. B., & Angel, S. (2019). Intensive care unit diaries: Developing a shared story strengthens relationships between critically ill patients and their relatives: A hermeneutic-phenomenological study. *International Journal of Nursing Studies, 92,* 90–96.

Nydahl, P., Ruhl, A. P., Bartoszek, G., Dubb, R., Filipovic, S., Flohr, H. J., . . . Needham, D. M. (2014). Early mobilization of mechanically ventilated patients: A 1-day point-prevalence study in Germany. *Critical Care Medicine, 42*(5), 1178–1186.

Ottenbacher, K. J., Smith, P. M., Illig, S. B., Linn, R. T., Ostir, G. V., & Granger, C. V. (2004). Trends in length of stay, living setting, functional outcome, and mortality following medical rehabilitation. *Journal of the American Medical Association, 292*(14), 1687–1695.

Paul, F., & Rattray, J. (2008). Short-and-long-term impact of critical illness on relatives: Literature review. *Journal of Advanced Nursing, 62*(3), 276–292.

Pennock, B. E., Crawshaw, L., Maher, T., Price, T., & Kaplan, P. D. (1994). Distressful events in the ICU as perceived by patients recovering from coronary artery bypass surgery. *Heart & Lung, 23,* 323–327.

Peris, A., Bonizzoli, M., Iozzelli, D., Migliaccio, M. L., Zagli, G., Bacchereti, A., . . . Belloni, L. (2011). Early intra-intensive care unit psychological intervention promotes recovery from post-traumatic stress disorders, anxiety and depression symptoms in critically ill patients. *Critical Care, 15*(1), R41. doi:10.1186/cc10003

Pochard, F., Azoulay, E., Chevret, S., Lemaire, F., Hubert, P., Canoui, P., . . . Dhainaut, J. F. (2001). Symptoms of anxiety and depression in family members of intensive care unit patients: Ethical hypothesis regarding decision-making capacity. *Critical Care Medicine, 29*(10), 1893–1897.

Prohaska, C. C., Sottile, P. D., Nordon-Craft, A., Gallagher, M. D., Burnham, E. L., Clark, B. J., . . . Moss, M. (2019). Patterns of utilization and effects of hospital-specific factors on physical, occupational, and speech therapy for critically ill patients with acute respiratory failure in the USA: Results of a 5-year sample. *Critical Care, 23*(1), 175.

Pun, B. T., Balas, M. C., Barnes-Daly, M. A., Thompson, J. L., Aldrich, J. M., Barr, J., . . . Ely, E. W. (2018). Caring for critically ill patients with the ABCDEF bundle: Results of the ICU liberation collaborative in over 15,000 Adults. *Critical Care Medicine, 47*(1), 3–14.

Reid, J. C., Unger, J., McCaskell, D., Childerhose, L., Zorko, D. J., & Kho, M. E. (2018). Physical rehabilitation interventions in the intensive care unit: A scoping review of 117 studies. *Journal of Intensive Care, 6,* 80.

Rotondi, A. J., Chelluri, L., Sirio, C., Mendelson, A., Schultz, R., Belle, S., . . . Pinsky, M. R. (2002). Patients recollection of stressful experiences while receiving prolonged mechanical ventilation in an intensive care unit. *Critical Care Medicine, 30,* 746–752.

Sakai, T., Hoshino, C., Yamaguchi, R., Hirao, M., Nakahara, R., & Okawa, A. (2020). Remote rehabilitation for patients with COVID-19. *Journal of Rehabilitation Medicine, 52*(9), jrm00095. doi:10.2340/16501977-2731

Schelling, G., Stoll, C., Haller, M., Briegel, J., Manert, W., Hummel, T., . . . Klaus, P. (1998). Health-related quality of life and posttraumatic stress disorder in survivors of the acute respiratory distress syndrome. *Critical Care Medicine, 26*(4), 651–659.

Schweickert, W. D., Pohlman, M. C., Pohlman, A. S., Nigos, C., Pawlik, A. J., Esbrook, C. L., . . . Kress, J. P. (2009). Early physical and occupational therapy in mechanically ventilated, critically ill patients: A randomised controlled trial. *Lancet, 373*(9678), 1874–1882.

Shahin, E. S. M., Dassen, T., & Halfens, R. J. G. (2009). Incidence, prevention, and treatment of pressure ulcers in intensive care patients: A longitudinal study. *International Journal of Nursing Studies, 46*(4), 413–421.

Simpson, R., & Robinson, L. (2020). Rehabilitation after critical illness in people with COVID-19 infection. *American Journal of Physical Medicine and Rehabilitation, 99*(6), 470–474. doi:10.1097/PHM.0000000000001443

Skoretz, S. A., Flowers, H. L., & Martino, R. (2010). The incidence of dysphagia following endotracheal intubation a systematic review. *Chest, 137*(3), 665–673.

Society of Critical Care Medicine. (2011). *Critical care units: A descriptive analysis* (2nd ed.). Society of Critical Care Medicine.

Stevens, R. D., Dowdy, D. W., Michaels, R. K., Mendez-Tellez, P. A., Pronovost, P. J., & Needham, D. M. (2007). Neuromuscular dysfunction acquired in critical illness: A systematic review. *Intensive Care Medicine, 33*(11), 1876–1891.

Stevens, R. D., Marshall, S. A., Cornblath, D. R., Hoke, A., Needham, D. M., De Jonghe, B., . . . Sharshar, T. (2009). A framework for diagnosing and classifying intensive care unit-acquired weakness. *Critical Care Medicine, 37*(10), S299–S308.

Stucky, K., Jutte, J. E., Warren, A. M., Jackson, J. C., & Merbitz, N. (2016). A survey of psychology practice in critical care settings. *Rehabilitation Psychology, 61*(2), 201–209.

Stucky, K. J., & Warren, A. M. (2019). Rehabilitation psychologists in critical care settings. In L. A. Brenner, S. Reid-Arndt, T. R. Elliott, R. G. Frank, & B. Caplan (Eds.), *The rehabilitation psychology handbook* (3rd ed., pp. 483–496). American Psychological Association.

Sukantarat, K., Greer, S., Brett, S., & Williamson, R. (2007). Physical and psychological sequelae of critical illness. *British Journal of Health Psychology, 12*(1), 65–74.

Tan, T., Brett, S. J., & Stokes, T. (2009). Rehabilitation after critical illness: Summary of NICE guidelines. *British Medical Journal, 338*, b822.

van den Born–van Zanten, S. A., Dongelmans, D. A., Dettling-Ihnenfeldt, D., Vink, R., & Van der Schaaf, M. (2016). Caregiver strain and posttraumatic stress symptoms of informal caregivers of intensive care unit survivors. *Rehabilitation Psychology, 61*(2), 179–185. http://dx.doi.org/10.1037/rep0000080

Van der Schaaf, M., Beelen, A., Dongelmans, D. A., Vroom, M. B., & Nollet, F. (2009). Functional status after intensive care: A challenge for rehabilitation professionals to improve outcome. *Journal of Rehabilitation Medicine, 41*, 360–366.

Walsh, T. S., Salisbury, L. G., Boyd, J., Ramsay, P., Merriweather, J., Huby, G., . . . Murray, G. D. (2012). A randomised controlled trial evaluating a rehabilitation complex intervention care discharge: The RECOVER study. *British Medical Journal, 2*(4), e001475.

Warren, A. M., Rainey, E., Weddle, R. J., Bennett, M., Roden-Foreman, K., & Foreman, M. L. (2016). The ICU experience: Psychological impact on family members of patients with and without traumatic brain injury. *Rehabilitation Psychology, 61*(2), 179–185.

Warren, A. M., Stucky, K., & Sherman, J. J. (2013). Rehabilitation psychology's role in the level I trauma center. *Journal of Trauma and Acute Care Surgery, 74*, 1357–1362.

Weinreich, M., Herman, J., Dickason, S., & Mayo, H. (2017). Occupational therapy in the intensive care unit: A systematic review. *Occupational Therapy in Health Care, 31*(3), 205–213.

More than 5 million patients are admitted annually to United States ICUs for intensive or invasive monitoring; support of airway, breathing, or circulation; stabilization of acute or life-threatening medical problems; comprehensive management of injury and/or illness; and maximization of comfort for dying patients.

SOCIETY OF CRITICAL CARE MEDICINE, 2020

Months ago, there was no clear indication that COVID-19 was coming. Today there is no clear indication of how or when it will end. An extraordinary ferment of courage, compassion, and collaboration will be essential to fuel an effective multifaceted response to this devastating pandemic.

COOK ET AL., 2020, p. E1

What is needed now, is not only high-quality ICU care, concentrated on providing adequate respiratory support to critically ill patients, but an identification of the source and degree of mental and spiritual suffering of patients as well as their families to provide the most ethical and person-centered care during this humanitarian crisis.

KOTFIS ET AL., 2020, p. 2

4   Contributions to Critical Care from Psychological Science and Practice

Nancy Merbitz, Joan Fleishman, Hannah Kamsky, Stephanie Sundborg, Jamie Lynne Tingey, Nancy Ciccolella, and Ann Marie Warren

Introduction

The multiple emotional, cognitive, and physical symptoms of patients who are critically ill in the intensive care unit (ICU) have been noted in health care literature as far back as the 1960s (e.g., Hackett et al., 1968; Spellman, 1960). Patients in critical care experience immense physical changes and losses while in an unfamiliar environment and without the activities and people that previously sustained them. Their diminished level of consciousness, delirium, and medical acuity all are barriers to participation in treatment planning and shared decision-making during ICU care. Orientation is disrupted in the absence of usual day–night cycles (Hopper et al., 2015; Wilcox et al., 2013). Ongoing sensory experiences in the ICU provide neither interactive opportunities nor aesthetic enjoyment, but instead a sensory overload of instrument noises, lights, the comings and goings of providers, and painful procedures superimposed upon ongoing physical discomfort (Hofhuis et al., 2008; Reade & Finfer, 2014). The combination of noisy ICU environment and its associated sleep

Nancy Merbitz, Joan Fleishman, Hannah Kamsky, Stephanie Sundborg, Jamie Lynne Tingey, Nancy Ciccolella, and Ann Marie Warren, *Contributions to Critical Care from Psychological Science and Practice* In: *Critical Care Psychology and Rehabilitation*. Edited by: Kirk J. Stucky and Jennifer E. Jutte, Oxford University Press. © Oxford University Press 2022. DOI: 10.1093/oso/9780190077013.003.0004 deprivation, invasive and painful medical procedures, and lack of privacy, autonomy, and control is a source of stress and potential trauma for patients and their families; this has been described as "medical dehumanization" (Leyens, 2014).

> In the midst of trying to correct organ failures, clinicians may neglect to carefully consider what the patient is experiencing: to be on the brink of death, be unable to speak, be stripped naked, have strangers enter the room and simultaneously do things to their bodies without explanation, have tubes inserted into multiple orifices, have their arms restrained, hear a cacophony of disorienting bedside alarms whose meaning lies beyond them, and to be poked, and prodded—all while family is torn away. Compounding these facts, patients often have no memory or understanding of how they ended up in this horrifying situation. (Wilson et al., 2019, p. 23)

The effects of prolonged immobilization, emotional trauma, and brain insults can persist for months or years afterward in physical and psychological (emotional and cognitive) morbidities known as post-intensive care syndrome (PICS), as detailed in a large and growing literature (McPeake & Mikkelsen, 2018; Needham et al., 2012; Rawal et al., 2017) that now includes attention to the impact on family (PICS-Family or PICS-F). Table 4.1 summarizes risk factors (British Psychological Society, 2020; Highfield et al., 2020; Jackson et al., 2016). The acute and longer term effects of critical illness have been receiving increased public attention during the prolonged crisis of COVID, highlighting where psychologists can make important contributions for patients, families, teams, and healthcare systems.

The psychological crisis of critical care

Stripped of the personal distinctions, roles, and abilities that contribute to their identity, patients in the ICU experience threat to their sense of self-continuity and embeddedness in a comprehensible world (Janoff-Bulman & Frantz, 1997; Lykkegaard & Delmar, 2013; Merbitz et al., 2016; Sideris, 2019; Wilson et al., 2019). As they come to understand where they are and how sick they are, they are challenged to find personal meaning in the midst of questions such as "why me?", "how can such things happen?", and "will I ever be whole?". Patients and their families may have acute symptoms such as panic, anxiety/fear, and acute stress reactions (Parker et al., 2015; Roberts et al., 2018; Wade et al., 2013).

TABLE 4.1.

Risk factors for psychological comorbidities after critical illness

Potentially modifiable risk factors	Static or preexisting risk factors
Barriers to communicating	Premorbid/comorbid psychopathology
Barriers to comprehending information	Prior health anxiety, health-related traumas
Feeling ignored, dismissed, or criticized	Repeat ICU admission
Witness to suffering of others	Other trauma history
Pain	Recent bereavement; illness of family/friends
Discomfort (positioning, thirst, hunger, etc.)	Preexisting cognitive impairment/dementia
Sleep deprivation	Female sex
Perceived lack of control and autonomy	Younger age
Duration and depth of sedation	Unemployment
Duration of mechanical ventilation	Type of illness (e.g., ARDS; traumatic injury)
Delirium, particularly memories of hallucinations/delusions, periods of unawareness and disorientation	Lower socioeconomic status, less education
Agitation and need for restraint	Likely risk during COVID-19: less availability of staff; staff in PPE
Medications used (e.g., benzodiazepines, vasopressors)	Likely risk during COVID-19: loved ones prohibited from visits

ARDS = acute respiratory distress syndrome

Crisis theory focuses on what happens when individuals face major disruptions to their established patterns of personal and social identity, representing a disequilibrium between environmental demands and perceived resources; intervention aims toward a new equilibrium with the most adaptive resolution possible (Jacobson, 1980; Moos & Holahan, 2007). Under conditions of threat with diminished resources and options, a crisis can evoke patterns of automatic response selected by evolution for survival (i.e., fight, flight, or freeze), which can be observed in the agitation, avoidant resistance, and/or passive withdrawal of patients who are critically ill (Caplan, 1964; Jacobson, 1980; Moos & Holahan, 2007; Shaw & Halliday, 1992; Sprangers et al., 2002). Sleep deprivation is known to have a host of detrimental physiological effects and probably interferes with the brain's processing of traumatic experiences (Germain et al., 2008).

Many will have persisting symptoms of depression and anxiety after the ICU, and as many as one in five may develop posttraumatic stress symptoms in the next year, meaning that each year approximately 1 million survivors develop posttraumatic stress symptoms after ICU admission (Righy et al., 2019). Barriers to psychological healing and resumption of meaningful social roles may include the persisting cognitive deficits after brain insults such as traumatic brain injury, stroke, hypoxia, sepsis, and delirium (Hopkins et al., 2017). Family members are at risk for persisting anxiety, depression, posttraumatic stress symptoms, and complicated grief (Needham et al., 2012) as well as decrements in physical, cognitive, and social functioning and quality of life (Davidson et al., 2017).

The ICU experience in the context of COVID-19

Circumstances of the current COVID-19 pandemic are likely to compound these acute and persisting effects (Tingey et al., 2020). Available data at the time of writing show that for patients with COVID-19, time in the ICU is at least twice the previous average of 3.3 ICU days (Ferguson et al., 2020; Hunter et al., 2014), and nearly 90% require mechanical ventilation (Cook et al., 2020; Devlin et al., 2020) compared to 20% to 40% of prepandemic patients in the ICU (Society of Critical Care Medicine, 2020). Kahn and colleagues (2020) found that the majority (73.6%) of patients with COVID-19 admitted to the ICU experienced delirium (i.e., altered mental status) for approximately 1 week; invasive mechanical ventilation was significantly associated with delirium. Delirium duration has been directly correlated with brain volume and white matter integrity at 3-month follow-up (Morandi et al., 2012).

As the COVID-19 crisis has rapidly developed, the "rules of engagement" for all clinicians in ICUs have changed due to the heightened risk of transmission. Family contact has been restricted to phone or video, mental health professionals have turned to telehealth, and clinician contact for direct care procedures has been altered by personal protective equipment (PPE) requirements (Marra et al., 2020). As some ventilated patients have reportedly remained in the ICU for weeks, the acute and chronic impacts of the ICU experience are predicted to be greater for patients with COVID-19 and their family members, according to multiple provider interviews conducted by an NBC medical reporter (Edwards, 2020).

Additional neurologic consequences for cognitive function are also anticipated from COVID-19; these may include direct central nervous system (CNS) viral infection and CNS para-infectious autoimmune reactions and definitely include the deficits that commonly accompany protracted critical illness. "The sheer volume of those suffering critical illness [during the pandemic] is likely to result in an increased burden of long-term cognitive impairment" (Needham et al., 2020, p. 670). Standards of ICU care to prevent or mitigate delirium and trauma have been progressing in recent years (Barr et al., 2013); however, during the pandemic such standards may be jettisoned by overburdened ICU teams struggling to save lives and contain infection among patients (Sher et al., 2020) (Figure 4.1). Kotfis and colleagues (2020) recently described ICU conditions during COVID-19 as "a delirium factory," and they cautioned:

> During such harrowing times . . . it would be easy to disregard patients' brains as not being an essential concern. If we follow the critical care literature, this would be a grave error. . . . The risk of complications such as acquired dementia and ICU-acquired weakness as well as depression and PTSD [posttraumatic stress disorder], the defining illnesses of post-intensive care syndrome (PICS), . . . will be greatly exacerbated if we allow patients to suffer unmitigated delirium. (Kotfis et al., 2020, p. 3)

The need for psychologists in ICU care

INTEGRATION OF PSYCHOLOGISTS INTO ICUS

For several decades, increasing numbers of psychologists have consulted to medical teams in hospitals and primary care due to greater recognition of the role of psychological factors in health and medical outcomes. Moreover, some medical specialties have incorporated psychologists as core members of their inpatient teams. ICUs offer opportunities for psychologists to bring a holistic, patient-centered perspective, informed by a working knowledge of factors that contribute to distress, maladaptation, and cognitive impairment. Some critical care teams have consulted or included psychologists for services to medical and surgical, pulmonary, cardiac, transplant, neonatal, pediatric, burn, and trauma ICUs, typically requesting their expertise in assessment of mental status and behavior (Stucky et al., 2016). Multiple fields of psychology contribute concepts and findings applicable in critical care for the support and education of patients, family, staff, and organizations (Ervin et al., 2018; Quenot et al., 2012).

When a psychologist is invited to contribute as an ICU team member, it may be with the unspoken request to support the humanity of the patients in the ICU and their families. As described in an early ICU Humanization effort in Brazil (Andreoli et al., 2001), the roles of the psychologist can include helping patients cope with their illness and its treatment as well as helping team members to interpret patients' subjective experiences, enhancing their capacity to sustain caring relationships with their patients. Thus, psychologists can encourage and guide teams in their

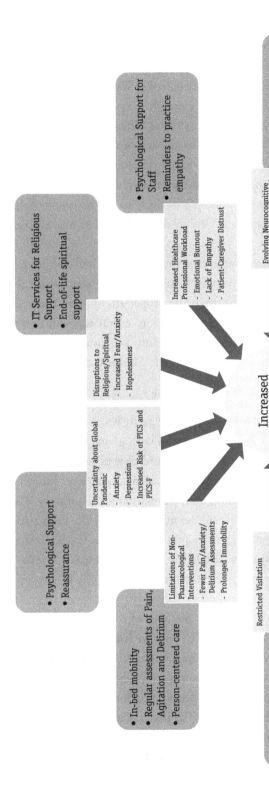

FIGURE 4.1. Potential factors contributing to ICU delirium during the SARS-CoV-2 pandemic.
Kotfis et al., 2020; http://creativecommons.org/licenses/by/4.0/

provision of trauma-informed care (TIC; Harris & Fallot, 2001). Psychologists can also support patients' and families' emotional and cognitive adaptation during crises (Efimova et al., 2015; Shulman & Shewbert, 2005). They assist in prevention, detection, and treatment of delirium (Jackson et al., 2014; Warren et al., 2014). They can encourage the team's understanding that, even when a patient is not frankly delirious, intermittent confusion can manifest as vague delusions, anxiety, mistrust, and dysphoria, coloring the patient's response to care and procedures.

An ICU psychology consult may request only clinical assessment of the patient without additional intervention, but intervention may also be requested when staff have had particular difficulty responding effectively to the behavior of distressed patients and families. If psychological intervention is delayed or unavailable,

> this results in an unnecessary burden for the immediate staff and frequently leads to an exacerbation of the patient's crisis. A standing psychological consult . . . would provide the means for giving proper attention to the patients' mind-body experience, while alleviating stressors which the staff is neither trained nor compensated to address. As a result, potential crisis situations can be minimized and in some cases prevented. (Shulman & Shewbert, 2005, p. 632)

Psychologists are well suited for this endeavor partly because they are not medical or nursing providers who are fully occupied with giving lifesaving treatment; they can be present with patients in difficult and chaotic situations, giving full attention to the psychological aspects of the patient experience. Frontline team members (physicians, nurses, clinical nursing assistants, respiratory therapists, rehabilitative therapists, social workers/case managers) have the most patient and family contact, and their approach to care profoundly affects the ICU experience; their ability to sustain performance and deliver care with compassion relies on personal, interpersonal, and organizational resources, to which the ICU psychologist can also contribute.

Stucky and Warren (2019) described a plethora of roles and tasks for rehabilitation psychologists, which—in addition to roles we have already described—may include assessment of psychological/neuropsychological function and psychosocial history, assessment of family dynamics, assistance to help patients and families process information from the team, and then preparation for, and assistance with, transition to step-down and other care levels. The psychologist can assist patients and/or families in writing the story of the patient's ICU experiences, facilitating entries into an ICU diary that may be reviewed to orient the patient and reduce post-ICU psychological morbidity (McIlroy et al., 2019). The British Psychological Society (2020) also provided detailed guidance for how psychologists may be utilized in the care of patients with COVID-19.

Psychological support to staff may take the form of one-to-one professional relationships (for teams fortunate enough to have an embedded psychologist), in-services or regular group meetings (varied topics, including self-care, empathy, and boundaries), and of course offloading some of the most taxing psychological needs of patient and family. Additional roles may include outpatient follow-up care, education of other hospital and community mental health providers (e.g., about PICS and PICS-F), and consultation/participation in program development and research. Warren and colleagues (2014) described three level 1 trauma centers where psychologists give direct inpatient and outpatient clinical care, provide psychological support for families of patients and treatment team members to reduce burnout, and engage in trauma research activities and injury prevention efforts.

The value of psychologists has been officially recognized in Brazil. For example, since 2005 a Ministerial Ordinance has required that each ICU must have a psychologist (Schneider & Moreira, 2017). In the United Kingdom, the latest edition of the Guidelines for the Provision of Intensive Care Services (Faculty of Intensive Care Medicine, 2019) gives extensive and detailed recommendations for the inclusion of psychologists in multiple aspects of ICU patient assessment, patient and family care, and post-ICU follow-up, as well as education and support to staff and involvement in organizational improvement (Wade & Howell, 2016).

If and when patients are medically stabilized, their rehabilitation may begin in the ICU with early mobilization, even while receiving mechanical ventilation. As in other rehabilitation settings, ICU rehabilitative efforts require teamwork and a therapeutic environment, with the additional challenge for patients and families to accommodate to the unique setting and culture of a critical care unit (Merbitz et al., 2016). With such endeavors comes the attendant need to optimize patient and family engagement (Lequerica & Kortte, 2010; Rozeboom et al., 2012; Stam et al., 2020). Korupolu and colleagues (2020) describe in-ICU rehabilitation for critically ill patients with COVID-19 in detail, with recommendations for team staffing to include psychologists. Critical illness survivors are less likely to receive inpatient rehabilitation afterward than are patients with traumatic injuries (Needham et al., 2012; Stucky & Warren, 2019); thus, the ICU may be their only opportunity for coordinated interdisciplinary rehabilitation that includes psychologists, since that is not the standard for subacute or home rehabilitation. As during inpatient rehabilitation, the psychologist can help patients, families, and providers understand each other and work toward mutual goals.

INVESTIGATING BENEFITS OF PSYCHOLOGIST INVOLVEMENT

Benefit to clinical care

There are very few quantitative investigations of outcomes after in-ICU psychological services; the most cited study and the only one involving a direct patient intervention included 209 patients in Italy (Peris et al., 2011): Posttraumatic stress symptoms at 1 year were significantly less frequent among those who received in-ICU psychological services compared with an equivalent sample of patients admitted and discharged prior to the study. As a staff intervention, weekly multidisciplinary team meetings including ICU psychologists were instituted in a Brazilian hospital to guide nurses' identification of patients at risk for worsening psychiatric status, to develop care plans, and to determine need for referral for specialist mental health services. Identification of patients at risk more than doubled in the first 3 months following institution of the weekly meetings (Guastelli et al., 2011).

There are several anecdotal, qualitative, or survey studies regarding psychological intervention in the ICU. Bennun (2001) provided an account of in-ICU psychotherapy with detailed case examples of two patients with very extended ICU stays, as well as an explication of psychological formulations to guide treatment: helping the patient focus on milestones passed and next immediate goals, giving patients the opportunity to describe themselves outside the ICU, eliciting and emphasizing a history of strengths and skills applicable to current circumstances, acknowledging past adverse experiences that may heighten present fears, reviewing the content of delusions during delirium, normalizing delirium as a medical condition, and reorienting.

Sharif and colleagues (2019) surveyed 33 physicians, nurses, and advanced practitioners a year after ICU psychologists were added; 78% agreed this led to increased recognition of delirium and 87% agreed that psychological consultation helped families understand delirium and have more realistic expectations of recovery. In a survey of ICU physicians and nurses, Piers and colleagues (2011) found a significant inverse correlation between the availability of a psychologist and an intention to leave one's job. Hosey and colleagues (2019) tracked ICU psychology consults in an academic medical center and identified reasons for consultation, which that included emotional distress (56%), rehabilitation therapy engagement (24%), family engagement (13%), cognitive disturbance (4%), and pain (4%). Psychotherapy was made available to 51 patients in a German cardiac care unit as they were undergoing heart transplants or implantation of ventricular assistive devices (Heilmann et al., 2011); there were a median of 10 contact hours for psychological services per patient, and families of almost half of all patients also made use of psychotherapy.

In a survey of several adult and pediatric French ICUs (Azoulay et al., 2001), families requested more information on diagnosis, prognosis, and/or treatment and also said they would like to receive help from a psychologist (48%). In the United Kingdom, Wade and Howell (2016) found that 23 of 135 surveyed ICUs reported that psychologists provided interventions to patients and families; they recommended that psychologists be part of the ICU multidisciplinary team, attend ward rounds, and be available for consultation on communication, sleep effects and sedation, anxiety, stress, mood, delirium, and family issues, plus contribute to development of holistic care plans for longer-stay patients in the ICU. The subsequent updated United Kingdom guidelines for critical care services included these recommendations (Faculty of Intensive Care Medicine, 2019).

Psychologists participate in applied research in critical care (e.g., Cooper et al., 2005; deRoon-Cassini et al., 2019; Stevenson et al., 2013). In addition to studying psychological variables, psychologists contribute to process improvement. For example, Pinto and colleagues in the United Kingdom (2011) describe psychologists applying the "small cycles of change" method (plan—do—study—act) in an initiative to prevent ICU pneumonia. Callahan and Griffen (2003) have guided applications of statistical process control (e.g., to reduce mortality from bloodborne infections).

Benefit to teams

The literature of social, cognitive, and organizational psychology informs psychologists' consultation to ICU teams and policymakers by addressing matters of team function, decision-making, safety, and leadership (Croskerry et al., 2013; Redelmeier & Ross, 2019). In their reviews of ICU teamwork, Reader and colleagues (2009, 2011) point to the well-established role of psychologists in consultation to high-risk industries such as aviation, where effective teamwork has been shown to be crucial for maintaining high reliability and safety. They note that the quality of teamwork in the ICU also affects patient safety: Poor communication during rounds and handoffs between shifts is linked to medical error, whereas ICUs with high levels of nurse–doctor collaboration have lower patient mortality rates and shorter length of stay. Bartunek (2011) describes intergroup problems among physicians, nurses, and administrators and recommends methods of socialization into cross-boundary communities of practice, fostering dual, superordinate identities with a common sense of purpose. Ervin and colleagues (2018) note that research on various health care teams demonstrates the importance of role clarity, psychological safety, and leader inclusiveness. They effectively argue that these are no less important in ICU teams.

Other authors have described the needs for and benefits of psychologists' services in assisting the team during discussions of end-of-life decision-making, participating in direct communication and/or consulting with providers. The last of these may include best practices in such communication as well as promoting provider self-care and peer support during and after these most difficult conversations (McCallister et al., 2015). Even when psychologists are available to palliative care teams, they may be infrequently utilized. Seaman and colleagues (2017) studied palliative teams consulting to ICUs of two large hospitals; consults were received an average of nearly 9 days after ICU admission (62% of the total ICU stay) and the mean duration of services was 4.6 days. Although psychologists were listed as team consultants, there were no psychologist visits documented, whereas the palliative social workers and chaplains had documented visits to 40% and 30%, respectively, of the referred ICU patients. However, Quenot and colleagues (2012) described benefits of including psychological facilitation in an intervention across several ICU teams to improve palliative and end-of-life care and reduce rates of provider burnout.

PROMOTING THE MENTAL HEALTH OF ICU HEALTH CARE PROFESSIONALS

Health care professionals are constantly exposed to stressful and potentially traumatizing events in the intensive care setting. Witnessing patients go through stressful and painful procedures such as debridement or ventilation liberation can have lasting effects. They can feel helpless when interventions are tried and fail. They have frequent exposure to patients who are at the end of life or who expire during their admission. They may experience moral distress regarding ethical decision-making around end-of-life care with differing perspectives on nonbeneficial care (previously referred to as medical futility) (Johnson-Coyle et al., 2016). ICU staff often are the recipients of communication from families who are struggling with their loved one's condition or prognosis. There can be stressful disagreements among staff; for example, nurses may disagree with physicians' continuing treatment because of their closer and sustained experience with patient suffering (Puntillo & McAdam, 2006). All clinicians in the ICU are at risk for psychological complications that have been described in overlapping concepts of vicarious or secondary trauma and PTSD, moral injury, compassion fatigue or burnout (as detailed in Nimmo and Huggard, 2013; Van Mol et al., 2015). These terms are used, sometimes interchangeably, to address the loss of compassion or numbing/distancing providers may experience as a direct result of the work they do (Van Mol et al., 2015).

As Remen noted (1996), "The expectation that we can be immersed in suffering and loss daily and not be touched by it is as unrealistic as expecting to be able to walk through water without getting wet" (p. 52). Most studies refer to the detrimental effects of this experience as burnout, which is often described as having three major components: emotional exhaustion, depersonalization, and lack of feelings of personal and professional accomplishment (Maslach & Jackson, 1986). Among physicians, burnout is not unique to the ICU; a study of 6,586 U.S. physicians found that 54.3% endorsed burnout symptoms, 10.5% reported a major medical error in the past 3 months, and 6.5% reported recent suicidal ideation (Tawfik et al., 2018). Indeed, an average of 300 to 400 physicians commit suicide each year (Goldman et al., 2017).

Burnout in the ICU has been specifically attributed to the external demands from the work environment that exceed the capacity of the individual provider (Moss et al., 2016). For both ICU physicians and nurses, independent risk factors for burnout include personal characteristics, organizational factors, the quality of working relationships with peers and colleagues, and end-of-life issues (reviewed in Pastores et al., 2019). Systematic reviews point to individual factors associated with burnout such as younger age, unmarried status, some personality features such as lower resilience, and fewer years of experience (Chuang et al., 2016). Perhaps most importantly, there has been a shift in focus beyond identifying person-specific characteristics related to burnout to include systemic issues such as the burdens placed by electronic medical records or unmanageable workloads (Lilly et al., 2019; Pastores et al., 2019). Organizational psychologist Anthony Montgomery and colleagues present a forceful case for organizational change:

> The most common responses have put the responsibility on healthcare professionals to take better care of themselves, become more resilient, and cope with stressors on their own. But such an individualistic approach can ignore the sources of chronic stressors in the workplace such as incivility, staff shortages, and austerity measures. (2019, p. 1)

> . . . Burnout is an occupational problem not a medical diagnosis. Healthcare organizations should assess burnout at departmental level and use it as a metric of safety of care. (2019, p. 3)

The onset of the novel coronavirus, with the United States currently having by far the most confirmed cases of COVID-19 worldwide, has added to risks for physician and health care worker burnout and distress in the ICU. Ripp and colleagues argue that, during the pandemic, "we are observing and anticipating enormous, unabated psychological stressors that necessitate the rapid development and scaling up of a robust model of wellbeing support for staff" (2020, p. 1). Providers of care to patients in the ICU with COVID-19 may be among the groups most affected by COVID-19, given their exposure to the most severely ill patients who also are more likely to die. In fact, a United Nations Policy Brief on mental health needs from COVID-19 identified first responders and frontline workers, particularly health care workers, "as a specific population of concern" (United Nations, 2020). A recent meta-analysis of mental health outcomes of health care workers in recent viral outbreaks (e.g., severe acute respiratory syndrome [SARS-CoV-1], Middle East respiratory syndrome [MERS], Ebola, and COVID-19 [SARS-CoV-2]) found that health care workers treating exposed patients had increased odds of both posttraumatic stress symptoms and psychological distress, whereas access to adequate PPE, access to psychological intervention, and clear communication and education regarding the virus all appeared to be protective factors (Kisely et al., 2020).

Studies of health care workers on the frontlines of the COVID-19 pandemic suggest that lack of PPE, fear of infection, separation from families, and increased work hours contributed to poor mental health outcomes (Kang et al., 2020). Research on health care workers in China showed elevated reports of depression (50.4%), anxiety (44.6%), insomnia (34%), and distress (71.5%) on the Impact of Event Scale-Revised (Lai et al., 2020). In this group, females were found to have the highest rates of depression, anxiety, and distress, although being a frontline health care worker was an independent risk factor for all variables. In Spain, specialists working with COVID-19 in respiratory medicine and geriatrics were found to have the highest levels of psychological impact (Romero et al., 2020). In Italy, considered one of the most affected countries, health care workers also reported PTSD symptoms (49.3%), severe depression (24.7%), anxiety (19.8%), and insomnia (8.3%). Worse outcomes were associated with female gender, younger age, being a frontline worker, and having a deceased, hospitalized, or quarantined colleague (Rossi et al., 2020). These studies support that COVID-19 has a direct effect on the psychological experience and emotional status of health care workers, particularly those working in frontline settings and in the critical care arena (the reader is referred to Chapter 8 for additional information).

INTERVENTION STRATEGIES TO REDUCE PROVIDER BURNOUT

Psychologists working in the ICU can inform intervention strategies as part of the interdisciplinary team, given their clinical skillset and appreciation for the potential psychological impacts of stressful events. Several interventions have addressed the adverse outcomes experienced at both an individual and organizational level (West et al., 2016). In a literature review, Lilly and colleagues (2019) describe countermeasures for burnout in critical care providers, including improving coping skills.

Recommended interventions include self-care, rest, exercise, meditation, and hobbies as well as ICU-specific environmental measures such as shift limits and increasing teamwork and collaboration among disciplines.

System- or organizational-level factors have been identified as targets of intervention, including telemedicine, changing staffing models, and including nurse practitioners, physician assistants, and residents/fellows as part of the staffing model for the ICU (Pastores et al., 2019). To combat physician burnout, Shanafelt and Noseworthy (2017) describe nine strategies that organizations can employ to reduce burnout: (a) acknowledge and assess the problem of burnout, (b) use the power of effective leadership, (c) develop and implement targeted interventions, (d) promote a workplace community, (e) use incentives wisely, (f) align the organization's values with the culture, (g) promote work–life integration, (h) provide resources for self-care and resilience, and (i) fund research related to the science of reducing burnout. Quenot and colleagues (2012) describe an ICU intervention developed with psychologists for team collaboration around palliative care. This included daily meetings of team and family, a section on relevant ethics in every patient's medical record, stress debriefings, and conflict prevention; over a 2-year period, reported burnout was reduced by 50%.

New research is emerging out of the recent pandemic to inform our understanding of how best to address burnout and psychological distress among frontline health care providers, including those working in critical care settings. Clinical researchers at the largest tertiary hospital in Hunan Province, China, developed a detailed psychological intervention plan for providers early in the pandemic: an online course to guide staff in coping with psychological problems, a psychological assistance hotline, and a support group to help cope with psychological problems and stress (Chen et al., 2020). Interestingly, staff did not participate in either individual or group psychological support interventions. Interviewed staff reported that what they needed was more rest and more PPE; they said psychological support should be directed toward the needs of the patients with COVID-19 or providing staff with strategies to cope with patients' emotional state. The intervention plan was subsequently revised after this feedback (Chen et al., 2020). Whether during an emerging viral outbreak or under usual circumstances, the provision of psychological support should be guided by input from critical care teams and tailored to their needs. Effective strategies to address burnout and psychological distress are likely to vary across settings, and psychologists should consider using collaborative approaches when designing interventions.

Shanafelt and colleagues (2020) exemplified this approach. At the onset of the COVID-19 pandemic in the United States, eight focus groups created with health

care professionals (including physicians, nurses, and advanced practice professionals) explored their greatest concerns, what messages and behaviors they wanted
from hospital leadership, and what support would be most helpful. Eight sources
of anxiety were identified: having access to PPE; being exposed and exposing others
outside of the hospital; lack of access to rapid testing; uncertainty about how the
organization would react in terms of support if they were found to be COVID-19
positive; access to childcare; support of personal and family basic needs; being able
to provide care if transferred to a new area (e.g., ICU); and lack of access to updated
information (Shanafelt et al., 2020). From these focus groups, five requests of the
health care organization emerged: (a) listen to the health care providers, (b) reduce
the risk, (c) provide training, (d) provide support if needed, and (e) provide medical care and subsequent related needs if a staff member contracts the virus and is
quarantined. While specific to COVID-19, this type of process could be transfer-
rable to psychologists seeking to develop intervention programs for any critical care
providers.

Albott and colleagues (2020) used a preexisting peer support model of Battle
Buddies, developed by the U.S. Army, to implement a psychological resilience
intervention for the anticipated needs of frontline workers treating patients with
COVID-19. This model begins with trained peer supports who focus on listening
and validating experiences, followed by unit-level collaboration to display hospital
leadership support; if needed, a mental health consultant assigned to each unit or
department is available to refer for additional evaluation and treatment (Abbott
et al., 2020). By using an existing model of psychological support, they were able to
rapidly scale this to a health care environment.

British researchers created a free online intervention to address the potential psychological and emotional health needs of health care workers within 3 weeks of the
U.K. COVID-19 outbreak, using both literature review of the evidence and peer-
based evaluation for content (Blake et al., 2020). Seven days after its release, the
site had been accessed over 17,633 times and had more than 50,000 social media
exposures. These forms of online intervention may prove to be relevant to critical
care providers, given the ease of access (please see Appendix A: Trauma-Informed
Care Practices in the ICU).

In summary, addressing the emotional health needs of critical care providers is complex and challenging but essential. The onset of COVID-19 has further
increased the need to support health care workers facing an unprecedented medical crisis. Psychologists have an important role in the study and implementation
of effective interventions, although a clear message from the literature is that the
needs of critical care providers should be considered and prioritized when designing

interventions. Ultimately, "Self-care is an ethical imperative. We have an obligation to our patients, as well as to ourselves, our colleagues, and our loved ones, not to be damaged by the work that we do" (Saakvitne & Pearlman, 1996).

THE UTILITY OF PSYCHOLOGICAL PRINCIPLES IN THE CARE OF ICU PATIENTS

Here we consider selected psychological principles as a source for developing creative interventions designed to effect change in the ICU system, including its patients, staff, and practices.

Rehabilitation psychology is rooted in the experience of people confronted with bodily and environmental challenges and, as such, is universally relevant to the human condition. It has particular origins in social psychology and counseling psychology. Its rich history of foundational principles and interdisciplinary practices was originally inspired by the challenges of rehabilitation for returning WWII veterans with disabling injuries and then by the crisis of the 1950s polio pandemic (Wright, 1959). This foundation is periodically revisited to keep us grounded as fellow travelers beside our patients (Dembo et al., 1975; Dunn & Elliott, 2005; Dunn et al., 2016; Keany & Glueckauf, 1993).

The foundational principles, not all of which are unique to rehabilitation psychology, are at the core of its theory and practice. Recognition of human dignity compels clinicians to offer encouragement to all patients and treat them with respect and dignity, regardless of their bodily limitations or other characteristics. This principle also motivates clinicians toward best practices through careful observation, self-monitoring, and exchange of information, including scientific literature. Recognizing the "insider/outsider" distinction helps clinicians avoid making assumptions about patients' experiences, abilities, priorities, and goals. Consideration of the person–environment relation reminds us to look for environmental influences on patients' behavior and avoid making unhelpful attributions about their dispositional characteristics.

The insider/outsider perspective

The distinction between the perspectives of patients and those of health care staff should be considered explicitly. Misattributions can take the form of projecting one's own perspective when information is limited regarding the person's actual point of view. One important example involves decisions about treatments and resource allocation in the ICU that are based, in part, on the outsider perspective when estimating future quality of life. In Gerhart and Corbet's (1995) study of life satisfaction among individuals with a spinal cord injury living with ventilator support, estimates of life satisfaction by health care staff were very discrepant from those of their patients, with staff underestimating the life satisfaction of such individuals. Regarding assumptions about older patients and benefits of ICU treatment, in a large general sample of traumatic injury survivors assessed in the ICU and 6 months after, Culp and colleagues (2019) found that older adult patients fared better than their younger adult counterparts, with less alcohol use, depression, and posttraumatic stress symptoms. Hofhuis and colleagues (2011) found good recovery of health-related quality of life in octogenarians surviving critical illness.

The person–environment relation

In psychological studies, the relation between person and environment is revealed as being dynamic and reciprocal. Within the ICU, patient behavior is partly a function of medical status, the physical and organizational environment, and staff behavior. As persons who are critically ill awaken in an unfamiliar setting, their behavior may present as grateful or demanding, cooperative or resistant, inattentive or hypervigilant, as well as suspicious, frightened, angry, or emotionally needy. As ICU staff struggle to optimize medical stability, their attributions about the behavior of their patients may focus on presumed internal dispositional traits rather than observable situational characteristics. This "fundamental attribution error" is discussed by Dunn and colleagues (2016) as a driving factor in the outsider's response to people with disabilities. Informally, the assumption may be stated like this: "When patients improve, it's because of my expertise, whereas patients who don't improve aren't motivated, have personality problems, are alcoholics, etc." (e.g., see Macciocchi & Eaton, 1995). This may serve staff self-protective functions, such as sparing them the effort to consider different, perhaps more effortful or sadly unavailable courses of action, and preserving a self-image of effectiveness.

Crosskerry and colleagues (2013) discuss biases affecting judgments and behaviors of health care staff, including the fundamental attribution error plus three others with particular relevance to ICU care:

1. Primacy effects: the information about a patient that is initially available is more easily recalled than subsequent information
2. The closely related confirmation bias: information encountered early in the course of assessment and treatment tends to continue shaping clinical judgments, resisting modification or disconfirmation (a pattern beautifully explicated by Sladeczek et al., 2006)

3. The just-world hypothesis: when confronted with others' tragedy, people look for explanations that include something they themselves could avoid through better behavior, which buttresses their belief in a just world where they can be safe (e.g., see Gruman & Sloan, 1983).

In addition to the social psychology lens of attribution, patients' behaviors and patient–staff interactions have been discussed through other psychological lenses. Caplan and Schechter (1993) bring a psychodynamic perspective to the overused and misused term "denial" and additionally provide a concise and pragmatic review of scenarios in which a patient's "difficult" behavior may be a logical, temporarily adaptive response to a demanding environment with little opportunity for control. Gans (1983) and Mullins (1989) startled the world of rehabilitation with their discussion and examples of hate, existential dread, and power struggles in rehabilitation— dynamic energies that can either derail the process or can be acknowledged and redirected.

The following examples illustrate the need for principled care:

- A woman experiencing prolonged, devastating effects of bone marrow transplant (graft-versus-host disease) was chastised during bedside rounds by her oncologist for "not trusting" him and losing her "will to live." The consulting psychologist witnessed this invalidating microaggression immediately after a supportive encounter with the patient but was not successful in conveying to the oncologist the power of this supposed "encouragement" to further depress his patient. Without trauma awareness and training in self-reflection, he was unable to perceive that he was bullying someone who confronted him with his limited power to heal.
- A man with hyponatremia and cognitive slowing was not participating in mobilization; rehabilitative therapists described "poor motivation," and the physician prescribed antidepressant medication. The patient felt these attributions added insult to injury: "I'm not depressed! I've always worked hard—ask my wife!" The psychologist discussed her assessment of the patient's status with the physician and the potential for antidepressant medication to worsen hyponatremia. The medication regimen was adjusted, the patient's sodium levels were normalized, and then the team witnessed the emergence of a very alert man, very determined to recover.
- ICU nurses caring for a man with acute tetraplegia and traumatic brain injury on mechanical ventilation misinterpreted his repeated demands to go home as "He doesn't want to live like this; he wants to be taken off the ventilator." When asked directly if he preferred to stop ventilatory support

and die, with appropriate palliative care during that process, he looked at the psychologist as though she had two heads and clearly mouthed, "I don't want to die; I want to go home!" When he was told "Well, if you leave here now you'll die, so the staff here think that's what you mean and patients do have the right to stop treatment," he replied, "Hell, no!" He was able to retain this conversation and did not ask again to leave; many months later he was home and independently driving a "sip-n-puff" power wheelchair.

- A male in his 60s fell into a snowdrift, became unconscious, and sustained severe frostbite, subsequently losing all fingers and toes. His chart showed a history of alcohol abuse. Staff discussions included recollections of intoxicated people who had passed out in freezing weather, whereas lab reports showed this patient tested negative for alcohol. During a psychological interview, the patient reported he had recently had knee surgery and couldn't get back up after he lost his footing. He struggled for hours before passing out. Efforts by the psychologist to give staff an accurate picture of this tragedy had mixed success, as the corrected information could not displace the staff's initial impressions. The patient was puzzled by staff's rather distant attitude in the ICU and later in rehabilitation as he struggled to learn the use of adaptive equipment.

PSYCHOLOGICAL PRINCIPLES OF LEARNING

If coping and adapting to critical illness or injury is a learning process, we should consider what is being taught during critical care. Applied behavior analysis (ABA) has informed inpatient and outpatient rehabilitation (e.g., Merbitz et al., 2003; Mozzoni & Bailey, 1996), as well as psychotherapy for patients with trauma histories (Kohlenberg & Tsai, 1991; Walser & Hayes, 2006), and also has some very apt formulations applicable to the ICU learning environment and its impact on patients. A central principle of ABA is that learning occurs within any and all environments, with or without any explicit intention to teach.

Antecedents and contingencies in critical care
Respondent conditioning
As detailed earlier in the chapter, the physical/sensory stimuli of the ICU are predominantly aversive, and social contacts are frequently paired with aversive procedures; thus, behavior in the ICU can be viewed as unconditioned responses to unconditioned stimuli (e.g., pain, noises, smells, confinement) and as conditioned responses (to previously neutral or positive stimuli paired with unconditioned,

noxious stimuli). The approach of staff may provoke a patient's withdrawal or agitation; while staff may intend to calm and reassure the patient, the success of that effort depends on the recency and quality of exposure to reassuring contact, so that it becomes more salient than the patient's experience with aversive contacts. In a typical ICU environment this could be difficult.

Operant conditioning

In addition, the ICU can be examined in terms of operant conditioning. Kanter and colleagues (2005) discussed many factors in the genesis of depression; of these, three are particularly apt for describing the ICU, and from Abreu and Santos (2008) we take a fourth. To each factor we have given an informal, layperson's explanation:

1. Lack of response-contingent reinforcement of behavior: From the patient's perspective, nothing much good is going on, and there is little if anything they can do to improve.
2. Too much punishment of behavioral responses: Moving hurts (or they may be restrained if they dislodge the tubes attached to them), visual inspection of the surrounding room is frightening, and staff's response to efforts to communicate may be negative (e.g., when patients get agitated when they are not understood or when their requests are not met).
3. Loss of effective operant behavior: Patients are weak and debilitated, often disoriented, and possibly unable to speak. They literally are unable to operate upon their environment to obtain much, if anything.
4. The presentation of noncontingent aversive stimulation: Unpleasant sensations and events are ubiquitous and unavoidable in the ICU and are unrelated to anything patients do or don't do.

The repeated, noncontingent presentation of aversive events occurring regardless of whatever the individual is or isn't doing is the formula for learned helplessness and depression, whereas the opportunity for agency, for exerting even some control, produces an active response and tends to preserve or improve mood. Thus, allowing patients to do any portion of their self-care and to exert some choice about the manner or timing of procedures (e.g., positioning, bathing) can have an outsized impact; by increasing reinforcement density and behavioral activation, engagement is maintained or restored.

Another antidote to the depression-promoting effects of the ICU is high-density reinforcement. Informally stated, ICU patients need frequent acts of random kindness. The randomness of kind actions is key, occurring not only when the patient is agitated, distressed, or withdrawn but also during periods of calm, or mobilization and efforts to recover independence. Such staff behavior fosters a nurturing (reinforcing) environment for patients, whether for recovery or simply for their sense of connectedness regardless of ultimate outcome, and to some extent counteracts the impact of prevalent aversive stimuli. ICU staff members' knowledge and practice of principles of respondent and operant conditioning can be transformative for patients and staff alike.

Conditioning and ventilator liberation

The emotional response when struggling to breathe can quickly move from anxiety to terror. "Having trouble taking a breath in, experiencing an unquenchable thirst for air, or feeling one's chest constricted immediately summons an existential fear, the fear of dying" (Demoule & Similowski, 2019, p. 1303). Rarely assessed specifically, when noted this reaction is commonly labeled as anxiety and is frequently cited as the reason for "failure to wean," sometimes with insufficient assessment for other etiologies. Heunks and van der Hoeven (2010) review a myriad of etiologies to investigate and remediations to deploy for delayed or failed ventilator liberation; they argue that anxiety is but one consideration and not necessarily the most likely. Psychologists who receive a consult to see a patient with delayed ventilator liberation may find themselves swimming upstream when noting that anxiety is not the only contributing factor.

That being said, anxiety during "weaning trials" does not always emanate solely or primarily from "traits" or "coping" of the individual patient but must be identified and addressed in the context of team treatment. For the patient with delayed liberation, to engage the patient's best efforts it is recommended that each trial session be lengthened gradually and predictably rather than extended to the limit of tolerance; in the latter case, the patient's anxious avoidance may be negatively reinforced (i.e., when an anxious response serves to end an aversive experience). When each event in a series of trials ends with success after a planned interval, this reinforces persistence and can build the patient's self-efficacy and trust in the process.

Discontinuation of ventilator support can be perceived as a threat to life, activating basic stress-response emotions as well as memories connected to past experiences of threat. A power differential is inherent as the health care professional initiates and controls the process. Telling a frightened patient struggling to breathe to "calm down" or overtly attributing a trial failure to the patient's anxiety constitutes punishment, and these microaggressions can be traumatizing. The psychologist working with patients in this circumstance knows that these moments may linger and fester in the patient's memory, affecting expectations, trust, and "motivation."

Informing ICU care with trauma psychology

Invalidating interactions with care providers, no matter how inadvertent, compound the trauma of critical illness or injury. Consider the regressive experience of having radically altered function and appearance, being in a state of complete dependence on others and likely disoriented. Patients in such a state look to the staff for clues about what has happened, who they are, and who they may become. The depersonalization of patients (e.g., when referred to by their diagnoses) reduces the immediacy of their suffering from an outsider perspective (e.g., Vaes & Muratore, 2013) and also reduces providers' and patients' shared experience of empathy and compassion.

The experience of trauma recapitulates developmental needs for safety, attention, validation, and self-coherence—what Kohut called "mirroring" (Banai et al., 2005; Street, 2008): the messages conveyed through word and deed that tell the patient "I'm caring for you; I see you; you are worthy and valuable; we will be by your side and help you through this unknown territory." Jacobson depicts the individual in crisis and disequilibrium as being especially receptive to outside influences. Moos and Holahan (2007) argue that this presents an opportunity for intervention by health care teams, but we also note heightened vulnerability in the ICU: Nonsupportive care and negative interactions in the context of critical illness and dependency may be uniquely traumatizing. Patients in the ICU and their families/support persons do not need any decrement of faith in others or themselves during this crisis. Their experiences and outcomes will benefit from care informed by trauma psychology. The authors regard the interdisciplinary field of trauma psychology, with its knowledge base of TIC for medical patients, as central to the humanization of critical care and central to this chapter.

THE NEUROBIOLOGY OF TRAUMA AND THE STRESS RESPONSE

Understanding the neurobiological impact of trauma is salient for all health care professionals working in ICUs. Whether from prior and/or acute trauma, this neurobiological impact shapes our patients' ability to process information and their ongoing behavioral and physical responses during critical illness and care. Bloom (2005) conceptualized trauma theory to capture the numerous short- and long-term effects of trauma described by neurosciences, psychology, and sociology and other disciplines. Trauma shapes human behavior, emotions, and information processing not only acutely, as in a crisis, but also developmentally. Development encompasses learned patterns and the structure and function of the brain. Thus, the patient's response reflects not only the real-time constraints and intrusions of critical illness and critical care but also previously established patterns and capabilities of the brain.

Research on the neurobiology of trauma has found that when individuals detect threat, a survival-oriented response is initiated in the brain. This flight, fight, freeze, or fright response emanates from the sympathetic nervous system, which prioritizes keeping us safe (Gunnar & Quevedo, 2007; McEwen, 2008). For example, when a threat is detected, cognitive resources are directed to the more primitive threat-detection brain structures such as the amygdala and associated threat-monitoring and threat-response pathways. However, the allocation of resources toward survival results in other important brain activities and functions receiving less attention. These limited cognitive resources can affect higher-order behaviors, such as freely exploring environments, decision-making, emotion regulation, goal setting, and flexibly adjusting to one's surroundings (Schore, 2005).

The ICU environment demands flexible coping. Patients with traumatic histories may be at a disadvantage in their recovery process as they may focus on perceived or misperceived threats and respond with established inflexible patterns of resistance, avoidance, or withdrawal. Along with clinicians' lifesaving efforts, there must be corresponding efforts to offer comfort, not only out of compassion but also for the sake of better outcomes. Quite simply, a reassured patient has a better chance to comprehend, cooperate, participate, and make decisions, and—if possible—is more likely to benefit from medical treatment.

PSYCHOLOGICAL TRAUMA HISTORY IS COMMON AMONG PATIENTS IN THE ICU

A close examination of the literature on trauma's association with physical and psychiatric conditions helps us anticipate the needs of our ICU patients. Premorbid psychiatric conditions predict greater distress during and after ICU care, including posttraumatic stress symptoms and PTSD (Patel et al., 2016; Ratzer et al., 2014). A history of adverse childhood experiences (ACEs) is common in the general population and must be considered as common among our ICU patients.

> We as providers need to recognize that many, many patients have a history of physical, sexual, and/or emotional abuse, as well as serious illnesses and negative experiences in the medical setting. . . . Trauma-informed care is the open-mindedness and compassion that all patients deserve, because anyone can have a history that impacts their encounter with the medical system. (Tello, 2019)

Findings of the National Comorbidity Survey in 1992 and later replications showed strong associations between lifetime frequencies of trauma and serious psychiatric disorders (Afifi et al., 2008; Green et al., 2010). In 1998, the first study of

ACEs (Felitti et al., 1998) examined associations of trauma with medical and mental disorders and found a significant association with negative social and health outcomes later in life. Approximately 66% of responders had experienced at least one of the following traumatic events: abuse (sexual, physical, and emotional), neglect (physical and emotional), and/or household dysfunction (e.g., living with a family member who has a mental illness or a drug problem or is incarcerated). Among these individuals, approximately 85% experienced more than one adverse event (Felitti et al., 1998). Moreover, nearly 13% had experienced four or more childhood adversities (Centers for Disease Control and Prevention, 2020).

Consideration for the health impact of ACEs among patients presenting to the ICU is pertinent, as prior trauma has been shown to be prevalent within health care populations (Cronholm et al., 2015; Green et al., 2015). A survey of ICU patients, which included veterans and civilians, revealed that 84% reported at least one traumatic experience (not related to war or prior critical illness) before their current episode of illness or injury (Patel et al., 2016). In contrast, the reported prevalence in the general population surveyed in the original ACEs study was 66% (Felitti et al., 1998). Another study found that an average of 3.66 prior traumatic events was reported (O'Donnell et al., 2010), highlighting the complex histories for many patients in the ICU.

The literature on ACEs and health outcomes shows linkages between ACEs and numerous negative health behaviors and outcomes, including substance abuse, physical inactivity, poor diet, alcohol use disorders, risky sexual behaviors, diabetes, obesity, asthma, cardiovascular disease and heart attack, cerebrovascular disease and stroke, chronic obstructive pulmonary disease, HIV, cancer, and early death (Anda et al., 2006, 2008; Brown et al., 2009; 2009, 2013; Dong et al., 2004; Felitti et al., 1998; Flaherty et al., 2013; Gilbert et al., 2015; National Center for Injury Prevention and Control, 2020; Schilling et al., 2007). Patients affected by trauma also tend toward a lower engagement in preventive care and treatment adherence (Kartha et al., 2008; Marsac et al., 2016; Sansone et al., 2014); thus, many services are delivered/received in emergency settings (Kobal et al., 2019). ACEs also are associated with higher adulthood rates of traumatic injuries from motor vehicle crashes, being stabbed or shot, interpersonal violence, and suicide attempts or completions, with injuries including traumatic brain injury, spinal cord injury, burns, and polytrauma (Guinn et al., 2019; McKibben et al., 2009; Peterson et al., 2019; Sotero et al., 2015; Thompson et al., 2002).

The health conditions and injuries reported at higher rates among people with ACEs are among the most common admission diagnoses and comorbidities seen in ICUs. In addition to traumatic injuries, these include acute myocardial infarction, heart failure, lung cancer, and septic shock, plus diabetes, chronic obstructive pulmonary disease, other cancers, end-stage renal disease, end-stage liver disease, HIV infection, and obesity (summarized in Esper & Martin, 2011). Thus, the literature suggests that trauma history is overrepresented in the population of patients in critical care compared to the general population. Whether we consider traumatic experiences that occurred before or after admission to the ICU, staff must understand the effects of prior trauma in order to optimize patient adaptation during and after the ICU.

SPECIFIC CHALLENGES IN PROVIDER INTERACTIONS WITH TRAUMATIZED PATIENTS

Dubay and colleagues (2018) advocate for a functional health care system that requires staff to understand the impact of trauma in their patients' lives to foster a meaningful response to care. As early adopters of TIC, they describe how the health care system can be retraumatizing to individuals with trauma histories, impeding their engagement in services and adherence to treatment.

For health care professionals, building trust with patients is necessary to address the complex medical needs (Daniel et al., 2018), yet providers have reported feeling unprepared to work with traumatized patients in terms of knowledge, skills, and practical resources to help (Elisseou et al., 2019; Green et al., 2015; Raja et al., 2015). They may not know how to respond to clues, such as a sad or flat affect or negative responses to particular procedures; conversely, persons with trauma history may perceive being ignored, overlooked, or dismissed (Green et al., 2012, 2015; Williamson & Kautz, 2016). Providers have reported feeling frustrated, overwhelmed, worried, and even drained when dealing with patients who have trauma histories (Green et al., 2015), although some report knowing about TIC and have positive attitudes about including TIC into their practice (Bruce et al., 2018). Providers who have a trauma-informed therapeutic alliance with their patients are less likely to experience burnout and are more likely to build relationships of trust and safety (Freeman et al., 2016, 2018; Magen & DeLisser, 2017). Fortunately, there appears to be growing consensus toward ensuring provider training and competence in TIC (Daniel et al., 2018; Marsac et al., 2016).

TIC PRACTICES

TIC is intended to minimize the detrimental impact of trauma during the provision of health care services and to promote development of policies for patients and families to feel safe (Bloom & Farragher, 2013; Fleishman et al., 2019). The Substance Abuse and Mental Health Services Administration (2014) proposed that trauma-informed organizations realize that trauma is prevalent among services users and staff, recognize the impact of trauma and how it manifests, and resist retraumatization by reviewing and altering their policies and practice.

Specific practices of "psychological first aid" are being advanced for TIC in the circumstance or immediate aftermath of traumatic events, and this has particular relevance for patients in critical care. Young (2006) recommended psychological first aid when an individual has an acute stress reaction in response to trauma (e.g., dissociative symptoms, anxiety, sleep disturbance). Psychological first aid is flexible and responsive to "the specific human needs and emotional style of an individual and his or her expressed needs at the moment of intervention" (Kantor & Beckett, 2011, p. 204). Principles of Effective PTSD Prevention (Hobfoll et al., 2007) have been adopted as a program of psychological first aid (e.g., Ng & Kantor, 2010). Key features include "contact and engagement, safety and comfort, stabilization, information gathering, practical assistance, connection with social supports, information on coping, and linkage with collaborative services" (Kantor & Beckert, 2011, p. 203).

TIC aligns with patient-centered care, which has been associated with increased patient knowledge, shared decision-making, and greater adherence to care (Levinson et al., 2010; Ozer & Kroll, 2002). Notably, the foundational principles of rehabilitation psychology parallel and predate the literature on TIC and patient-centered care. In addition to the uncompromising value of humans for their intrinsic worth rather than their comparative status, there was an early insistence in rehabilitation psychology on person-first language, and emphasis on identifying individuals' assets, honoring the insider experience of patients, examining the total life space to understand individuals' behavior, and using that knowledge to expand the scope of services and resources (e.g., Dembo et al., 1975; Keany & Gleuckauf, 1993; McCarthy, 2011).

TIC IN INTENSIVE CARE SETTINGS

Principles of TIC, patient-centered care, and rehabilitation psychology can guide the training and support of ICU staff, who are encouraged to apply TIC as a "universal precaution" (Racine et al., 2019) to optimize the adaptation of patients, family, friends, and providers. There are vast opportunities to evaluate ICU practices and apply a trauma-informed lens to the experience of both patients and health care professionals (see Machtinger et al., 2015; Sperlich et al., 2017). Ashana and colleagues (2020) argue that TIC will improve the care of individuals with prior trauma, reducing the impact of critical illness as a retraumatizing event. Still, few publications address TIC in this work, and more research is needed (Dubay et al., 2018). TIC has been explored and utilized in the neonatal ICU (Coughlin, 2016; Marcellus &

Cross, 2016; Sanders & Hall, 2017), and there is growing awareness of the need for it in acute medical rehabilitation (Freeman et al., 2016; Merbitz et al., 2016).

We do know that the likelihood of emotional and cognitive morbidities post-ICU is lessened by successful efforts to reduce the following: pain and discomfort (Daoust et al., 2020; Kalfon et al., 2019); delirium and threats to brain integrity (Hopkins et al., 2017; Wilcox et al., 2013); and fear, distress, and isolation (Ely, 2017; Ratzer et al., 2014; Wade et al., 2013). Wilson and colleagues (2019) list dehumanizing aspects of intensive care and several practices to preserve patients' humanity. These, along with evolving critical care standards summarized in the ABCDEFGH bundle (i.e., ICU liberation bundle) (Table 4.2; Davidson et al., 2013; Inoue et al., 2019; Vasilevskis et al., 2010), align well with the principles of patient-centered care and TIC.

Prior to the COVID crisis, critical care physicians, nurses, and other ICU team members rightly took pride in the progress they had made toward humanizing the ICU and optimizing outcomes via best practices such as the ICU liberation bundle:

Consistent implementation [of this bundle] shifts ICU culture from the harmful inertia of sedation and restraints to an animated ICU filled with patients who are awake, cognitively engaged, and mobile with family members engaged as partners with the ICU team at the bedside. In so doing, patients are liberated from iatrogenic aspects of care that threaten her or his sense of self-worth and human dignity. (Ely, 2017, p 321)

TABLE 4.2.

ABCDEFGH bundle in critical care

Evidence-based guide to optimize ICU patient recovery and outcomes

A	Airway management; assess, prevent, and manage pain
B	Breathing trials; daily interruptions of mechanical ventilation, spontaneous awakening trials, and spontaneous breathing trials
C	Choice of analgesia and sedation; coordination of care and communication
D	Delirium assessment, prevention, and management
E	Early mobility and exercise
F	Family involvement, follow-up referrals, and functional reconciliation
G	Good handoff communication
H	Handout materials on PICS and PICS-F

PICS = postintensive care syndrome; PICS-F = postintensive care syndrome—family

Source: Ely, 2017; Inoue et al., 2019

Devlin and colleagues (2020) note the strong evidence behind the ICU bundle, and during the pandemic they caution against abandoning a set of tools that "would seem to be tailor made to reduce duration of mechanical ventilation and shorten the ICU stay" (p. 2).

Given that delirium is associated with persisting symptoms of traumatic stress, TIC includes efforts toward delirium prevention or mitigation. For the confused or simply terrified patient in the ICU, the kind faces of staff convey regard and a shared humanity. When the patient with delirium has intermittent periods of improved clarity, very basic explanations of delirium can help to normalize their experience as something that happens to many people who are very sick, a temporary medical condition, not an indication that they've gone "crazy" or become someone completely different.

A recent and fascinating randomized controlled trial (Xue et al., 2020) even found that patients who received education about delirium prior to cardiac surgery had less than half the incidence of delirium afterward, plus significantly fewer hours on mechanical ventilation and fewer hours in the ICU. Apparently knowledge is power, mitigating the force of deliriogenic factors such as general anesthesia. This raises the question: Could all conscious patients arriving in the ICU benefit from straightforward information about delirium.

When discussing nonpharmacologic interventions for delirium, LaHue and colleagues (2020) recommend standard measures to maintain the diurnal light–dark cycle: minimize nighttime disruptions; provide physical mobilization, cognitive stimulation, and reorientation; and ensure the availability of eyeglasses and hearing aids. Noting the absence of family visits during the COVID-19 crisis, they also emphasize enabling use of communication devices to facilitate phone calls and virtual visits. Highfield and colleagues have provided detailed recommendations for communicating with patients while they are delirious (Box 4.1), which are likely to ease distress during that frightening experience.

Conclusion

As they witness patient and family suffering, ICU clinicians are challenged to remain engaged intellectually and empathically in order to contribute to the healing and well-being of their patients and bring a renewed passion to their work. Concepts and principles from psychological science and practice help clinicians to contact aspects of others' realities without being engulfed and flooded, or withdrawing (Kearney et al., 2009). Viewing the ICU as a learning environment may prompt creative and effective strategies to identify modifiable features related to personal interactions

BOX 4.1.
COMMUNICATING WITH PATIENTS HAVING DELIRIUM AND DISTRESS

Antecedents/Unit atmosphere
Be person-centered: warm, genuine, accepting, understanding, nonjudgmental.Build rapport: Be open, honest and listening to gain trust.Acknowledge that the ICU is distressing, and that discussing worries is difficult.

Address root causes of agitation by proactively identifying unmet needs (e.g., pain, thirst).

Responding to patients who are confused and/or in distress
Have open, visible body language and give hallucinating patients lots of personal space.

Use a caring tone of voice and manner when discussing worries and fears.

Use slow speech, simple vocabulary, and short sentences.

If a verbal patient is speaking rapidly, then slow down the pace of conversation.

Talk to patients with hallucinations and delusions as rational people with unusual experiences.

If challenged by patients to confirm a delusion, then say it seems unlikely to you, but you are open to learning otherwise.Acknowledge the stress and unusual experiences; emphasize helping the patient feel calm and safe.

What not to do
Make gestures that look like ordering/criticizing (e.g., pointing, arm-folding, and finger-wagging).

Allow your voice to sound frustrated or irritable or use phrases that sound patronizing or sarcastic.

Laugh at hallucinations and delusions, or contradict, dismiss, or minimize.

Adapted from Highfield et al., 2020

and processes of care. Awareness of ubiquitous tendencies toward bias improves clinicians' treatment of all patients in spite of differing appearance, abilities, histories, and perspectives. Applying principles of TIC guides the ICU milieu toward safety, trustworthiness, choice, collaboration, and empowerment.

Staff messages, verbal and nonverbal alike, convey that the patient's struggle with critical illness or injury in the ICU is a worthy one, with recognition given to every milestone. When progress doesn't materialize, the team continues to convey that the patient is a person of significance and is not alone. For ICU staff to do this, they themselves need to receive parallel messages from each other and from their leadership. Psychologists can assist in the compelling, international movement to humanize the ICU for patients, families, and health care providers.

References

Abreu, P. R., & Santos, C. E. (2008). Behavioral models of depression: A critique of the emphasis on positive reinforcement. *International Journal of Behavioral Consultation and Therapy, 4*(2), 130–135. http://dx.doi.org/10.1037/h0100838

Afifi, T. O., Enns, M. W., Cox, B. J., Asmundson, G. J., Stein, M. B., & Sareen, J. (2008). Population attributable fractions of psychiatric disorders and suicide ideation and attempts associated with adverse childhood experiences. *American Journal of Public Health, 98*(5), 946–952. https://doi.org/10.2105/ajph.2007.120253

Albott, C. S., Wozniak, J. R., McGlinch, B. P., Wall, M. H., Gold, B. S., & Vinogradov, S. (2020). Battle buddies: Rapid deployment of a psychological resilience intervention for health care workers during the coronavirus disease 2019 pandemic. *Anesthesia and Analgesia, 131*(1), 43–54. https://doi.org/10.1213/ANE.0000000000004912

Anda, R., Brown, D., Dube, S., Bremner, J., Felitti, V., & Giles, W. (2008). Adverse childhood experiences and chronic obstructive pulmonary disease in adults. *American Journal of Preventive Medicine, 34*(5), 396–403. https://doi.org/10.1016/j.amepre.2008.02.002

Anda, R., Felitti, F., Bremner, V., Walker, J., Whitfield, D., Perry, C., ... Giles, S. (2006). The enduring effects of abuse and related adverse experiences in childhood. *European Archives of Psychiatry and Clinical Neuroscience, 256*(3), 174–186. https://doi.org/10.1007/s00406-005-0624-4

Andreoli, P. B. A., Novaes, M. A. F. P., Karam, C. H., & Knobel, E. (2001). The ICU humanization program: Contributions from the psychologist team [Meeting abstract]. *Critical Care, 5*(Suppl. 3), P80. http://dx.doi.org/10.1186/cc1413

Ashana, D., Lewis, C., & Hart, J. (2020). Dealing with "difficult" patients and families: Making a case for trauma-informed care in the intensive care unit. *Annals of the American Thoracic Society, 17*(5), 541–544. https://doi.org/10.1513/AnnalsATS.201909-700IP

Azoulay, E., Pochard, F., Chevret, S., Lemaire, F., Mokhtari, M., Le Gall, J. R., ... Schlemmer, B. (2001). Meeting the needs of intensive care unit patient families: A multicenter study. *American Journal of Respiratory and Critical Care Medicine, 163*(1), 135–139. https://doi.org/10.1164/ajrccm.163.1.2005117

Banai, E., Mikulincer, M., & Shaver, P. R. (2005). "Self object" needs in Kohut's self psychology: Links with attachment, self-cohesion, affect regulation, and adjustment. *Psychoanalytic Psychology, 22*(2), 224–260. https://doi.org/10.1037/0736-9735.22.2.224

Barr, J., Fraser, G. L., Puntillo, K., Ely, E. W., Gélinas, C., Dasta, J. F., ... American College of Critical Care Medicine. (2013). Clinical practice guidelines for the management of pain, agitation, and delirium in adult patients in the intensive care unit. *Critical Care Medicine, 41*(1), 263–306. https://doi.org/10.1097/ccm.0b013e3182783b72

Bartunek, J. M. (2011). Intergroup relationships and quality improvement in healthcare. *BMJ Quality & Safety, 20*(1), 162–166. https://doi.org/10.1136/bmjqs.2010.046169

Bennun, I. (2001). Intensive care unit syndrome: A consideration of psychological interventions. *British Journal of Medical Psychology, 74*(3), 369–377. https://doi.org/ 10.1348/000711201161046

Blake, H., Bermingham, F., Johnson, G., & Tabner, A. (2020). Mitigating the psychological impact of COVID-19 on healthcare workers: A digital learning package. *International Journal of Environmental Research and Public Health, 17*(9), 2997. https://doi.org/10.3390/ijerph17092997

Bloom, S. L. (2005). Neither liberty nor safety: The impact of fear on individuals, institutions, and societies, part III. *Psychotherapy and Politics International, 3*(2), 96–111. https://doi.org/10.1002/ppi.23

Bloom, S. L., & Farragher, B. J. (2013). *Restoring sanctuary: A new operating system for trauma-informed systems of care.* Oxford University Press.

British Psychological Society. (2020). Meeting the psychological needs of people recovering from severe coronavirus (Covid-19). https://www.bps.org.uk/sites/www.bps.org.uk/files/Policy/Policy%20-%20Files/Meeting%20the%20psychological%20needs%20of%20people%20recovering%20from%20severe%20coronavirus.pdf

Brown, D., Anda, R., Tiemeier, H., Felitti, V., Edwards, V., Croft, J., & Giles, W. (2009). Adverse childhood experiences and the risk of premature mortality. *American Journal of Preventive Medicine, 37*(5), 389–396. https://doi.org/10.1016/j.amepre.2009.06.021

Brown, M. J., Thacker, L.R., & Cohen, S. A. (2013). Association between adverse childhood experiences and diagnosis of cancer. *PLoS One, 8*(6), E65524. https://doi.org/10.1371/journal.pone.0065524

Bruce, M. M., Kassam-Adams, N., Rogers, M., Anderson, K. M., Sluys, K. P., & Richmond, T. S. (2018). Trauma providers' knowledge, views, and practice of trauma-informed care. *Journal of Trauma Nursing, 25*(2), 131–138. https://doi.org/10.1097/JTN.0000000000000356

Callahan, C. D., & Griffen, D. L. (2003). Applying statistical process control techniques to emergency medicine: A primer for providers. *Academic Emergency Medicine, 10,* 883–890.

Caplan, G. (1964). *Principles of preventive psychiatry.* New York: Basic Books.

Caplan, B., & Shechter, J. (1993). Reflections on the "depressed", "unrealistic", "inappropriate", "manipulative", "unmotivated", "noncompliant", "denying", "maladjusted", "regressed", etc. patient. *Archives of Physical Medicine and Rehabilitation, 74*(10), 1123–1124.

Centers for Disease Control and Prevention. (2020). *Adverse childhood experiences.*https://www.cdc.gov/violenceprevention/acestudy/index.html

Chen, Q., Liang, M., Li, Y., Guo, J., Fei, D., Wang, L., . . . Wang, J. (2020). Mental health care for medical staff in China during the COVID-19 outbreak. *Lancet Psychiatry, 7*(4), e15–e16. https://doi.org/10.1016/S2215-0366(20)30078-X

Chuang, C. H., Tseng, P. C., Lin, C. Y., Lin, K. H., & Chen, Y. Y. (2016). Burnout in the intensive care unit professionals: A systematic review. *Medicine, 95*(50), e5629. https://doi.org/10.1097/MD.0000000000005629

Ciccolella, N. (April 21, 2020). Personal communication.

Cook, D. J., Marshall, J. C., & Fowler, R. A. (2020). Critical illness in patients with COVID-19: Mounting an effective clinical and research response. *Journal of the American Medical Association, 323*(16), 1559–1560. https://doi.org/10.1001/jama.2020.5775

Cooper, D., Farmery, K., Johnson, M., Harper, C., & Clarke, F. (2005). Changing personnel behavior to promote quality care practices in an intensive care unit. *Therapeutics and Clinical Risk Management, 1*(4), 321–332.

Coughlin, M. (2016). *Trauma-informed care in the NICU: Evidenced-based practice guidelines for neonatal clinicians.* Springer Publishing Company.

Croskerry, P., Singhal, G., & Mamede, S. (2013). Cognitive debiasing 2: Impediments to and strategies for change. *BMJ Quality & Safety, 22*(2), ii65–ii72. https://doi.org/10.1136/bmjqs-2012-001713

Cronholm, P., Forke, C., Wade, R., Bair-Merritt, M., Davis, M., Harkins-Schwarz, M., . . . Fein, J. (2015). Adverse childhood experiences: Expanding the concept of adversity. *American Journal of Preventive Medicine, 49*(3), 354–361. https://doi.org/10.1016/j.amepre.2015.02.001

Culp, B. L., Roden-Foreman, J. W., Thomas, E. V., McShan, E. E., Bennett, M. M., Martin, K. R., Powers, M. B., Foreman, M. L., Petrey, L. B., & Warren, A. M. (2019). Better with age? A comparison of geriatric and non-geriatric trauma patients' psychological outcomes six months post-injury. *Cognitive Behavioral Therapy, 48*(5), 406–418.

Daniel, H., Bornstein, S. S., & Kane, G. C. (2018). Addressing social determinants to improve patient care and promote health equity: An American College of Physicians Position paper. *Annals of Internal Medicine, 168*(8), 577–578. https://doi.org/10.7326/M17-2441

Daoust, R., Paquet, J., Boucher, V., Pelletier, M., Gouin, É., & Émond, M. (2020). Relationship between pain, opioid treatment, and delirium in older emergency department patients. *Academic Emergency Medicine, 27*(8), 708–716. https://doi.org/10.1111/acem.14033

Davidson, J. E., Harvey, M. A., Schuller, J., & Black, G. (2013). Post-intensive care syndrome: What it is and how to help prevent it. *American Nurse Today, 8*(5), 32. https://doi.org/10.1183/20734735.0013-2019

Davidson, J., McDuffie, M., & Campbell, K. (2017). Family-centered care. In S. Goldsworthy, R. Kleinpell, & G. E. Speed (Eds.), *International best practices in critical care* (pp. 311–368). World Federation of Critical Care Nursing.

Dembo, T., Leviton, G., & Wright, B. (1975). Adjustment to misfortune: A problem of social-psychological rehabilitation. *Rehabilitation Psychology, 22*(1), 1–100. https://doi.org/10.1037/h0090832

Demoule, A., & Similowski, T. (2019). Respiratory suffering in the ICU: Time for our next great cause. *American Journal of Respiratory and Critical Care Medicine, 199*(11), 1302–1304. https://doi.org/10.1164/rccm.201812-2248ED

deRoon-Cassini, T. A., Hunt, J. C., Geier, T. J., Warren, A. M., Ruggiero, K. J., Scott, K., . . . Zatzick, D. (2019). Screening and treating hospitalized trauma survivors for posttraumatic stress disorder and depression. *Journal of Trauma and Acute Care Surgery, 87*(2), 440–450. https://doi.org/10.1097/TA.0000000000002370

Devlin, J. W., O'Neal Jr, H. R., Thomas, C., Daly, M. A. B., Stollings, J. L., Janz, D. R., . . . Lin, J. C. (2020). Strategies to optimize ICU liberation (A to F) bundle performance in critically ill adults with coronavirus disease 2019. *Critical Care Explorations, 2*(6), e0139. https://doi.org/10.1097/CCE.0000000000000139

Dong, M., Giles, W., Felitti, V., Dube, S., Williams, J., Chapman, D., & Anda, R. (2004). Insights into causal pathways for ischemic heart disease: Adverse childhood experiences study. *Circulation, 110*(13), 1761–1766. https://doi.org/10.1161/01.CIR.0000143074.54995.7F

Dubay, L., Burton, R. A., & Epstein, M. (2018). *Early adopters of trauma-informed care: An implementation analysis of the Advancing Trauma-Informed Care grantees.* Urban Institute. https://www.chcs.org/media/early_adopters_of_trauma-informed_care-evaluation.pdf

Dunn, D., Ehde, D., & Wegener, S. (2016). The foundational principles as psychological lodestars: Theoretical inspiration and empirical direction in rehabilitation psychology. *Rehabilitation Psychology, 61*(1), 1–6. https://doi.org/10.1037/rep0000082

Dunn, D. S., & Elliott, T. R. (2005). Revisiting a constructive classic: Wright's physical disability: A psychosocial approach. *Rehabilitation Psychology, 50*(2), 183. https://doi.org/10.1037/0090-5550.50.2.183

Edwards, E. (2020). "Post intensive-care syndrome": Why some COVID-19 patients may face problems even after recovery. NBC News. March 28, 2020. https://www.nbcnews.com/health/health-news/post-intensive-care-syndrome-why-some-covid-19-patients-may-n1166611

Efimova, O., Salakhova, V., Mikhaylova, I., Gnedova, S., Chertushkina, T., & Agadzhanova, E. (2015). Theoretical Review of Scientific Approaches to Understanding Crisis Psychology. *Mediterranean Journal of Social Sciences, Mediterranean Journal of Social Sciences, 6*(2), 241–249. doi:10.5901/mjss.2015.v6n2s3p241

Elisseou, S., Puranam, S., & Nandi, M. (2019). A novel, trauma-informed physical examination curriculum for first-year medical students. *MedEdPORTAL, 15*(1), 10799. https://doi.org/10.15766/mep_2374-8265.10799

Ely, E. W. (2017). The ABCDEF bundle: Science and philosophy of how ICU liberation serves patients and families. *Critical Care Medicine, 45*(2), 321. https://doi.org/10.1097/CCM.0000000000002175

Ervin, J. N., Kahn, J. M., Cohen, T. R., & Weingart, L. R. (2018). Teamwork in the intensive care unit. *American Psychologist, 73*(4), 468–477. https://doi.org/10.1037/amp0000247

Esper, A., & Martin, G. (2011). The impact of comorbid conditions on critical illness. *Critical Care Medicine, 39*(12), 2728–2735. http://dx.doi.org/10.1097/CCM.0b013e318236f27e

Faculty of Intensive Care Medicine (2019). *Guidelines for the Provision of Intensive Care Services (GPICS)* (2nd ed.). https://www.ficm.ac.uk/sites/default/files/gpics-v2.pdf

Harris, M. E., & Fallot, R. D. (2001). *Using trauma theory to design service systems*. Jossey-Bass/Wiley.

Felitti, V. J., Anda, R. F., Nordenberg, D., Williamson, D. F., Spitz, A. M., Edwards, V., . . . Marks, J. S. (1998). Relationship of childhood abuse and household dysfunction to many of the leading causes of death in adults: The Adverse Childhood Experiences (ACE) study. *American Journal of Preventive Medicine, 14*(4), 245–258. http://dx.doi.org/10.1016/S0749-3797(98)00017-8

Ferguson, N., Laydon, D., Nedjati Gilani, G., Imai, N., Ainslie, K., Baguelin, M., Bhatia, S., Boonyasiri, A., Cucunuba Perez, Z., Cuomo-Dannenburg, G., Dighe, A., Dorigatti, I., Fu, H., Gaythorpe, K., Green, W., Hamlet, A., Hinsley, W., Okell, L., Van Elsland, S., . . . Ghani, A. (2020). Impact of non-pharmaceutical interventions (NPIs) to reduce COVID19 mortality and healthcare demand. Imperial College COVID-19 Response Team. https://doi.org/10.25561/77482

Flaherty, E. G., Thompson, R., Dubowitz, H., Harvey, E. M., English, D. J., Proctor, L. J., & Runyan, D. K. (2013). Adverse childhood experiences and child health in early adolescence. *JAMA Pediatrics, 167*(7), 622–629. http://dx.doi.org/10.1001/jamapediatrics.2013.22

Fleishman, J., Kamsky, H., & Sundborg, S. (May 31, 2019). Trauma-Informed Nursing Practice. *OJIN: The Online Journal of Issues in Nursing, 24*(2). doi:10.3912/OJIN.Vol24No02Man03.

Freeman Williamson, L., & Kautz, D. (2016). Trauma-informed care is the best clinical practice in rehabilitation nursing. *Rehabilitation Nursing, 43*(2), 73–80. https://doi.org/10.1002/rnj.311

Gans, J. S. (1983). Hate in the rehabilitation setting. *Archives of Physical Medicine and Rehabilitation, 64*(4), 176–179.

Gerhart, K. A., & Corbet, B. (1995). Uninformed consent: Biased decision making following spinal cord injury. *HEC Forum, 7*, 110–121. https://doi.org/10.1007/BF01439238

Germain, A., Buysse, D., & Nofzinger, E. (2008). Sleep-specific mechanisms underlying post-traumatic stress disorder: Integrative review and neurobiological hypotheses. *Sleep Medicine Reviews, 12*(3), 185–195. https://doi.org/10.1016/j.smrv.2007.09.003

Gilbert, L., Breiding, M., Merrick, M., Thompson, W., Ford, D., Dhingra, S., & Parks, S. (2015). Childhood adversity and adult chronic disease: An update from ten states and the District of Columbia, 2010. *American Journal of Preventive Medicine, 48*(3), 345–349. https://doi.org/10.1111/10.1016/j.amepre.2014.09.006

Goldman, M. L., Shah, R. N., & Bernstein, C. A. (2017). Depression and suicide among physician trainees: Recommendations for a national response. *JAMA Psychiatry, 72*(5), 411–412. https://doi.org/10.1001/jamapsychiatry.2014.3050

Green, B. L., Saunders, P. A., Power, E., Dass-Brailsford, P., Schelbert, K. B., Giller, E., . . . Mete, M. (2015). Trauma-informed medical care: CME communication training for primary care providers. *Family medicine, 47*(1), 7–14.

Green, B., Kaltman, S., Chung, J., Holt, M., Jackson, S., & Dozier, M. (2012). Attachment and health care relationships in low-income women with trauma histories: A qualitative study. *Journal of Trauma & Dissociation: Trauma, Attachment, and Intimate Relationships, 13*(2), 190–208. https://doi.org/10.1080/15299732.2012.642761

Green, J. G., McLaughlin, K. A., Berglund, P. A., Gruber, M. J., Sampson, N. A., Zaslavsky, A. M., & Kessler, R. C. (2010). Childhood adversities and adult psychiatric disorders in the national comorbidity survey replication I: Associations with first onset of DSM-IV disorders. *Archives of General Psychiatry, 67*(2), 113–123.

Gruman, J. C., & Sloan, R. P. (1983). Disease as justice: Perceptions of the victims of physical illness. *Basic and Applied Social Psychology, 4*(1), 39–46. https://doi.org/10.1207/s15324834basp0401_4

Guastelli, L. R., Silva, A. L. M., Neto, A. M., Araújo, C. M. P., Blaya, R. P., Camargo, A. L. L., & Silva, E. (2011). Integral patient care: Mental health in a critical patient service. *Critical Care, 15*(2), P47. https://doi.org/10.1186/cc10195

Guenther, R. (March 16, 2020). Personal communication.

Guinn, A. S., Ports, K. A., Ford, D. C., Breiding, M., & Merrick, M. T. (2019). Associations between adverse childhood experiences and acquired brain injury, including traumatic brain injuries: 2014 BRFSS North Carolina. *Injury Prevention, 25*(6), 514–520. https://doi.org/10.1136/injuryprev-2018-042927

Gunnar, M., & Quevedo, K. (2007). The neurobiology of stress and development. *Annual Review of Psychology, 58*, 145–173. https://doi.org/10.1146/annurev.psych.58.110405.085605

Hackett, T., Cassem, N., & Wishnie, H. (1968). The coronary-care unit: An appraisal of its psychologic hazards. *New England Journal of Medicine, 279*(25), 1365–1370. https://doi.org/10.1056/NEJM196812192792504

Heilmann, C., Kuijpers, N., Beyersdorf, F., Berchtold-Herz, M., Trummer, G., Stroh, A. L., . . . Fritzsche, K. (2011). Supportive psychotherapy for patients with heart transplantation or ventricular assist devices. *European Journal of Cardio-Thoracic Surgery, 39*(4), e44–e50. https://doi.org/10.1016/j.ejcts.2010.11.074

Heunks, L., & Van Der Hoeven, J. (2010). Clinical review: The ABC of weaning failure—a structured approach. *Critical Care, 14*(6), 245. https://doi.org/10.1186/cc9296

Highfield, J., Beadman, M., & Wade, D. (2020). Psychology: Person-centered care a key to successful recovery. In C. Boulanger & D. McWilliams (Eds.), *Passport to successful ICU discharge* (pp. 135–154). Springer.

Hobfoll, S. E., Watson, P. J., Bell, C. C., & Bryant, R. (2007). Five essential elements of immediate and mid-term mass trauma intervention: Empirical evidence. *Psychiatry, 70*(4), 283. https://doi.org/10.1521/psyc.2007.70.4.283

Hofhuis, J. G., Spronk, P. E., van Stel, H. F., Schrijvers, A. J., Rommes, J. H., & Bakker, J. (2008). Experiences of critically ill patients in the ICU. *Intensive and Critical Care Nursing, 24*(5), 300–313. http://dx.doi.org/10.1016/j.iccn.2008.03.004

Hofhuis, J. G., van Stel, H. F., Schrijvers, A. J., Rommes, J. H., & Spronk, P. E. (2011). Changes of health-related quality of life in critically ill octogenarians: A follow-up study. *Chest, 140*(6), 1473–1483.

Hopper, K., Fried, T., & Pisani, M. (2015). Health care worker attitudes and identified barriers to patient sleep in the medical intensive care unit. *Heart and Lung, 44*(2), 95–99. https://doi.org/10.1016/j.hrtlng.2015.01.011

Hopkins, R. O., Wade, D., & Jackson, J. C. (2017). What's new in cognitive function in ICU survivors. *Intensive Care Medicine, 43*(2), 223–225. https://doi.org/10.1007/s00134-016-4550-x

Hosey, M. M., Ali, M. K., Mantheiy, E. C., Albert, K., Wegener, S. T., & Needham, D. M. (2019). Psychology consultation patterns in a medical intensive care unit: A brief report. *Rehabilitation Psychology, 64*(3), 360. https://doi.org/10.1037/rep0000264

Hunter, A., Johnson, L., & Coustasse, A. (2014). Reduction of intensive care unit length of stay: The case of early mobilization. *Health Care Manager, 33*(2), 128–135. https://doi.org/10.1097/HCM.0000000000000006

Inoue, S., Hatakeyama, J., Kondo, Y., Hifumi, T., Sakuramoto, H., Kawasaki, T., . . . Kenmotsu, Y. (2019). Post-intensive care syndrome: Its pathophysiology, prevention, and future directions. *Acute Medicine & Surgery, 6*(3), 233–246. https://doi.org/10.1002/ams2.415

Jackson, J. C., Jutte, J. E., Hunter, C. H., Ciccolella, N., Warrington, H., Sevin, C., & Bienvenu, O. J. (2016). Posttraumatic Stress Disorder (PTSD) after critical illness: A conceptual review of distinct clinical issues and their implications. *Rehabilitation Psychology, 61*, 132–140. http://dx.doi.org/10.1037/rep0000085

Jackson, J. C., Santoro, M. J., Ely, T. M., Boehm, L., Kiehl, A. L., Anderson, L. S., & Ely, E. W. (2014). Improving patient care through the prism of psychology: Application of Maslow's hierarchy to sedation, delirium, and early mobility in the intensive care unit. *Journal of Critical Care, 29*(3), 438–444. https://doi.org/10.1016/j.jcrc.2014.01.009

Jacobson, G. F. (1980). Crisis theory. *New Directions for Mental Health Services, 1980*(6), 1–10.

Janoff-Bulman, R., & McPherson Frantz, C. (1997). The impact of trauma on meaning: From meaningless world to meaningful life. In M. J. Power & C. R. Brewin (Eds.), *The transformation of meaning in psychological therapies: Integrating theory and practice* (pp. 91–106). John Wiley & Sons Inc.

Johnson-Coyle, L., Opgenorth, D., Bellows, M., Dhaliwal, J., Richardson-Carr, S., & Bagshaw, S. M. (2016). Moral distress and burnout among cardiovascular surgery intensive care unit healthcare professionals: A prospective cross-sectional survey. *Canadian Journal of Critical Care Nursing, 27*(4), 27–36.

Kalfon, P., Alessandrini, M., Boucekine, M., Renoult, S., Geantot, M. A., Deparis-Dusautois, S., . . . Julien, A. (2019). Tailored multicomponent program for discomfort reduction in critically ill patients may decrease post-traumatic stress disorder in general ICU survivors at 1 year. *Intensive Care Medicine, 45*(2), 223–235. https://doi.org/10.1007/s00134-018-05511-y

Kang, L., Li, Y., Hu, S., Chen, M., Yang, C., Yang, B. X., . . . Liu, Z. (2020). The mental health of medical workers in Wuhan, China dealing with the 2019 novel coronavirus. *Lancet Psychiatry, 7*(3), e14. https://doi.org/10.1016/S2215-0366(20)30047-X

Kanter, J. W., Cautilli, J. D., Busch, A. M., & Baruch, D. E. (2005). Toward a comprehensive functional analysis of depressive behavior: Five environmental factors and a possible sixth and seventh. *Behavior Analyst Today, 6*(1), 65. https://doi.org/10.1037/h0100920

Kantor, E. M., & Beckert, D. R. (2011). Psychological first aid. In F. J. Stoddard, A. Pandya, & C. L. Katz (Eds.), *Disaster psychiatry: Readiness, evaluation, and treatment* (pp. 203–212). American Psychiatric Publishing, Inc.

Kartha, A., Brower, V., Saitz, R., Samet, J., Keane, T., & Liebschutz, J. (2008). The impact of trauma exposure and post-traumatic stress disorder on healthcare utilization among primary care patients. *Medical Care, 46*(4), 388–393. https://doi.org/10.1097/mlr.0b013e31815dc5d2

Keany, K. C., & Glueckauf, R. L. (1993). Disability and value change: An overview and reanalysis of acceptance of loss theory. *Rehabilitation Psychology, 38*(3), 199. https://doi.org/10.1037/h0080297

Kearney, M. K., Weininger, R. B., Vachon, M. L., Harrison, R. L., & Mount, B. M. (2009). Self-care of physicians caring for patients at the end of life: Being connected . . . a key to my survival. *Journal of the American Medical Association, 301*(11), 1155–1164. https://doi.org/10.1001/jama.2009.352

Khan, S. H., Lindroth, H., Perkins, A. J., Jamil, Y., Wang, S., Roberts, S., Farber, M., Rahman, O., Gao, S., Marcantonio, E. R., Boustani, M., Machado, R., & Khan, B. A. (2020). Delirium incidence, duration and severity in critically ill patients with COVID-19. medRXiv. https://doi.org/10.1101/2020.05.31.20118679

Kisely, S., Warren, N., McMahon, L., Dalais, C., Henry, I., & Siskind, D. (2020). Occurrence, prevention, and management of the psychological effects of emerging virus outbreaks on health-care workers: Rapid review and meta-analysis. *British Medical Journal, 369*, M1642. https://doi.org/10.1136/bmj.m1642

Koball, A. M., Rasmussen, C., Olson-Dorff, D., Klevan, J., Ramirez, L., & Domoff, S. E. (2019). The relationship between adverse childhood experiences, healthcare utilization, cost of care and medical comorbidities. *Child Abuse & Neglect, 90*, 120–126. https://doi.org/10.1016/j.chiabu.2019.01.021

Kohlenberg, R. J., & Tsai, M. (1991). *Functional analytic psychotherapy: Creating intense and curative therapeutic relationships.* Springer Science & Business Media.

Korupolu, R., Francisco, G. E., Levin, H., & Needham, D. M. (2020). Rehabilitation of critically ill COVID-19 survivors. *Journal of the International Society of Physical and Rehabilitation Medicine, 3*(2), 45–52. https://doi.org/10.4103/jisprm.jisprm_8_20

Kotfis, K., Roberson, S. W., Wilson, J. E., Dabrowski, B. T., & Ely, E. W. (2020). COVID-19: ICU delirium management during SARS-CoV-2 pandemic. *Critical Care, 24*, 176, https://doi.org/10.1186/s13054-020-02882-x

LaHue, S. C., James, T. C., Newman, J. C., Esmaili, A. M., Ormseth, C. H., & Ely, E. W. (2020). Collaborative delirium prevention in the age of COVID-19. *Journal of the American Geriatrics Society, 68*(5), 947. https://doi.org/10.1111/jgs.16480

Lai, J., Ma, S., Wang, Y., Cai, Z., Hu, J., Wei, N., . . . Tan, H. (2020). Factors associated with mental health outcomes among health care workers exposed to coronavirus disease

2019. *JAMA Network Open Psychiatry, 3*(3), e203976–e203976. https://doi.org/10.1016/S2215-0366(20)30047-X

Lequerica, A. H., & Kortte, K. (2010). Therapeutic engagement: A proposed model of engagement in medical rehabilitation. *American Journal of Physical Medicine & Rehabilitation, 89*(5), 415–422. https://doi.org/10.1097/PHM.0b013e3181d8ceb2

Levinson, W., Lesser, C. S., & Epstein, R. M. (2010). Developing physician communication skills for patient-centered care. *Health Affairs, 29*(7), 1310–1318. https://doi.org/10.1377/hlthaff.2009.0450

Leyens, J. P. (2014). Humanity forever in medical dehumanization. In P. G. Bain, J. Vaes, & J. P. Leyens (Eds.), *Humanness and dehumanization* (pp. 175–193). Psychology Press.

Lilly, C., Cucchi, E., Marshall, N., & Katz, A. (2019). Battling intensivists' burnout: A role for workload management. *Chest, 156*(5), 1001–1007. https://doi.org/10.1016/j.chest.2019.04.103

Lykkegaard, K., & Delmar, C. (2013). A threat to the understanding of oneself: Intensive care patients' experiences of dependency. *International Journal of Qualitative Studies on Health and Well-being, 8*(1), 20934. https://doi.org/10.3402/qhw.v8i0.20934

Macciocchi, S. N., & Eaton, B. (1995). Decision and attribution bias in neurorehabilitation. *Archives of Physical Medicine and Rehabilitation, 76*, 521–524. http://dx.doi.org/10.1016/S0003-9993(95)80505-2

Machtinger, E. L., Cuca, Y. P., Khanna, N., Rose, C. D., & Kimberg, L. S. (2015). From treatment to healing: The promise of trauma-informed primary care. *Women's Health Issues, 25*(3), 193–197. https://doi.org/10.1016/j.whi.2015.03.008

Magen, E., & DeLisser, H. M. (2017). Best practices in relational skills training for medical trainees and providers: An essential element of addressing adverse childhood experiences and promoting resilience. *Academic Pediatrics, 17*(7), S102–S107. https://doi.org/10.1016/j.acap.2017.03.006

Marcellus, L., & Cross, S. (2016). Trauma-informed care in the NICU: Implications for early childhood development. *Neonatal Network, 35*(6), 359–366. https://doi.org/10.1891/0730-0832.35.6.359

Marra, A., Buonanno, P., Vargas, M., Iacovazzo, C., Ely, E. W., & Servillo, G. (2020). How COVID-19 pandemic changed our communication with families: Losing nonverbal cues. *Critical Care, 24*(1), 1–2. https://doi.org/10.1186/s13054-020-03035-w

Marsac, M. L., Kassam-Adams, N., Hildenbrand, A. K., Nicholls, E., Winston, F. K., Leff, S. S., & Fein, J. (2016). Implementing a trauma-informed approach in pediatric health care networks. *JAMA Pediatrics, 170*(1), 70–77. https://doi.org/10.1001/jamapediatrics.2015.2206

Maslach, C., & Jackson, S. E. (1986). *Maslach Burnout Inventory: Manual* (2nd ed.). Consulting Psychologists Press.

McCallister, J. W., Gustin, J. L., Wells-Di Gregorio, S., Way, D. P., & Mastronarde, J. G. (2015). Communication skills training curriculum for pulmonary and critical care fellows. *Annals of the American Thoracic Society, 12*(4), 520–525. https://doi.org/10.1513/AnnalsATS.201501-039OC

McCarthy, H. (2011). A modest festschrift and insider perspective on Beatrice Wright's contributions to rehabilitation theory and practice. *Rehabilitation Counseling Bulletin, 54*(2), 67–81. https://doi.org/10.1177/0034355210386971

McEwen, B. S. (2008). Central effects of stress hormones in health and disease: Understanding protective and damaging effects of stress mediators. *European Journal of Pharmacology, 583*, 174–185. https://doi.org/10.1016/j.ejphar.2007.11.071

McIlroy, P. A., King, R. S., Garrouste-Orgeas, M., Tabah, A., & Ramanan, M. (2019). The effect of ICU diaries on psychological outcomes and quality of life of survivors of critical illness and their relatives: A systematic review and meta-analysis. *Critical Care Medicine, 47*(2), 273–279. https://doi.org/10.1097/CCM.0000000000003547

McKibben, J. B., Ekselius, L., Girasek, D. C., Gould, N. F., Holzer III, C., Rosenberg, M., . . . Gielen, A. C. (2009). Epidemiology of burn injuries II: Psychiatric and behavioural perspectives. *International Review of Psychiatry, 21*(6), 512–521. https://doi.org/10.3109/09540260903343794

McPeake, J., & Mikkelsen, M. E. (2018). The evolution of post intensive care syndrome. *Critical Care Medicine, 46*(9), 1551–1552. https://doi.org/10.1097/CCM.0000000000003232

Merbitz, C., Miller, T., & Hansen, N. (2003). Cueing and logical problem solving in brain trauma rehabilitation: Frequency patterns in clinician and patient behaviors. *European Journal of Behavior Analysis, 4*(1–2), 45–57. https://doi.org/10.1080/15021149.2003.11434215

Merbitz, N., Westie, K., Dammeyer, J., Butt, L., & Schneider, J. (2016). After critical care: Challenges in the transition to inpatient rehabilitation. *Rehabilitation Psychology, 61*(2), 186–200. https://doi.org/10.1037/rep0000072

Montgomery, A., Panagopoulou, E., Esmail, A., Richards, T., & Maslach, C. (2019). Burnout in healthcare: The case for organisational change. *British Medical Journal, 366*, L4774. https://doi.org/10.1136/bmj.l4774

Moos, R. H., & Holahan, C. J. (2007). Adaptive tasks and methods of coping with illness and disability. In E. Martz, H. Livneh, & B. Wright (Eds.), *Coping with chronic illness and disability* (pp. 107–126). Springer.

Morandi, A., Pandharipande, P. P., Jackson, J. C., Bellelli, G., Trabucchi, M., & Ely, E. W. (2012). Understanding terminology of delirium and long-term cognitive impairment in critically ill patients. *Best Practice & Research Clinical Anaesthesiology, 26*(3), 267–276. http://dx.doi.org/10.1016/j.bpa.2012.08.001

Moss, M., Good, V. S., Gozal, D., Kleinpell, R., & Sessler, C. N. (2016). An official critical care societies collaborative statement: Burnout syndrome in critical care health care professionals: A call for action. *American Journal of Critical Care, 25*(4), 368–376. https://doi.org/10.4037/ajcc2016133

Mozzoni, M., & Bailey, J. (1996). Improving training methods in brain injury rehabilitation. *Journal of Head Trauma Rehabilitation, 11*(1), 1–17. http://dx.doi.org/10.1097/00001199-199602000-00003

Mullins, L. L. (1989). Hate revisited: Power, envy, and greed in the rehabilitation setting. *Archives of Physical Medicine and Rehabilitation, 70*(10), 740–744.

Needham, D., Davidson, J., Cohen, H., Hopkins, R., Weinert, C., Wunsch, H., . . . Harvey, M. (2012). Improving long-term outcomes after discharge from intensive care unit: Report from a stakeholders' conference. *Critical Care Medicine, 40*(2), 502–509. https://doi.org/10.1097/CCM.0b013e318232da75

Needham, E. J., Chou, S. H. Y., Coles, A. J., & Menon, D. K. (2020). Neurological implications of COVID-19 infections. *Neurocritical Care, 1*(1), 1–5. https://doi.org/10.1007/s12028-020-00978-4

Ng, A. T., & Kantor, E. M. (2010). Psychological first aid. In F. J. Stoddard, Jr., C. Katz, & J. Merlino (Eds.), *Hidden impact: What you need to know for the next disaster: A practical mental health guide for clinicians* (pp. 115–122). Jones & Bartlett Learning.

Nimmo, A., & Huggard, P. (2013). A systematic review of the measurement of compassion fatigue, vicarious trauma, and secondary traumatic stress in physicians. *Australasian Journal of Disaster and Trauma Studies, 2013*(1), 37–44.

O'Donnell, M., Creamer, M., Holmes, A., Ellen, S., Mcfarlane, A., Judson, R., . . . Bryant, R. (2010). Posttraumatic stress disorder after injury: Does admission to intensive care unit increase risk? *Journal of Trauma: Injury, Infection, and Critical Care, 69*(3), 627–632. https://doi.org/10.1097/TA.0b013e3181bc0923

Ozer, M., & Kroll, T. (2002). Patient-centered rehabilitation: Problems and opportunities. *Critical Reviews in Physical and Rehabilitation Medicine, 14*(3–4), 273–289. http://dx.doi.org/10.1615/CritRevPhysRehabilMed.v14.i34.30

Parker, A. M., Sricharoenchai, T., Raparla, S., Schneck, K., Bienvenu, O. J., & Needham, D. M. (2015). Post-traumatic stress disorder in critical illness survivors: A meta-analysis. *Critical Care Medicine, 43*(5), 1121–1129. http://dx.doi.org/10.1097/CCM.0000000000000882

Pastores, S. M., Kvetan, V., Coopersmith, C. M., Farmer, J. C., Sessler, C., Christman, J. W., . . . Kapu, A. N. (2019). Workforce, workload, and burnout among intensivists and advanced practice providers: A narrative review. *Critical Care Medicine, 47*(4), 550–557. https://doi.org/10.1097/CCM.0000000000003637

Patel, M. B., Jackson, J. C., Morandi, A., Girard, T. D., Hughes, C. G., Thompson, J. L., . . . Beckham, J. C. (2016). Incidence and risk factors for intensive care unit-related post-traumatic stress disorder in veterans and civilians. *American Journal of Respiratory and Critical Care Medicine, 193*(12), 1373–1381. http://dx.doi.org/10.1186/cc14635

Peris, A., Bonizzoli, M., Iozzelli, D., Migliaccio, M. L., Zagli, G., Bacchereti, A., . . . Belloni, L. (2011). Early intra-intensive care unit psychological intervention promotes recovery from post traumatic stress disorders, anxiety and depression symptoms in critically ill patients. *Critical Care, 15*(1), R41. http://dx.doi.org/10.1186/cc10003

Peterson, K. A., Zhou, L., & Watzlaf, V. J. (2019). A comprehensive review of quality of life surveys for trauma-affected communities. *Perspectives in Health Information Management, 16*(Winter), 1e–14.

Piers, R. D., Azoulay, E., Ricou, B., Ganz, F. D., Decruyenaere, J., Max, A., . . . Depuydt, P. (2011). Perceptions of appropriateness of care among European and Israeli intensive care unit nurses and physicians. *Journal of the American Medical Association, 306*(24), 2694–2703. http://dx.doi.org/10.1001/jama.2011.1888

Pinto, A., Burnett, S., Benn, J., Brett, S., Parand, A., Iskander, S., & Vincent, C. (2011). Improving reliability of clinical care practices for ventilated patients in the context of a patient safety improvement initiative. *Journal of Evaluation in Clinical Practice, 17*(1), 180–187. https://doi.org/10.1111/j.1365-2753.2010.01419.x

Puntillo, K. A., & McAdam, J. L. (2006). Communication between physicians and nurses as a target for improving end-of-life care in the intensive care unit: Challenges and opportunities for moving forward. *Critical Care Medicine, 34*(11), S332–S340. https://doi.org/10.1097/01.CCM.0000237047.31376.28

Quenot, J. P., Rigaud, J. P., Prin, S., Barbar, S., Pavon, A., Hamet, M., . . . Moutel, G. (2012). Suffering among carers working in critical care can be reduced by an intensive communication strategy on end-of-life practices. *Intensive Care Medicine, 38*(1), 55–61. https://doi.org/10.1007/s00134-011-2413-z

Racine, N., Killam, T., & Madigan, S. (2019). Trauma-informed care as a universal precaution: Beyond the adverse childhood experiences questionnaire. *JAMA Pediatrics, 174*(1), 1–2. http://dx.doi.org/10.1001/jamapediatrics.2019.3866

Raja, S., Hasnain, M., Hoersch, M., Gove-Yin, S., & Rajagopalan, C. (2015). Trauma informed care in medicine: Current knowledge and future research directions. *Family & Community Health, 38*(3), 216–226. https://doi.org/10.1097/FCH.0000000000000071

Remen, R. N. (1996). *Kitchen table wisdom: Stories that heal.* Berkeley Publishing Group/ Penguin Group.

Ratzer, M., Romano, E., & Elklit, A. (2014). Posttraumatic stress disorder in patients following intensive care unit treatment: A review of studies regarding prevalence and risk factors. *Journal of Treatment and Trauma, 3*, 1–15. http://dx.doi.org/10.4172/2167-1222.1000190

Rawal, G., Yadav, S., & Kumar, R. (2017). Post-intensive care syndrome: An overview. *Journal of Translational Internal Medicine, 5*(2), 90–92. http://dx.doi.org/10.1515/jtim-2016-0016

Reade, M. C., & Finfer, S. (2014). Sedation and delirium in the intensive care unit. *New England Journal of Medicine, 370*, 444–454. http://dx.doi.org/10.1056/NEJMra1208705

Reader, T. W., & Cuthbertson, B. H. (2011). Teamwork and team training in the ICU: Where do the similarities with aviation end? *Critical Care, 15*(6), 313. http://dx.doi.org/10.1186/cc10353

Reader, T. W., Flin, R., Mearns, K., & Cuthbertson, B. H. (2009). Developing a team performance framework for the intensive care unit. *Critical Care Medicine, 37*(5), 1787–1793. http:// dx.doi.org/10.1097/CCM.0b013e31819f0451

Redelmeier, D., & Ross, A. (2019). Practicing medicine with colleagues: Pitfalls from social psychology science. *Journal of General Internal Medicine, 34*(4), 624–626. http://dx.doi.org/ 10.1007/s11606-019-04839-5

Righy, C., Rosa, R., Da Silva, R., Kochhann, R., Migliavaca, C., Robinson, C., . . . Falavigna, M. (2019). Prevalence of post-traumatic stress disorder symptoms in adult critical care survivors: A systematic review and meta-analysis. *Critical Care, 23*(1), 213. http://dx.doi.org/ 10.1186/s13054-019-2489-3

Ripp, J., Peccoralo, L., & Charney, D. (2020). Attending to the emotional well-being of the health care workforce in a New York City health system during the COVID-19 pandemic. *Academic Medicine, 95*(8), 1136–1139. https://doi.org/10.1097/ACM.0000000000003414

Roberts, M. B., Glaspey, L. J., Mazzarelli, A., Jones, C. W., Kilgannon, H. J., Trzeciak, S., & Roberts, B. W. (2018). Early interventions for the prevention of posttraumatic stress symptoms in survivors of critical illness: A qualitative systematic review. *Critical Care Medicine, 46*(8), 1328–1333. https://doi.org/10.1097/CCM.0000000000003222

Romero, C. S., Catalá, J., Delgado, C., Ferrer, C., Errando, C., Iftimi, A., . . . Otero, M. (2020). COVID-19 psychological impact in 3109 healthcare workers in Spain: The PSIMCOV group. *Psychological Medicine*, 1–14. https://doi.org/10.1017/S0033291720001671

Rossi, R., Socci, V., Pacitti, F., Di Lorenzo, G., Di Marco, A., Siracusano, A., & Rossi, A. (2020). Mental health outcomes among frontline and second-line health care workers during the coronavirus disease 2019 (COVID-19) pandemic in Italy. *JAMA Network Open, 3*(5), e2010185– e2010185. https://doi.org/10.1001/jamanetworkopen.2020.10185

Rozeboom, N., Parenteau, K., & Carratturo, D. (2012). Rehabilitation starts in the intensive care unit. *Critical Care Nursing Quarterly, 35*(3), 234–240. https://doi.org/10.1097/ CNQ.0b013e3182542d8c

Saakvitne, K., & Pearlman, L. A. (1996). *Transforming the pain: A workbook on vicarious trauma-tization*. W.W. Norton & Company.

Sanders, M. R., & Hall, S. L. (2017). Trauma-informed care in the newborn intensive care unit: Promoting safety, security and connectedness. *Journal of Perinatology, 38*(1), 3–10. https://doi.org/10.1038/jp.2017.124

Sansone, R. A., Bohinc, R. J., & Wiederman, M. W. (2014). A cross-sectional survey of child-hood trauma and compliance with general health care among adult primary care outpatients. *Primary Care Companion for CNS Disorders, 16*(6). https://doi.org/10.4088/PCC.14m01692

Schilling, E., Aseltine, R., & Gore, S. (2007). Adverse childhood experiences and mental health in young adults: A longitudinal survey. *BMC Public Health, 7*, 30. https://doi.org/10.1186/1471-2458-7-30

Schneider, A. M. & Moreira, M. C. (2017). Intensive Care Psychologist: Reflections about Professional Insertion, Professional Qualification and Practice at the Hospital. *Trends in Psychology, 25*(3), 1241–1255. doi:10.9788/TP2017.3-15En

Schore, A. (2005). Back to basics: Attachment, affect regulation, and the developing right brain: Linking developmental neuroscience to pediatrics. *Pediatrics in Review, 26*(6), 204–217. https://doi.org/10.1542/pir.26-6-204

Seaman, J. B., Barnato, A. E., Sereika, S. M., Happ, M. B., & Erlen, J. A. (2017). Patterns of pal-liative care service consultation in a sample of critically ill ICU patients at high risk of dying. *Heart & Lung, 46*(1), 18–23. https://doi.org/10.1016/j.hrtlng.2016.08.008

Shanafelt, T. D., & Noseworthy, J. H. (2017). Executive leadership and physician well-being: Nine organizational strategies to promote engagement and reduce burnout. *Mayo Clinic Proceedings, 92*(1), 129–146. https://doi.org/10.1016/j.mayocp.2016.10.004

Shanafelt, T., Ripp, J., & Trockel, M. (2020). Understanding and addressing sources of anxiety among health care professionals during the COVID-19 pandemic. *Journal of the American Medical Association, 323*(21), 2133–2134. https://doi.org/10.1001/jama.2020.5893

Sharif, A., Hall, E., & Khalid, M. I. (2019). ICU Psychology: What do the frontline providers think? *Critical Care Medicine, 47*(1), 352. https://doi.org/10.1097/01.ccm.0000551496.75464.95

Shaw, M. C., & Halliday, P. H. (1992). The family, crisis and chronic illness: an evolutionary model. *Journal of Advanced Nursing, 17*(5), 537–543.

Sher, Y., Rabkin, B., Maldonado, J. R., & Mohabir, P. (2020). A case report of Covid-19-associated hyperactive ICU delirium with proposed pathophysiology and treatment. *Psychosomatics, 61*(5), 544–550. https://doi.org/10.1016/j.psym.2020.05.007

Shulman, N. M., & Shewbert, A. L. (2005). A model of crisis intervention in critical and intensive care units of general hospitals. In A. R. Roberts (Ed.), *Crisis intervention handbook: Assessment, treatment, and research* (pp. 412–429). Oxford University Press.

Sideris, T. (2019). From post-traumatic stress disorder to absolute dependence in an intensive care unit: Reflections on a clinical account. *Medical Humanities, 45*(1), 37–44. https://doi.org/10.1136/medhum-2017-011435

Sladeczek, I. E., Dumont, F., Martel, C. A., & Karagiannakis, A. (2006). Making sense of client data: Clinical experience and confirmationism revisited. *American Journal of Psychotherapy, 60*(4), 375–391. https://doi.org/10.1176/appi.psychotherapy.2006.60.4.375

Society of Critical Care Medicine (2020). Critical care statistics. https://www.sccm.org/Communications/Critical-Care-Statistics

Sotero, M., Chino, M., Ramona, D. B., Shan, G., & Shen, J. (2015). The effects of adverse childhood experiences on subsequent injury in young adulthood: Findings from the National Longitudinal Study of Adolescent and Adult Health. Digital Scholarship@UNLV. https://digitalscholarship.unlv.edu/thesesdissertations/2432

Spellman, N. T. (1960). Prevention of immobility complications through early rehabilitation. *Rehabilitation, 6,* 7–9.

Sperlich, M., Seng, J., Li, Y., Taylor, J., & Bradbury-Jones, C. (2017). Integrating trauma-informed care into maternity care practice: Conceptual and practical issues. *Journal of Midwifery & Women's Health, 62*(6), 661–672. https://doi.org/10.1111/jmwh.12674

Sprangers, M., Tempelaar, R., Van den Heuvel, W., & M de Haes, H. (2002). Explaining quality of life with crisis theory. *Psycho-Oncology, 11*(5), 419–426.

Stam, H., Stucki, G., & Bickenbach, J. (2020). Covid-19 and post intensive care syndrome: A call for action. *Journal of Rehabilitation Medicine, 52*(4). https://doi.org/10.2340/16501977-2677

Stevenson, J. E., Colantuoni, E., Bienvenu, O. J., Sricharoenchai, T., Wozniak, A., Shanholtz, C., . . . Needham, D. M. (2013). General anxiety symptoms after acute lung injury: Predictors and correlates. *Journal of Psychosomatic Research, 75,* 287–293. https://doi.org/10.1016/j.jpsychores.2013.06.002

Street, H. G. (2008). Self psychology at work in trauma therapy. Unpublished master's thesis, Smith College, Northampton, MA. https://scholarworks.smith.edu/theses/1266

Stucky, K., Jutte, J. E., Warren, A. M., Jackson, J. C., & Merbitz, N. (2016). A survey of psychology practice in critical-care settings. *Rehabilitation Psychology, 61*(2), 201.

Stucky, K., & Warren, A.M. (2019). Rehabilitation psychologists in critical care settings. In L. A. Brenner, S. A. Reid-Arndt, T. R. Elliot, R. G., Frank, & B. Caplan (Eds.), *Handbook of rehabilitation psychology* (3rd ed., pp. 483–496). American Psychological Association.

Substance Abuse and Mental Health Services Administration. (2014). *Concept of trauma and guidance for a trauma-informed approach.* https://samhsa.gov

Tawfik, D. S., Profit, J., Morgenthaler, T. I., Satele, D. V., Sinsky, C. A., Dyrbye, L. N., . . . Shanafelt, T. D. (2018). Physician burnout, well-being, and work unit safety grades in relationship to reported medical errors. *Mayo Clinic Proceedings, 93*(11), 1571–1580. https://doi.org/10.1016/j.mayocp.2018.05.014

Tello, M. (2019). Trauma-informed care: What it is, and why it's important. Harvard Health Blog. https://www.health.harvard.edu/blog/trauma-informed-care-what-it-is-and-why-its-important-2018101613562

Thompson, M., Arias, I., Basile, K., & Desai, S. (2002). The association between childhood physical and sexual victimization and health problems in adulthood in a nationally representative sample of women. *Journal of Interpersonal Violence, 17*(10), 1115–1129. http://dx.doi.org/10.1177/088626002236663

Tingey, J. L., Bentley, J. A., & Hosey, M. M. (2020). COVID-19: Understanding and mitigating trauma in ICU survivors. *Psychological Trauma: Theory, Research, Practice, and Policy, 12*(S1), S100–S104. http://dx.doi.org/10.1037/tra0000884

United Nations. (2020). Policy brief: COVID-19 and the need for action on mental health. https://www.cmhnetwork.org/wp-content/uploads/2020/05/un_policy_brief-covid_and_mental_health_final.pdf

Vaes, J., & Muratore, M. (2013). Defensive dehumanization in the medical practice: A cross-sectional study from a health care worker's perspective. *British Journal of Social Psychology*, *52*(1), 180–190. http://dx.doi.org/10.1111/bjso.12008

Van Mol, M. M., Kompanje, E. J., Benoit, D. D., Bakker, J., & Nijkamp, M. D. (2015). The prevalence of compassion fatigue and burnout among healthcare professionals in intensive care units: A systematic review. *PloS One*, *10*(8), e0136955. https://doi.org/10.4037/ajcc2016133

Vasilevskis, E. E., Ely, E. W., Speroff, T., Pun, B. T., Boehm, L., & Dittus, R. S. (2010). Reducing iatrogenic risks: ICU-acquired delirium and weakness—crossing the quality chasm. *Chest*, *138*(5), 1224–1233. https://doi.org/10.1378/chest.10-0466

Wade, D., Hardy, R., Howell, D., & Mythen, M. (2013). Identifying clinical and acute psychological risk factors for PTSD after critical care: A systematic review. *Minerva Anestesiologica*, *79*(8), 944–963.

Wade, D., & Howell, D. (2016). What can psychologists do in intensive care? *ICU Management & Practice*, *16*(4), 242–244.

Walser, R. D., & Hayes, S. C. (2006). Acceptance and commitment therapy in the treatment of posttraumatic stress disorder: Theoretical and applied issues. In V. M. Follette & J. I. Ruzek (Eds.), *Cognitive-behavioral therapies for trauma* (2nd ed., pp. 146–172). Guilford Press.

Warren, A. M., Stucky, K., & Sherman, J. J. (2014). Rehabilitation psychology's role in the level 1 trauma center. *Journal of Trauma Nursing*, *21*(3), 1357–1362. https://doi.org/10.1097/01586154-201305000-00025

West, C. P., Dyrbye, L. N., Erwin, P. J., & Shanafelt, T. D. (2016). Interventions to prevent and reduce physician burnout: A systematic review and meta-analysis. *Lancet*, *388*(10057), 2272–2281. https://doi.org/10.1017/S0033291720001671

World Health Organization. (2020). Naming the coronavirus disease (COVID-19) and the virus that causes it. https://www.who.int/emergencies/diseases/novel-coronavirus-2019/technical-guidance/naming-the-coronavirus-disease-(covid-2019)-and-the-virus-that-causes-it

Wilcox, M. E., Brummel, N. E., Archer, K., Ely, E. W., Jackson, J. C., & Hopkins, R. O. (2013). Cognitive dysfunction in ICU patients: Risk factors, predictors, and rehabilitation interventions. *Critical Care Medicine*, *41*(9), S81–S98. https://doi.org/10.1097/CCM.0b013e3182a16946

Wilson, M., Beesley, S., Grow, A., Rubin, E., Hopkins, R., Hajizadeh, N., & Brown, S. (2019). Humanizing the intensive care unit. *Critical Care*, *23*(1), 32. http://dx.doi.org/10.1186/s13054-019-2327-7

Wright, B. A. (Ed.). (1959). *Psychology and rehabilitation*. American Psychological Association. https://doi.org/10.1037/10539-000

Young, B. (2006). The immediate response to disaster. Guidelines for adult psychological first aid. In E. C. Ritchie, J. P., Watson, & M. J. Friedman (Eds.), *Interventions following mass violence and disasters: Strategies for mental health practice*. Guilford Press.

Xue, X., Wang, P., Wang, J., Li, X., Peng, F., & Wang, Z. (2020). Preoperative individualized education intervention reduces delirium after cardiac surgery: A randomized controlled study. *Journal of Thoracic Disease*, *12*(5), 2188. https://doi.org/10.21037/jtd.2020.04.26

5 Psychological Morbidity After Critical Illness
O. Joseph Bienvenu and Megan M. Hosey

Stresses of critical illness and intensive care: a rationale for prevention

Patients with critical illnesses receiving intensive care face a number of severe psychic and physical stressors, including dyspnea, endotracheal intubation and other invasive procedures, systemic inflammation, hypothalamic–pituitary–adrenal axis strain, endogenous and exogenous catecholamine surges, delirium, a reduced ability to communicate, and restricted autonomy. Cognitive impairment, anxiety, and depressive symptoms are evident in over half of patients within 96 hours of discharge from the intensive care unit (ICU; Karnatovskaia et al., 2019). In addition, survivors often must deal with long-term cognitive and physical impairments (Herridge et al., 2003, 2011; Needham et al., 2012) as well as negative impacts on family, finances, and other factors (Cheung et al., 2006; Unroe et al., 2010). These potential stressors appear to increase the risk of psychiatric disturbances substantially.

This chapter describes the substantial burden of and risk factors for distress-related psychiatric morbidity in patients who survive critical illnesses. This knowledge serves as the motivation to develop new approaches that can ameliorate or even prevent long-term distress in survivors. Therefore, the chapter also contains information about early attempts to reduce, prevent, and manage long-term psychological morbidity.

O. Joseph Bienvenu and Megan M. Hosey, *Psychological Morbidity After Critical Illness* In: *Critical Care Psychology and Rehabilitation*. Edited by: Kirk J. Stucky and Jennifer E. Jutte, Oxford University Press. © Oxford University Press 2022. DOI: 10.1093/oso/9780190077013.003.0005

Long-term distress-related psychological morbidity after critical illness

POSTTRAUMATIC STRESS PHENOMENA

Posttraumatic stress disorder (PTSD) and related symptoms are perhaps the most vivid psychological distress phenomena experienced by survivors of critical illness. Survivors often have intrusive memories and nightmares related to their critical illness and ICU experiences, including fearing they will die, experiencing noxious physical stimuli like deep suctioning of endotracheal tubes, and having frightening hallucinations and paranoid delusional thoughts (e.g., that staff are trying to kill them). Many critical illness survivors try to avoid hospitals, germs, or television shows involving medical care—anything that could increase the risk of or remind them of being critically ill (Jackson et al., 2016).

Several narrative and systematic reviews have addressed PTSD phenomena in critical illness survivors (Davydow, Desai, et al., 2008; Davydow, Gifford, et al., 2008; Griffiths et al., 2007; Jackson et al., 2007; Wade et al., 2013), including recent meta-analyses (Parker et al., 2015; Righy et al., 2019). Though the prevalence of substantial PTSD symptoms or PTSD diagnoses varies by setting and assessment method, it appears that approximately 20% of critical illness survivors are affected (Davydow, Gifford, et al., 2008; Parker et al., 2015; Righy et al., 2019), higher than the 12% prevalence in survivors of acute coronary syndromes (Edmondson et al., 2012). However, patients who survive acute respiratory distress syndrome (ARDS) and/or septic shock may have higher prevalence rates (Bienvenu, Gellar, et al., 2013; Davydow, Desai, et al., 2008; Davydow, Gifford, et al., 2008; Griffiths et al., 2007). PTSD phenomena are associated with worse quality of life and, in one study, with a need for more frequent medical rehospitalizations (Davydow, Desai, et al., 2008; Davydow, Gifford, et al., 2008; Davydow et al., 2014; Parker et al., 2015).

To some extent, risk factors for PTSD in critical illness survivors overlap with risk factors for PTSD in other settings (Brewin et al., 2000). For example, patients with a history of anxiety, depression, or other mental health issues are at increased risk for PTSD given critical illness and intensive care, and certain personality traits (e.g., pessimism) likely also increase risk (Bienvenu, Gellar, et al., 2013; Davydow, Gifford, et al., 2008; Myhren et al., 2010; Parker et al., 2015). Less education may also be a risk factor (Davydow, Gifford, et al., 2008; Parker et al., 2015).

Interestingly, severity of critical illness is not associated with PTSD in survivors (Davydow, Gifford, et al., 2008; Parker et al., 2015). Neither is ICU length of stay (Davydow, Gifford, et al., 2008; Parker et al., 2015), except perhaps in ARDS survivors, for whom results are inconsistent (Bienvenu, Gellar, et al., 2013; Davydow, Desai, et al., 2008; Huang et al., 2016; Kapfhammer et al., 2004). The reason for this lack of relation with severity is unclear, though it is important to recognize that all of the patients in these studies were critically ill (i.e., clinicians judged the patients to need intensive care). Thus, all had a high level of medical stress.

The relations between in-ICU delirium and subsequent PTSD symptoms deserve special attention. Perhaps surprisingly, the duration of delirium in the ICU has not been associated with later PTSD symptoms in most studies that have explored this issue (Bienvenu, Gellar, et al., 2013; Girard et al., 2007; Jackson et al., 2010, 2014; Patel et al., 2016; Wolters et al., 2016), with two exceptions (Bashar et al., 2018; Denke et al., 2018). It is understandable that most investigators have employed duration of delirium as a potential risk factor, since delirium is so common in critically ill patients. That is, an investigator should be concerned about both statistical power and generalizability if addressing whether the presence of in-ICU delirium is associated with PTSD. In one study of this topic, the presence of in-ICU delirium was associated with later PTSD symptoms (Warlan et al., 2016). Further, in a study investigating the relations between delirium and PTSD symptoms in a broader sample of hospitalized patients, Grover and colleagues (2019) noted that both severity of delirium and particular delirium symptoms (e.g., motor agitation) were associated with later PTSD symptoms. In addition, several indirect lines of evidence suggest that something about in-ICU delirium increases risk for PTSD phenomena in survivors:

1. Agitation and need for physical restraint (markers of hyperactive delirium) are associated with later PTSD symptoms (Jones et al., 2007).
2. High doses of benzodiazepines and opioids, which increase the risk of delirium, are associated with later PTSD symptoms (Bienvenu, Gellar, et al., 2013; Davydow, Gifford, et al., 2008; Girard et al., 2007; Jones et al., 2007; Parker et al., 2015; Wade et al., 2012).
3. Early post-ICU memories of nightmarish psychotic experiences (e.g., frightening, vivid visual hallucinations and delusions of being imprisoned, tortured, sexually assaulted, etc.—evidence of having been delirious without prior psychosis) are associated with later PTSD symptoms (Davydow, Gifford, et al., 2008; Jones et al., 2001, 2003, 2007, 2010; Parker et al., 2015; Rattray et al., 2004, 2005; Weinert & Sprenkle, 2008). It is notable that a need for higher in-ICU sedative doses and later memories of frightening psychotic experiences appear to be more common in patients with pre–critical illness histories of anxiety and depression (Jones et al., 2007); thus, causal relations are not straightforward.

Notably, psychological distress early in the recovery period is a powerful predictor of later PTSD symptoms (Rattray et al., 2005; Samuelson et al., 2007). In fact, to identify those at highest risk for long-term distress, it may be as useful to assess in-ICU or early post-ICU psychiatric morbidity as it is to determine pre–critical illness psychiatric history (Milton et al., 2018).

MEASUREMENT OF PTSD PHENOMENA IN CRITICAL ILLNESS SURVIVORS

Most studies of critical illness survivors have employed questionnaire measures with thresholds for clinically significant PTSD symptoms. That is, most studies have not employed clinicians to perform structured or semistructured psychiatric interviews with the patients. It is reasonable to ask: How well do questionnaires perform versus more rigorous diagnostic assessments?

The first clinical psychometric validation study of a PTSD assessment tool in critical illness survivors compared results of a modified version of the Post-Traumatic Stress Syndrome 10-Questions Inventory (PTSS-10) (Weisaeth, 1989a, 1989b, 1993) to psychiatrists' diagnoses of PTSD using the Structured Clinical Interview for DSM-IV (SCID-IV) (First et al., 1996) in survivors of ARDS (Stoll et al., 1999). The authors modified the PTSS-10 in two ways. First, in Part A, they added questions regarding memories of the patient's time in the ICU, specifically nightmares, severe anxiety or panic, severe pain, and shortness of breath or feelings of suffocation. Part B of the modified instrument resembles the original version of the PTSS-10, covering sleep disturbance, nightmares, depression, hyperalertness, emotional and social withdrawal (emotional numbing and inability to care for others), irritability, moodiness, guilt, avoidance of reminders of the trauma, and muscle tension. The authors changed the wording of the ninth item to be more directly relevant to a patient's ICU experience ("fear of places and situations which remind me of the intensive care unit"). Patients rate each of the 10 items on a 7-point scale reflecting symptom frequency; the potential total score ranges from 10 to 70. As the authors noted, the original PTSS-10 was based on an earlier conception of PTSD (Schelling & Kapfhammer, 2013), and some items are less relevant to a more modern conception of PTSD (e.g., depressed mood, muscle tension) (Bienvenu, Williams, et al., 2013). Nevertheless, this modified form of the PTSS-10 performed well psychometrically, with high internal consistency (Cronbach's $\alpha = 0.89$), test–retest reliability (intraclass correlation coefficient $\alpha = 0.89$), and construct validity (a monotonic relation between the number of Part A "traumatic memories" and Part B scores, Spearman's $\rho = 0.48$). In addition, the authors demonstrated high criterion validity of the Part B score versus psychiatrists' diagnoses of DSM-IV PTSD, with a sensitivity of 0.77 and specificity of 0.98 at a threshold of 35. (Table 5.1 may be helpful as a reminder of some psychometric terms.)

TABLE 5.1.

Measurement terms and their meanings

Sensitivity	The ability of a screening test to correctly classify a person with a condition as affected. It has values between 0 and 1, with higher values indicating greater sensitivity.
Specificity	The ability of a screening test to correctly classify a person without a condition as unaffected. It has values between 0 and 1, with higher values indicating greater specificity.
Receiver operating characteristic (ROC) curve	An ROC analysis plots screening test scores against sensitivity and specificity values.
Area under the ROC curve (AUC)	A measure of classification performance across screening test scores. It has values between 0 and 1, with higher values indicating greater screening tool performance

Later, Twigg and colleagues (2008) expanded the PTSS-10 to create the PTSS-14, since the PTSS-10 focused mostly on hyperarousal symptoms (five items) with only one item addressing re-experiencing or intrusion phenomena (i.e., nightmares) and one item addressing avoidance and numbing (withdrawal from others). The PTSS-14 adds another intrusion item ("Upsetting, unwanted thoughts or images of my time on the intensive care unit"), as well as an additional avoidance item ("Avoid places, people or situations that remind me of the intensive care unit") and two "numbness" items ("Feeling numb [e.g., cannot cry, unable to have loving feelings]" and "Feeling as if my plans or dreams of the future will not come true"). Patients rate each of the 14 items on a 7-point scale, reflecting symptom frequency; the potential total score ranges from 14 to 98. The authors validated the PTSS-14 against a previously validated diagnostic questionnaire, the Posttraumatic Stress Diagnostic Scale (PDS) (Foa, 1995). The authors reported high internal consistency (α ranged between 0.84 and 0.89), high test–retest reliability (intraclass correlation coefficient as high as 0.90), high concurrent validity (Pearson's r as high as 0.86 with the PDS symptom severity score and as high as 0.71 with the Impact of Event Scale [IES] total score), and high predictive validity (Pearson's r as high as 0.85 with the PDS symptom severity score and as high as 0.71 with the IES total score). A receiver operating characteristic (ROC) analysis indicated very good sensitivity (as high as 0.86) and specificity (as high as 0.97) at a threshold of 45. The area under the ROC curve (AUC) ranged from 0.82 to 0.95. (Table 5.1 may be helpful to readers unfamiliar with the terms ROC and AUC.)

Bienvenu and colleagues (2013) validated the revised version of the IES, the IES-R (Weiss & Marmar, 1997), against the DSM-IV version of the "gold standard" structured clinical interview for PTSD, the Clinician-Administered PTSD Scale (CAPS) (Blake et al., 1995), in ARDS survivors. The IES-R is a 22-item questionnaire; patients rate each item on a 5-point severity scale. The developers recommend using a mean score for either the total score or for subscales (in either case, the potential mean score range is between 0 and 4). The internal consistency of the IES-R was high in the study ($\alpha = 0.96$). The IES-R total score and the CAPS total severity score were strongly correlated (Pearson's $r = 0.80$). Using CAPS data, 13% of the survivors had PTSD at the time of assessment, and 27% had at least partial PTSD. In a ROC analysis with CAPS PTSD or partial PTSD as criterion variables, the AUC ranged from 0.95 to 0.97. At an IES-R threshold (total mean score) of 1.6, with the same criterion variables, sensitivities ranged from 0.80 to 1.0, specificities from 0.85 to 0.91, positive predictive values from 0.50 to 0.75, negative predictive values from 0.93 to 1.0, positive likelihood ratios from 6.5 to 9.0, negative likelihood ratios from 0.0 to 0.2, and efficiencies from 0.87 to 0.90. A minimal (clinically) important difference for the IES-R is 0.2 points (Chan et al., 2016). Notably, the IES-R is recommended as a core outcome measure for clinical research in acute respiratory failure survivors (Needham et al., 2017).

Recently, Hosey and colleagues (2019) assessed an abbreviated form of the IES-R, the IES-6, in more than 1,000 ARDS survivors. The IES-6 had high internal consistency ($\alpha = 0.86$ to 0.91), convergent validity with anxiety and depression measures ($r = 0.32$ to 0.52), and criterion validity versus the DSM-IV version of the CAPS in a subsample (AUC = 0.95; at a threshold of 1.75, the sensitivity and specificity were 0.88 and 0.85, respectively).

It is important to note that none of the above studies included a DSM-5 criterion measure. Nevertheless, the PTSS-14 and IES-R are reasonable tools, aimed at the same core PTSD construct (Bienvenu et al., 2013).

DEPRESSIVE PHENOMENA

Depressive phenomena have also received substantial attention in the critical illness outcomes literature; depressive mood states are relatively common in survivors (Bienvenu & Jones, 2017; Davydow et al., 2009; Rabiee et al., 2016). Loss of energy, poor concentration, and sleep difficulties are particularly common in this population, but many patients also report low mood and anhedonia (loss of interest and pleasure) (Bienvenu & Jones, 2017).

Though the prevalence of depressive symptoms or depression-related diagnoses varies by setting and assessment method, it appears that about 30% of critical illness survivors are affected (Bienvenu & Jones, 2017; Davydow et al., 2009; Rabiee et al., 2016); this is comparable to the prevalence of depression in patients with cardiac disease (Huffman et al., 2013). Depressive phenomena in critical illness survivors are associated with worse quality of life, impaired physical function, and increased risk for mortality (Bienvenu et al., 2012; Bienvenu & Jones, 2017; Davydow et al., 2009; Hatch et al., 2018).

Risk factors for depressed mood in critical illness survivors overlap, to some extent, with risk factors for depression in other settings. For example, patients with a history of depression or other mental health issues are at increased risk for depressive mood states following critical illness and intensive care (Bienvenu & Jones, 2017; Davydow et al., 2009; Hopkins et al., 2010; Rabiee et al., 2016). In addition, women, the less educated, and the underemployed may be at increased risk (Bienvenu et al., 2012; Bienvenu & Jones, 2017; Davydow et al., 2009; Hopkins et al., 2010).

As with PTSD, severity of critical illness is not associated with later depressive symptoms in survivors, and neither is ICU length of stay (Bienvenu & Jones, 2017; Davydow et al., 2009; Rabiee et al., 2016). Though studied less frequently than in PTSD, early memories of nightmares, hallucinations, and persecutory delusions have been associated with later depressive phenomena in survivors (Bienvenu & Jones, 2017; Rabiee et al., 2016).

Also, like PTSD, psychological distress early in the recovery period is a powerful predictor of later depressive symptoms, and depressive phenomena tend to co-occur with other psychiatric distress phenomena (Bienvenu et al., 2015; Bienvenu & Jones, 2017; Davydow et al., 2009; Rabiee et al., 2016; Rattray et al., 2005; Samuelson et al., 2007). Comorbidity is associated with both reduced quality of life and psychiatric treatment seeking (Bienvenu et al., 2015; Wang et al., 2017).

GENERAL OR NONSPECIFIC ANXIETY PHENOMENA

Our Johns Hopkins group conducted a systematic review and meta-analysis of general or nonspecific anxiety phenomena in critical illness survivors (Nikayin et al., 2016). In 27 eligible unique patient cohorts (total $n = 2,880$), we found that the prevalence of clinically important anxiety symptoms was 32% between 2 and 3 months after the critical illness, 40% at 6 months, and 34% at 12 to 14 months after illness. These prevalences, estimated using the most commonly used anxiety and depression symptom measure in this field, the Hospital Anxiety and Depression Scale (HADS) questionnaire (anxiety subscale) (Turnbull et al., 2016; Zigmond & Snaith, 1983), are substantially higher than the 21% general population prevalence in a representative European sample (Hinz & Brähler, 2011). As with depressive phenomena, anxiety symptoms were more common in patients who had psychiatric distress during the index admission as well as in those who remembered frightening nightmares, persecutory delusions, and hallucinations during the ICU stay (Nikayin et al., 2016; Rattray et al., 2005; Samuelson et al., 2007).

To date, the nature of these general or nonspecific anxiety phenomena remains unclear. For example, we are unsure whether these reflect illness anxiety, posttraumatic stress, or other symptoms.

MEASUREMENT OF ANXIETY AND DEPRESSIVE PHENOMENA IN CRITICAL ILLNESS SURVIVORS

Most psychometric studies of measures of anxiety and depressive phenomena in critical illness survivors have not employed clinical interviews as external validators, perhaps because there are so many categories of clinically relevant anxiety and depressive diagnoses. Nevertheless, there are exceptions. For example, Weinert and Meller (2006) examined the measurement properties of the Center for Epidemiologic Studies Depression Scale (CES-D) (Radloff, 1977) versus DSM-IV diagnoses as ascertained using the SCID-IV. With the CES-D, patients rate each of the 20 items on a 4-point scale reflecting symptom frequency; the potential total score ranges from 0 to 60. The CES-D performed well discriminating major depressive episodes (MDEs, AUC 0.94) and MDEs or depressive disorder not otherwise specified (DD NOS, AUC 0.91). A threshold of 16 seemed optimal to maximize sensitivity and specificity.

As noted previously, the HADS is the most commonly used measure in research in this field (Turnbull et al., 2016). A potential advantage of the HADS is that it emphasizes nonphysical symptoms of anxiety and depression, since it was developed for use in a general hospital setting (Zigmond & Snaith, 1983). In addition, clinical researchers have validated the HADS in numerous general medical and psychiatric populations as a measure of clinically significant anxiety and depression symptoms, consistent with a variety of psychiatric disorders, including adjustment disorders (Bjelland et al., 2002). A threshold of 8 on either subscale appears to maximize sensitivity and specificity (Bjelland et al., 2002). The psychometric structure of the HADS appears as expected in critical illness survivors (Jutte et al., 2015), and the subscales show convergent validity with other measures of mental distress in this population (Jutte et al., 2015; Pfoh et al., 2016). The minimal (clinically) important difference for either subscale is 2 to 2.5 points (Chan et al., 2016).

WHICH CAME FIRST—THE PSYCHIATRIC MORBIDITY OR THE CRITICAL ILLNESS?

Some may wonder whether the immense stress of critical illness and intensive care underlies the development or worsening of mental distress, or whether psychiatric morbidity is simply constant before and after critical illness. Indeed, as noted previously, a pre-illness history of psychiatric morbidity is a risk factor for post–critical illness psychiatric morbidity.

In a particularly large and generalizable study, Wunsch and colleagues (2014) examined linked data from longitudinal medical databases in Denmark. The study included more than 24,000 patients who were critically ill and required mechanical ventilation as well as two matched comparison cohorts—hospitalized patients who were not critically ill and persons in the general population who were not hospitalized during the same period. The results were striking. Briefly, psychiatric diagnoses in the prior 5 years were weakly associated with becoming critically ill compared to simply being hospitalized (prevalence ratio 1.3). In addition, psychiatric diagnoses in the prior 5 years were more common in persons who became critically ill than in the nonhospitalized population (prevalence ratio 2.6). Also, being prescribed a psychiatric medication in the prior 5 years was associated with hospitalization, intensive care or otherwise (prevalence ratio 1.4). However, after a hospitalization, critically ill patients requiring mechanical ventilation were substantially more likely to receive a new psychiatric diagnosis than patients who were hospitalized but did not require intensive care (adjusted hazard ratio 3.4) or persons in the general population who were not hospitalized (hazard ratio 22!). In addition, critically ill patients requiring mechanical ventilation were substantially more likely to be prescribed a psychoactive medication than were hospitalized patients who did not require intensive care (adjusted hazard ratio 2.4) or persons in the general population who were not hospitalized (hazard ratio 21!). To summarize this important study, the authors found that being diagnosed with a psychiatric illness and being prescribed a psychiatric medication were associated with a moderately increased risk for hospitalization. However, being hospitalized, especially with a critical illness, was associated with a markedly increased risk for receiving a new psychiatric diagnosis and/or a prescription for a psychoactive medication. Thus, critical illnesses do lead to new or worsening mental distress beyond that of being ill enough to require hospitalization. Critical illness and intensive care are indeed huge stressors.

THE INTERPLAY OF PHYSICAL PHENOMENA AND PSYCHIATRIC MORBIDITY IN CRITICAL ILLNESS SURVIVORS

As our understanding of psychiatric morbidity associated with medical phenomena increases, the lines between "psychological" and "physical" symptomatology blur. Critical illness survivors report breathlessness, fatigue, pain, sleep disturbance, and body image concerns (Altman et al., 2017; Kemp et al., 2019; Neufeld et al., 2020; Tansey et al., 2007), and these symptoms are highly correlated with psychiatric symptoms. For example, Neufeld and colleagues (2020) found that more than two thirds of ARDS survivors experienced clinically significant symptoms of fatigue, which strongly co-occurred with symptoms of anxiety and depression. Taken together, this suggests that effective post-ICU treatment must focus not only on reduction of psychiatric symptoms but also promotion of healthy behaviors (e.g., sleep hygiene, energy conservation, breathlessness management, and behavioral pain management).

Prevention of long-term distress-related psychiatric morbidity after critical illness

This section summarizes the emerging literature on prevention of long-term distress-related psychiatric morbidity after critical illness, focusing on in-ICU psychological interventions, in-ICU family presence, and ICU diaries. This is an emerging field, and we have much to learn about what might be effective and for whom (Bienvenu, 2019).

IN-ICU PSYCHOLOGICAL INTERVENTIONS

With few exceptions, most ICUs do not have "built-in" mental health experts. Thus, it is reasonable to wonder what the benefits of such expertise might be for improving long-term mental health outcomes. As a first step, investigators identified ways to measure and treat acute symptoms in the ICU. For example, Chlan (2004) validated a visual analog scale to measure acute anxiety in patients receiving mechanical ventilation. Subsequently, Chlan and colleagues (2013) conducted a randomized controlled clinical trial and found that allowing patients to choose the type and duration of music played during mechanical ventilation reduced acute anxiety symptoms and need for sedation when compared to those without access to music. Indeed, calming music or nature sounds and mind–body interventions generally appear to reduce anxiety and correlated physiologic parameters (e.g., heart rate), but it is unclear whether these acute interventions improve longer-term outcomes (Wade et al., 2016).

In one promising early study of an in-ICU clinical psychologist intervention, the investigators reported longer-term outcomes (Peris et al., 2011). Briefly, they examined mental health outcomes (HADS and IES-R) in critically ill patients with major trauma before and after introduction of a clinical psychological service. Patients were included if they required mechanical ventilation, had no preexisting psychiatric illness or medications, and could be interviewed during the ICU stay. The intervention involved emotional support and coping strategies provided to family members and patients when the latter became conscious, including education, counseling, and stress management with cognitive restructuring. At 1-year follow-up, the 86 patients in the pre-intervention group had a significantly higher prevalence of clinically significant PTSD symptoms (IES-R mean score ≥ 1.5, 57%) than the 123 patients in the intervention group (21%). There was also a trend for lower prevalences of severe anxiety and depression symptoms in the intervention group. In addition, patients in the pre-intervention group were prescribed anxiolytics or antidepressants significantly more often (42%) than patients in the intervention group (8%) (Peris et al., 2011).

In the ambitious Psychological Outcomes Following a Nurse-Led Preventive Psychological Intervention for Critically Ill Patients (POPPI) trial, the investigators assessed whether ICU nurses could deliver similarly helpful psychological care for their patients (Wade et al., 2019). The investigators noted that many ICUs do not have access to psychologists, but cognitive-behavioral therapy techniques can be effective when delivered by non-experts. The intervention included promotion of a therapeutic environment and psychological support delivered by trained ICU nurses for orally communicative, acutely stressed patients. The therapeutic environment included sleep optimization, noise reduction, improved patient orientation, and family involvement (implemented with varying levels of success). The psychological support sessions (up to three per patient) included emotional expression, normalization, psychoeducation, cognitive reappraisal, and "homework" tasks. The researchers' primary outcome of interest was PTSD symptoms at 6-month follow-up. Unfortunately, patients in the intervention group had similar mental health outcomes as patients in the control conditions (historical control and simultaneous control), despite a reduction in state anxiety while in the ICU. The investigators considered possible reasons that the intervention was ineffective, including that it was administered too early (patients were too ill and still in the midst of the traumatic experience) or that it was too difficult for ICU nurses to deliver in a real-world setting (Wade et al., 2019).

FAMILY PRESENCE IN THE ICU

Globally, steps have been taken to reduce family and visitor restrictions in the ICU with positive results. More flexible visiting hours have been associated with lower rates of delirium and anxiety in critically ill patients (Nassar et al., 2018). The effective integration of family members as part of the patient's ICU team is an area of significant research interest (Haines et al., 2017). There is hope that ICU staff can guide family to help patients remain cognitively stimulated, actively participate in activities of daily living, and self-manage anxiety and distress symptoms. Early evidence suggests that ICU patients see more added benefit than stress with family at the bedside (Gonzalez et al., 2004). In addition, having family members at the bedside during an ICU stay may increase patients' endurance during ventilator weaning trials (Happ et al., 2007). Most important for our purposes, in-ICU social support may improve patients' long-term mental health outcomes (Deja et al., 2006).

ICU DIARIES

The idea for ICU diaries emerged from European ICU follow-up clinics, where clinicians realized that patients who had survived critical illnesses often had little knowledge regarding what occurred while they were critically ill, and this was associated with emotional distress. Though the rationales for ICU diaries vary, they include allowing patients to "fill in the blanks" in their memories as well as to contextualize distorted memories and better comprehend the care received.

As noted previously, a large proportion of critically ill patients experience delirium. Thus, survivors' memories of what occurred in intensive care are often colored both by being on the verge of death and simultaneous acute brain dysfunction. Given that context, it is not surprising that patients have distorted memories of things that did occur (e.g., clinicians placing urinary catheters perceived as sexual assault), as well as things that did not actually occur (e.g., children without faces floating by). When patients are no longer delirious, these memories can remain quite vivid and "real." Thus, when considering psychotherapy with such patients, it is useful for the provider to know what actually occurred in order to help patients optimally process the events and sort out truth from fiction. To this end, ICU diaries can be a valuable tool.

In a typical ICU diary, clinicians (especially bedside nurses) and family members write in plain language what happened, typically on at least a daily basis, while the patient is critically ill. Many ICU diaries include photographs of the patient, of the ICU room, and of staff members. In contrast to in-ICU psychological interventions, ICU diaries are meant for patient use when the patient is in a more recovered state (no longer acutely ill, no longer delirious, and able to process the information).

Christina Jones and European colleagues (2010) conducted the first large-scale study of long-term PTSD prevention using ICU diaries. Many of the sites (but not all) had established ICU diary programs, so one might look at this study as an effectiveness trial. The investigators included mechanically ventilated patients who were in the ICU for at least 3 days. They randomized patients to receive their ICU diaries at 1-month follow-up (the intervention group) or 3-month follow-up (the control group). Both groups completed the PTSS-14 at 1-month and 3-month follow-up; the primary outcome was critical illness–related PTSD measured with the PDS at

3-month follow-up. As hypothesized, patients who received ICU diaries at 1-month follow-up had a lower prevalence of PTSD at 3-month follow-up compared to those in the control group (5% vs. 13%, $p = .02$). Perhaps just as important, the investigators noted that patients with more severe PTSD symptoms at 1-month follow-up accounted for the preventive effect. That is, ICU diaries were only effective in reducing PTSD symptoms in patients who had a high symptom burden at 1-month follow-up. Interestingly, ICU diaries may also be beneficial to family members' mental health (e.g., Jones et al., 2012; also see Chapter 12).

It should be noted that in a subsequent, very large multisite trial in France, Maité Garrouste-Orgeas and colleagues (2019) were unable to replicate their own (2012) or Jones and colleagues' (2010) findings of a preventive effect for ICU diaries. Specifically, at 3-month follow-up, patients in the intervention group had a similar prevalence of substantial PTSD symptoms (30%) as patients in the control group (34%). The investigators considered possible reasons why the intervention was ineffective, including less patient use of the diary than expected and lack of a formal turnover of the diary (i.e., an in-person explanation of the purpose and the contents of the diary). The authors also noted that, as with other interventions (Cox et al., 2018), including patients at higher risk for long-term psychological distress may be warranted (Garrouste-Orgeas et al., 2019).

Treatment of psychiatric morbidity after hospital discharge

Early research about psychological interventions to reduce anxiety, depression, and PTSD in critical illness survivors is promising and innovative. Some institutions have opened critical care follow-up clinics, often with peer support groups, which include mental health specialists working alongside ICU clinicians to provide patients with an understanding of their ICU stay and to initiate screening for physical and neuropsychiatric sequelae (see Chapter 13; Haines et al., 2019).

Unfortunately, many critical illness survivors have difficulty attending in-person follow-up visits on a regular basis. Thus, clinical researchers have begun testing telemedicine and M-health interventions to overcome this particular barrier to care. Cox and colleagues (2014) conducted a pilot study of a telephone-based mindfulness training intervention and reported that the intervention was acceptable, feasible, and promising in terms of psychiatric symptom reduction. In a subsequent multicenter trial, Cox and colleagues (2018) tested the efficacy of a telephone- and internet-based coping skills training program, compared with an education program. As in Jones and colleagues' (2010) ICU diary study, the intervention only seemed to have a beneficial effect in patients with higher baseline distress (Cox et al., 2018). Thus, offering the intervention to all critical illness survivors would not seem as prudent as offering it to patients with substantial distress. Recently, Parker and colleagues (2020) conducted a pilot study of a mobile application to deliver a combined behavioral activation and physical rehabilitation intervention; the authors reported that their application prototype was both useable and acceptable. Efficacy remains to be established.

It is exciting to see the development of additional interventions tailored to the needs of critical illness survivors. Recently, Murray and colleagues (2020) described a cognitive-behavioral therapy intervention specifically for patients with post–critical illness PTSD. We look forward to seeing efficacy and effectiveness studies in the future.

Conclusion

Critical illness and intensive care are huge potential stressors, and long-term psychological distress is common in survivors. Risk factors for long-term distress include prior psychiatric history and memories of frightening in-ICU experiences. Mental health clinicians have an important role in prevention and treatment for this growing population, with several possible time points at which to intervene (Figure 5.1).

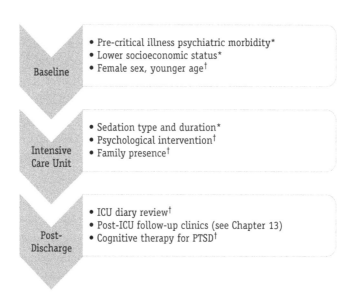

Baseline
- Pre-critical illness psychiatric morbidity*
- Lower socioeconomic status*
- Female sex, younger age[†]

Intensive Care Unit
- Sedation type and duration*
- Psychological intervention[†]
- Family presence[†]

Post-Discharge
- ICU diary review[†]
- Post-ICU follow-up clinics (see Chapter 13)
- Cognitive therapy for PTSD[†]

* Consistent associations in prior studies; [†]Limited or inconsistent associations in prior studies

FIGURE 5.1. Factors associated with long-term psychiatric outcomes in critical illness survivors.

References

Altman, M. T., Knauert, M. P., & Pisani, M. A. (2017). Sleep disturbance after hospitalization and critical illness: A systematic review. *Annals of the American Thoracic Society, 14*(9), 1457–1468.

Bashar, F. R., Vahedian-Azimi, A., Hajiesmaeili, M., Salesi, M., Farzanegan, B., Shojaei, S., . . . Miller, A. C. (2018). Post-ICU psychological morbidity in very long ICU stay patients with ARDS and delirium. *Journal of Critical Care, 43*, 88–94.

Bienvenu, O. J. (2019). What do we know about preventing or mitigating post-intensive care syndrome. *Critical Care Medicine, 47*(11), 1671–1672.

Bienvenu, O. J., Colantuoni, E., Mendez-Tellez, P. A., Dinglas, V. D., Shanholtz, C., Husain, N., . . . Needham, D. M. (2012). Depressive symptoms and impaired physical function after acute lung injury: A 2-year longitudinal study. *American Journal of Respiratory and Critical Care Medicine, 185*(5), 517–524.

Bienvenu, O. J., Colantuoni, E., Mendez-Tellez, P. A., Shanholtz, C., Dennison-Himmelfarb, C. R., Pronovost, P. J., & Needham, D. M. (2015). Cooccurrence of and remission from general anxiety, depression, and posttraumatic stress disorder symptoms after acute lung injury: A 2-year longitudinal study. *Critical Care Medicine, 43*(3), 642–653.

Bienvenu, O. J., Gellar, J., Althouse, B. M., Colantuoni, E., Sricharoenchai, T., Mendez-Tellez, P. A., . . . Needham, D. M. (2013). Post-traumatic stress disorder symptoms after acute lung injury: A 2-year prospective longitudinal study. *Psychological Medicine, 43*(12), 2657–2671.

Bienvenu, O. J., & Jones, C. (2017). Psychological impact of critical illness. In O. J. Bienvenu, C. Jones, & R. O. Hopkins (Eds.), *Psychological and cognitive impact of critical illness* (pp. 69–104). Oxford University Press.

Bienvenu, O. J., Needham, D. M., & Hopkins, R. O. (2013). Response. *Chest, 144*(6), 1974–1975.

Bienvenu, O. J., Williams, J. B., Yang, A., Hopkins, R. O., & Needham, D. M. (2013). Posttraumatic stress disorder in survivors of acute lung injury: Evaluating the Impact of Event Scale-Revised. *Chest, 144*(1), 24–31.

Bjelland, I., Dahl, A. A., Haug, T. T., & Neckelmann, D. (2002). The validity of the Hospital Anxiety and Depression Scale. An updated literature review. *Journal of Psychosomatic Research, 52*(2), 69–77.

Blake, D. D., Weathers, F. W., Nagy, L. M., Kaloupek, D. G., Gusman, F. D., Charney, D. S., & Keane, T. M. (1995). The development of a Clinician-Administered PTSD Scale. *Journal of Traumatic Stress, 8*(1), 75–90.

Brewin, C. R., Andrews, B., & Valentine, J. D. (2000). Meta-analysis of risk factors for posttraumatic stress disorder in trauma-exposed adults. *Journal of Consulting and Clinical Psychology, 68*(5), 748–766.

Chan, K. S., Aronson Friedman, L., Bienvenu, O. J., Dinglas, V. D., Cuthbertson, B. H., Porter, R., . . . Needham, D. M. (2016). Distribution-based estimates of minimal important difference for hospital anxiety and depression scale and impact of event scale-revised in survivors of acute respiratory failure. *General Hospital Psychiatry, 42*, 32–35.

Cheung, A. M., Tansey, C. M., Tomlinson, G., Diaz-Granados, N., Matté, A., Barr, A., . . . Herridge, M. S. (2006). Two-year outcomes, health care use, and costs of survivors of acute respiratory distress syndrome. *American Journal of Respiratory and Critical Care Medicine, 174*(5), 538–544.

Chlan, L. L. (2004). Relationship between two anxiety instruments in patients receiving mechanical ventilatory support. *Journal of Advanced Nursing, 48*(5), 493–499.

Chlan, L. L., Weinert, C. R., Heiderscheit, A., Tracy, M. F., Skaar, D. J., Guttormson, J. L., & Savik, K. (2013). Effects of patient-directed music intervention on anxiety and sedative exposure in critically ill patients receiving mechanical ventilatory support: A randomized clinical trial. *Journal of the American Medical Association, 309*(22), 2335–2344.

Cox, C. E., Hough, C. L., Carson, S. S., White, D. B., Kahn, J. M., Olsen, M. K., . . . Porter, L. S. (2018). Effects of a telephone- and web-based coping skills training program compared with an education program for survivors of critical illness and their family members: A randomized clinical trial. *American Journal of Respiratory and Critical Care Medicine, 197*(1), 66–78.

Cox, C. E., Porter, L. S., Buck, P. J., Hoffa, M., Jones, D., Walton, B., . . . Greeson, J. M. (2014). Development and preliminary evaluation of a telephone-based mindfulness training intervention for survivors of critical illness. *Annals of the American Thoracic Society, 11*(2), 173–181.

Davydow, D. S., Desai, S. V., Needham, D. M., & Bienvenu, O. J. (2008). Psychiatric morbidity in survivors of the acute respiratory distress syndrome: A systematic review. *Psychosomatic Medicine, 70*(4), 512–519.

Davydow, D. S., Gifford, J. M., Desai, S. V., Bienvenu, O. J., & Needham, D. M. (2009). Depression in general intensive care unit survivors: A systematic review. *Intensive Care Medicine, 35*(5), 796–809.

Davydow, D. S., Gifford, J. M., Desai, S. V., Needham, D. M., & Bienvenu, O. J. (2008). Posttraumatic stress disorder in general intensive care unit survivors: A systematic review. *General Hospital Psychiatry, 30*(5), 421–434.

Davydow, D. S., Hough, C. L., Zatzick, D., & Katon, W. J. (2014). Psychiatric symptoms and acute care service utilization over the course of the year following medical-surgical ICU admission: A longitudinal investigation. *Critical Care Medicine, 42*(12), 2473–2481.

Deja, M., Denke, C., Weber-Carstens, S., Schröder, J., Pille, C. E., Hokema, F., . . . Kaisers, U. (2006). Social support during intensive care unit stay might improve mental impairment and consequently health-related quality of life in survivors of severe acute respiratory distress syndrome. *Critical Care, 10*, R147.

Denke, C., Balzer, F., Menk, M., Szur, S., Brosinsky, G., Tafelski, S., . . . Deja, M. (2018). Long-term sequelae of acute respiratory distress syndrome caused by severe community-acquired pneumonia: Delirium-associated cognitive impairment and post-traumatic stress disorder. *Journal of International Medical Research, 46*(6), 2265–2283.

Edmondson, D., Richardson, S., Falzon, L., Davidson, K. W., Mills, M. A., & Neria, Y. (2012). Posttraumatic stress disorder prevalence and risk of recurrence in acute coronary syndrome patients: A meta-analytic review. *Public Library of Science One, 7*(6), e38915.

First, M. B., Spitzer, R. L., Gibbon, M., & Williams, J. B. W. (1996). *Structured clinical interview for DSM-IV Axis I disorders*. American Psychiatric Press, Inc.

Foa, E. B. (1995). *Posttraumatic Stress Diagnostic Scale Manual*. National Computer Systems Inc.

Garrouste-Orgeas, M., Coquet, I., Périer, A., Timsit, J. F., Pochard, F., Lancrin, F., . . . Misset, B. (2012). Impact of an intensive care unit diary on psychological distress in patients and relatives. *Critical Care Medicine, 40*(7), 2033–2040.

Garrouste-Orgeas, M., Flahault, C., Vinatier, I., Rigaud, J. P., Thieulot-Rolin, N., Mercier, E., . . . Timsit, J. F. (2019). Effect of an ICU diary on posttraumatic stress disorder symptoms among patients receiving mechanical ventilation: A randomized clinical trial. *Journal of the American Medical Association, 322*(3), 229–239.

Girard, T. D., Shintani, A. K., Jackson, J. C., Gordon, S. M., Pun, B. T., Henderson, M. S., . . . Ely, E. W. (2007). Risk factors for post-traumatic stress disorder symptoms following critical illness requiring mechanical ventilation: A prospective cohort study. *Critical Care, 11*(1), R28.

Gonzalez, C. E., Carroll, D. L., Elliott, J. S., Fitzgerald, P. A., & Vallent, H. J. (2004). Visiting preferences of patients in the intensive care unit and in a complex care medical unit. *American Journal of Critical Care, 13*(3), 194–198.

Griffiths, J., Fortune, G., Barber, V., & Young, J. D. (2007). The prevalence of posttraumatic stress disorder in survivors of ICU treatment: A systematic review. *Intensive Care Medicine, 33*(9), 1506–1518.

Grover, S., Sahoo, S., Chakrabarti, S., & Avasthi, A. (2019). Post-traumatic stress disorder (PTSD) related symptoms following an experience of delirium. *Journal of Psychosomatic Research, 123*, 109725.

Haines, K. J., Kelly, P., Fitzgerald, P., Skinner, E. H., & Iwashyna, T. J. (2017). The untapped potential of patient and family engagement in the organization of critical care. *Critical Care Medicine, 45*(5), 899–906.

Haines, K. J., McPeake, J., Hibbert, E., Boehm, L. M., Aparanji, K., Bakhru, R. N., . . . Sevin, C. M. (2019). Enablers and barriers to implementing ICU follow-up clinics and peer support groups following critical illness: The Thrive Collaboratives. *Critical Care Medicine, 47*(9), 1194–1200.

Happ, M. B., Swigart, V. A., Tate, J. A., Arnold, R. M., Sereika, S. M., & Hoffman, L. A. (2007). Family presence and surveillance during weaning from prolonged mechanical ventilation. *Heart and Lung, 36*(1), 47–57.

Hatch, R., Young, D., Barber, V., Griffiths, J., Harrison, D. A., & Watkinson, P. (2018). Anxiety, depression, and posttraumatic stress disorder after critical illness: A UK-wide prospective cohort study. *Critical Care, 22*(1), 310.

Herridge, M. S., Cheung, A. M., Tansey, C. M., Matte-Martyn, A., Diaz-Granados, N., Al-Saidi, F., . . . Slutsky, A. S. (2003). One-year outcomes in survivors of the acute respiratory distress syndrome. *New England Journal of Medicine, 348*(8), 683–693.

Herridge, M. S., Tansey, C. M., Matté, A., Tomlinson, G., Diaz-Granados, N., Cooper, A., . . . Cheung, A. M. (2011). Functional disability 5 years after acute respiratory distress syndrome. *New England Journal of Medicine, 364*(14), 1293–1304.

Hinz, A., & Brähler, E. (2011). Normative values for the Hospital Anxiety and Depression Scale (HADS) in the general German population. *Journal of Psychosomatic Research, 71*, 74–78.

Hopkins, R. O., Key, C. W., Suchyta, M. R., Weaver, L. K., & Orme, J. F., Jr. (2010). Risk factors for depression and anxiety in survivors of acute respiratory distress syndrome. *General Hospital Psychiatry, 32*(2), 147–155.

Hosey, M. M., Leoutsakos, J. S., Li, X., Dinglas, V. D., Bienvenu, O. J., Parker, A. M., . . . Neufeld, K. J. (2019). Screening for posttraumatic stress disorder in ARDS survivors: Validation of the Impact of Event Scale-6 (IES-6). *Critical Care, 23*(1), 276.

Huang, M., Parker, A. M., Bienvenu, O. J., Dinglas, V. D., Colantuoni, E., Hopkins, R. O., & Needham, D. M. (2016). Psychiatric symptoms in acute respiratory distress syndrome survivors: A 1-year national multicenter study. *Critical Care Medicine, 44*(5), 954–965.

Huffman, J. C., Celano, C. M., Beach, S. R., Motiwala, S. R., & Januzzi, J. L. (2013). Depression and cardiac disease: Epidemiology, mechanisms, and diagnosis. *Cardiovascular Psychiatry and Neurology, 2013*, 695925.

Jackson, J. C., Girard, T. D., Gordon, S. M., Thompson, J. L., Shintani, A. K., Thomason, J. W., . . . Ely, E. W. (2010). Long-term cognitive and psychological outcomes in the awakening and breathing controlled trial. *American Journal of Respiratory and Critical Care Medicine, 182*(2), 183–191.

Jackson, J. C., Hart, R. P., Gordon, S. M., Hopkins, R. O., Girard, T. D., & Ely, E. W. (2007). Post-traumatic stress disorder and post-traumatic stress symptoms following critical illness in medical intensive care unit patients: Assessing the magnitude of the problem. *Critical Care, 11*(1), R27.

Jackson, J. C., Jutte, J. E., Hunter, C. H., Ciccolella N., Warrington, H., Sevin, C., & Bienvenu, O. J. (2016). Posttraumatic stress disorder (PTSD) after critical illness: A conceptual review of distinct clinical issues and their implications. *Rehabilitation Psychology, 61*(2), 132–140.

Jackson, J. C., Pandharipande, P. P., Girard, T. D., Brummel, N. E., Thompson, J. L., Hughes, C. G., . . . Ely, E. W. (2014). Depression, post-traumatic stress disorder, and functional disability in survivors of critical illness in the BRAIN-ICU study: A longitudinal cohort study. *Lancet Respiratory Medicine, 2*(5), 369–379.

Jones, C., Bäckman, C., Capuzzo, M., Egerod, I., Flaatten, H., Granja, C., . . . Griffiths, R. D. (2010). Intensive care diaries reduce new-onset posttraumatic stress disorder following critical illness. *Critical Care, 14*(5), R168.

Jones, C., Bäckman, C., Capuzzo, M., Flaatten, H., Rylander, C., & Griffiths, R. D. (2007). Precipitants of post-traumatic stress disorder following intensive care: A hypothesis-generating study of diversity in care. *Intensive Care Medicine, 33*(6), 978–985.

Jones, C., Bäckman, C., & Griffiths, R. D. (2012). Intensive care diaries and relatives' symptoms of posttraumatic stress disorder after critical illness: A pilot study. *American Journal of Critical Care, 21*(3), 172–176.

Jones, C., Griffiths, R. D., Humphris, G., & Skirrow, P. M. (2001). Memory, delusions, and the development of acute posttraumatic stress disorder-related symptoms after intensive care. *Critical Care Medicine, 29*(3), 573–580.

Jones, C., Skirrow, P., Griffiths, R. D., Humphris, G. H., Ingleby, S., Eddleston, J., . . . Gager, M. (2003). Rehabilitation after critical illness: A randomized controlled trial. *Critical Care Medicine, 31*(10), 2456–2461.

Jutte, J. E., Needham, D. M., Pfoh, E. R., & Bienvenu, O. J. (2015). Psychometric evaluation of the Hospital Anxiety and Depression Scale 3 months after acute lung injury. *Journal of Critical Care, 30*(4), 793–798.

Kapfhammer, H. P., Rothenhäusler, H. B., Krauseneck, T., Stoll, C., & Schelling, G. (2004). Posttraumatic stress disorder and health-related quality of life in long-term survivors of acute respiratory distress syndrome. *American Journal of Psychiatry, 161*(1), 45–52.

Karnatovskaia, L. V., Schulte, P. J., Philbrick, K. L., Johnson, M. M., Anderson, B. K., Ognjen, G., & Clark, M. M. (2019). Psychocognitive sequelae of critical illness and correlation with 3 months follow-up. *Journal of Critical Care, 52*, 166–171.

Kemp, H. I., Laycock, H., Costello, A., & Brett, S. J. (2019). Chronic pain in critical care survivors: A narrative review. *British Journal of Anaesthesia, 123*(2), e372–e384.

Milton, A., Schandl, A., Soliman, I. W., Meijers, K., van den Boogaard, M., Larsson, I. M., . . . Sackey, P. V. (2018). Development of an ICU discharge instrument predicting psychological morbidity: A multinational study. *Intensive Care Medicine, 44*(12), 2038–2047.

Murray, H., Grey, N., Wild, J., Warnock-Parkes, E., Kerr, A., Clark, D. M., & Ehlers, A. (2020). Cognitive therapy for post-traumatic stress disorder following critical illness and intensive care unit admission. *Cognitive Behaviour Therapist, 13*(e13), 1–17.

Myhren, H., Ekeberg, O., Tøien, K., Karlsson, S., & Stokland, O. (2010). Posttraumatic stress, anxiety and depression symptoms in patients during the first year post intensive care unit discharge. *Critical Care, 14*(1), R14.

Nassar, A. P., Jr., Besen, B. A. M. P., Robinson, C. C., Falavigna, M., Teixeira, C., & Rosa, R. G. (2018). Flexible versus restrictive visiting policies in ICUs: A systematic review and meta-analysis. *Critical Care Medicine, 46*(7), 1175–1180.

Needham, D. M., Davidson, J., Cohen, H., Hopkins, R. O., Weinert, C., Wunsch, H., . . . Harvey, M. A. (2012). Improving long-term outcomes after discharge from intensive care unit: Report from a stakeholders' conference. *Critical Care Medicine, 40*(2), 502–509.

Needham, D. M., Sepulveda, K. A., Dinglas, V. D., Chessare, C. M., Friedman, L. A., Bingham, C. O., 3rd, & Turnbull, A. E. (2017). Core outcome measures for clinical research in acute respiratory failure survivors: An international modified Delphi consensus study. *American Journal of Respiratory and Critical Care Medicine, 196*(9), 1122–1130.

Neufeld, K. J., Leoutsakos, J. S., Yan, H., Lin, S., Zabinski, J. S., Dinglas, V. D., . . . Needham, D. M. (2020). Fatigue symptoms during the first year following ARDS. *Chest, 58*(3), 999–1007.

Nikayin, S., Rabiee, A., Hashem, M. D., Huang, M., Bienvenu, O. J., Turnbull, A. E., & Needham, D. M. (2016). Anxiety symptoms in survivors of critical illness: A systematic review and meta-analysis. *General Hospital Psychiatry, 43*, 23–29.

Parker, A. M., Nelliot, A., Chessare, C. M., Malik, A. M., Koneru, M., Hosey, M. M., . . . Needham, D. M. (2020). Usability and acceptability of a mobile application prototype for a combined behavioural activation and physical rehabilitation intervention in acute respiratory failure survivors. *Australian Critical Care, 33*(6), 511–517.

Parker, A. M., Sricharoenchai, T., Raparla, S., Schneck, K. W., Bienvenu, O. J., & Needham, D. M. (2015). Posttraumatic stress disorder in critical illness survivors: A meta-analysis. *Critical Care Medicine, 43*(5), 1121–1129.

Patel, M. B., Jackson, J. C., Morandi, A., Girard, T. D., Hughes, C. G., Thompson, J. L., . . . Pandharipande, P. P. (2016). Incidence and risk factors for intensive care unit-related post-traumatic stress disorder in veterans and civilians. *American Journal of Respiratory and Critical Care Medicine, 193*(12), 1373–1381.

Peris, A., Bonizzoli, M., Iozzelli, D., Migliaccio, M. L., Zagli, G., Bacchereti, A., . . . Belloni, L. (2011). Early intra-intensive care unit psychological intervention promotes recovery from post-traumatic stress disorders, anxiety and depression symptoms in critically ill patients. *Critical Care, 15*(1), R41.

Pfoh, E. R., Chan, K. S., Dinglas, V. D., Cuthbertson, B. H., Elliott, D., Porter, R., . . . Needham, D. M. (2016). The SF-36 offers a strong measure of mental health symptoms in survivors of acute respiratory failure: A tri-national analysis. *Annals of the American Thoracic Society, 13*(8), 1343–1350.

Rabiee, A., Nikayin, S., Hashem, M. D., Huang, M., Dinglas, V. D., Bienvenu, O. J., . . . Needham, D. M. (2016). Depressive symptoms after critical illness: A systematic review and meta-analysis. *Critical Care Medicine, 44*(9), 1744–1753.

Radloff, L. S. (1977). The CES-D Scale: A self-report depression scale for research in the general population. *Applied Psychological Measurement, 1*(3), 385–401.

Rattray, J. E., Johnston, M., & Wildsmith, J. A. W. (2004). The intensive care experience: Development of the ICE questionnaire. *Journal of Advanced Nursing, 47*(1), 64–73.

Rattray, J. E., Johnston, M., & Wildsmith, J. A. W. (2005). Predictors of emotional outcomes of intensive care. *Anaesthesia, 60*(11), 1085–1092.

Righy, C., Rosa, R. G., da Silva, R. T. A., Kochhann, R., Migliavaca, C. B., Robinson, C. C., . . . Falavigna, M. (2019). Prevalence of post-traumatic stress disorder symptoms in adult critical care survivors: A systematic review and meta-analysis. *Critical Care, 23*(1), 213.

Samuelson, K. A., Lundberg, D., & Fridlund, B. (2007). Stressful memories and psychological distress in adult mechanically ventilated intensive care patients—a 2-month follow-up study. *Acta Anesthesiologica Scandinavica, 51*(6), 671–678.

Schelling, G., & Kapfhammer, H. P. (2013). Surviving the ICU does not mean that the war is over. *Chest, 144*(1), 1–3.

Stoll, C., Kapfhammer, H. P., Rothenhäusler, H. B., Haller, M., Briegel, J., Schmidt, M., . . . Schelling, G. (1999). Sensitivity and specificity of a screening test to document traumatic experiences and to diagnose post-traumatic stress disorder in ARDS patients after intensive care treatment. *Intensive Care Medicine, 25*(7), 697–704.

Tansey, C. M., Louie, M., Loeb, M., Gold, W. L., Muller, M. P., de Jager, J., . . . Herridge, M. S. (2007). One-year outcomes and health care utilization in survivors of severe acute respiratory syndrome. *Archives of Internal Medicine, 167*(12), 1312–1320.

Turnbull, A. E., Rabiee, A., Davis, W. E., Nasser, M. F., Venna, V. R., Lolitha, R., . . . Needham, D. M. (2016). Outcome measurement in ICU survivorship research from 1970 to 2013: A scoping review of 425 publications. *Critical Care Medicine, 44*(7), 1267–1277.

Twigg, E., Humphris, G., Jones, C., Bramwell, R., & Griffiths, R. D. (2008). Use of a screening questionnaire for post-traumatic stress disorder (PTSD) on a sample of UK ICU patients. *Acta Anaesthesiologica Scandinavica, 52*(2), 202–208.

Unroe, M., Kahn, J. M., Carson, S. S., Govert, J. A., Martinu, T., Sathy, S. J., . . . Cox, C. E. (2010). One-year trajectories of care and resource utilization for recipients of prolonged mechanical ventilation: A cohort study. *Annals of Internal Medicine, 153*(3), 167–175.

Wade, D., Hardy, R., Howell, D., & Mythen, M. (2013). Identifying clinical and acute psychological risk factors for PTSD after critical care: A systematic review. *Minerva Anestesiologica, 79*(8), 944–963.

Wade, D. M., Howell, D. C., Weinman, J. A., Hardy, R. J., Mythen, M, G., Brewin, C. R., . . . Raine, R. R. (2012). Investigating risk factors for psychological morbidity three months after intensive care: A prospective cohort study. *Critical Care, 16*(5), R192.

Wade, D. F., Moon, Z., Windgassen, S. S., Harrison, A. M., Morris, L., & Weinman, J. A. (2016). Non-pharmacological interventions to reduce ICU-related psychological distress: A systematic review. *Minerva Anestesiologica, 82*(4), 465–478.

Wade, D. M., Mouncey, P. R., Richards-Belle, A., Wulff, J., Harrison, D. A., Sadique, M. Z., . . . Rowan, K. M. (2019). Effect of a nurse-led preventive psychological intervention on symptoms of posttraumatic stress disorder among critically ill patients: A randomized clinical trial. *Journal of the American Medical Association, 321*(7), 665–675.

Wang, S., Mosher, C., Perkins, A. J., Gao, S., Lasiter, S., Khan, S., . . . Khan, B. (2017). Post-intensive care unit psychiatric comorbidity and quality of life. *Journal of Hospital Medicine, 12*(10), 831–835.

Warlan, H., Howland, L., & Connelly, C. (2016). Detection of posttraumatic stress symptoms in patients after discharge from intensive care. *American Journal of Critical Care, 25*(6), 509–515.

Weinert, C., & Meller, W. (2006). Epidemiology of depression and antidepressant therapy after acute respiratory failure. *Psychosomatics, 47*(5), 399–407.

Weinert, C. R., & Sprenkle, M. (2008). Post-ICU consequences of patient wakefulness and sedative exposure during mechanical ventilation. *Intensive Care Medicine, 34*(1), 82–90.

Weisaeth, L. (1989a). A study of behavioural responses to an industrial disaster. *Acta Psychiatrica Scandinavica, 355*(Suppl), 13–24.

Weisaeth, L. (1989b). Torture of a Norwegian ship's crew. The torture, stress reactions and psychiatric after-effects. *Acta Psychiatrica Scandinavica, 355*(Suppl), 63–72.

Weisaeth, L. (1993). Torture of a Norwegian ship's crew: Stress reactions, coping and psychiatric after-effects. In J. P. Wilson & B. Raphael (Eds.), *International handbook of traumatic stress syndromes* (pp. 743–750). Plenum Press.

Weiss, D. S., & Marmar, C. R. (1997). The Impact of Event Scale-Revised. In J. P. Wilson & T. M. Keane (Eds.), *Assessing psychological trauma and PTSD: A practitioner's handbook* (pp. 399–411). Guilford Press.

Wolters, A. E., Peelen, L. M., Welling, M. C., Kok, L., de Lange, D. W., Cremer, O. L., . . . Veldhuijzen, D. S. (2016). Long-term mental health problems after delirium in the ICU. *Critical Care Medicine, 44*(10), 1808–1813.

Wunsch, H., Christiansen, C. F., Johansen, M. B., Olsen, M., Ali, N., Angus, D. C., & Sørensen, H. T. (2014). Psychiatric diagnoses and psychoactive medication use among nonsurgical critically ill patients receiving mechanical ventilation. *Journal of the American Medical Association, 311*(11), 1133–1142.

Zigmond, A. S., & Snaith, R. P. (1983). The Hospital Anxiety and Depression Scale. *Acta Psychiatrica Scandinavica, 67*(6), 361–370.

6 Neurocognitive Disorders

Ramona O. Hopkins and Kirk J. Stucky

Introduction

This chapter discusses the prevalence, characteristics, risk factors, assessment, management, and the short- and long-term neurologic outcomes for survivors of critical illness and critically ill survivors of COVID-19 including neurocognitive disorders. Although the psychologist's role in caring for survivors of critical illness will be discussed, there is also coverage of integrative concepts that require collaboration among members of the interdisciplinary team. Interventions to improve outcomes, including environmental management, tracking mental status, pharmacologic interventions, family intervention and support, and rehabilitation interventions, are also discussed.

There are many reasons why patients are admitted to, and treated in, the intensive care unit (ICU), including individuals who require close monitoring and support for critical organ systems such as the cardiovascular, respiratory, neurologic, and renal system. Severe medical illness (e.g., sepsis); neurologic injury, including traumatic brain injury (TBI); cardiovascular disease (e.g., stroke, heart attack); and acute respiratory distress syndrome (ARDS) are diseases and disorders often requiring treatment in the ICU (Smith & Nielsen, 1999). While some of these disorders directly injure the brain (e.g., brain trauma, stroke), others injure the brain through a variety of pathophysiologic mechanisms such as hypoxia, glucose dysregulation

Ramona O. Hopkins and Kirk J. Stucky, *Neurocognitive Disorders* In: *Critical Care Psychology and Rehabilitation.*
Edited by: Kirk J. Stucky and Jennifer E. Jutte, Oxford University Press. © Oxford University Press 2022.
DOI: 10.1093/oso/9780190077013.003.0006

(hypoglycemia, hyperglycemia, and glucose variability), and neuroinflammation. In critical illness the damage caused by pathophysiologic processes associated with the condition can be exacerbated by iatrogenic factors. The proper medical management of TBI and stroke can reduce the risk of secondary injury to the brain and other organ systems. Similarly, cognitive impairment following critical illness may be inevitable in 20% to 40% of survivors, but with proper recognition and treatment the severity and extent of the cognitive impairments may be reduced. This review will focus on cognitive outcomes of critical illness survivors treated in the ICU for acute respiratory failure, sepsis, and other medical or surgical conditions.

History and background

The increasing prevalence of critical illness, coupled with improvements in its treatment, has resulted in a substantial increase in the number of ICU survivors (Elliott et al., 2014). Some survivors will recover and return to their pre-illness baseline level of function; however, one third to one half of all survivors are not so fortunate and will develop postintensive care syndrome (PICS) (Elliott et al., 2014; Needham et al., 2012). PICS includes new or worsening morbidities in physical function, cognitive impairments, and psychological disorders (e.g., depression, anxiety, and posttraumatic stress disorder [PTSD]) that contribute to impairments in daily functioning. Cognitive impairment in survivors of critical illness was first described over 20 years ago in patients with ARDS (Hopkins et al., 1999). Over the past two decades numerous studies have identified cognitive impairments as a common morbidity of critical illness (Hopkins et al., 2005; Needham et al., 2016; Needham, Dinglas, Bienvenu, et al., 2013; Needham, Dinglas, Morris, et al., 2013; Pandharipande et al., 2013). The cognitive impairments that develop during critical illness may improve to some degree in the first 6 to 12 months in some patients, but for others these impairments remain severe and may persist for months to years afterward (Hopkins et al., 2005; Pandharipande et al., 2013). The finding of adverse cognitive outcomes in survivors of critical illnesses is supported by several large prospective multicenter studies (Hopkins et al., 2005; Needham et al., 2016; Needham, Dinglas, Bienvenu, et al., 2013; Needham, Dinglas, Morris, et al., 2013; Pandharipande et al., 2013).

New or worsening cognitive impairments can occur after critical illness across broad cognitive domains. Decline in global intellectual function, impaired memory (Hopkins et al., 2005; Mikkelsen et al., 2012) and executive function are the most frequently documented impairments (Pandharipande et al., 2013). Impaired attention, visuospatial impairments, and slow mental processing speed also occur but are less frequently reported, often due to variability in neuropsychological tests used to measure cognitive function (Rawal et al., 2017). The prevalence of cognitive impairments ranges from almost 100% of survivors at hospital discharge to 20% to 40% of survivors at 1 and 2 years after leaving the hospital, suggesting that the cognitive impairments improve over time in some patients (Hopkins et al., 2005; Needham et al., 2016). A systematic review of studies that reported cognitive impairments (the definition of cognitive impairment varied by study) found the prevalence ranged from a mean of 35% (95% confidence interval [CI], 25–41%) to a mean of 81% (95% CI 71–91%) (Honarmand et al., 2020). The prevalence of cognitive impairments was higher in ARDS survivors (82%) compared to 42% in a mixed ICU population (Honarmand et al., 2020). Cognitive impairments can occur in one or multiple cognitive domains, range in severity from mild to severe, and are similar to those documented following TBI and dementia (Pandharipande et al., 2013). Across various neurocognitive disorders (e.g., TBI, stroke, critical illness), an individual's cognitive and behavioral presentation may be similar, but there are likely distinct differences in etiology, mechanisms of injury, and risk factors based on the disorder.

Cognitive impairments during or following critical illness can occur in isolation but typically co-occur with physical, psychological, and functional disabilities. One study found that cognitive impairments were associated with depression, anxiety, and PTSD; furthermore, severe psychological symptoms were associated with worse cognitive impairments (Bruck et al., 2018). A study by Marra and colleagues (2018) found that cognitive impairments occurred alone in 17% of ICU survivors, co-occurred in 10% of patients with depression, 4% with disability in activities of daily living (ADLs), and 6% of survivors with both depression and disability in ADLs. At 12 months post-ICU discharge, cognitive impairments were present in 16% of patients, co-occurred in 10% with depression, 2% with disability in ADLs, and 10% of patients who had both depression and disability in ADLs. Higher educational attainment predicted greater odds of being PICS free (having no impairments in physical, cognitive, or psychological disorders) at 3 and 12 months. Conversely, higher clinical frailty scores at ICU admission predicted lower odds of being PICS free (Marra et al., 2018); that is, greater frailty was associated with developing physical, psychological, and/or cognitive impairments.

Cognitive impairments are associated with reduced quality of life (Hopkins et al., 2005) and functional declines affecting personal ADLs (Iwashyna et al., 2010). These cognitive impairments have significant real-world consequences, including problems driving, inability to return to work (Kamdar et al., 2017, 2020), and impaired instrumental ADLs such as paying bills and managing multiple medications (Hopkins et al., 2017), similar to the functional disabilities that occur following TBI or dementia. In a study of 922 ARDS survivors who were employed prior to their critical illness, 44% were jobless at 12-month follow-up (Kamdar et al., 2017). After accounting for death and retirement, 68% of these survivors had not returned to work by 12 months. Delay in returning to work was associated with older age, longer ICU length of stay, and being nonwhite (Kamdar et al., 2017). Inability to work contributed to financial distress related to joblessness, loss of or change in health insurance, and inability to pay large medical bills or co-payments (Hauschildt et al., 2020). Financial distress is associated with adverse psychological outcomes, including depression and anxiety, and impaired physical health and social relationships (Hauschildt et al., 2020). These issues, in concert with the burden of critical illness on patients and families, create a daunting future.

Pathophysiology

The pathophysiology of cognitive impairments after critical illness is complex and to date has not been fully elucidated. A detailed review of the pathophysiology of cognitive impairment is beyond the scope of this chapter; for a comprehensive review of mechanisms of brain injury in critical illness see Sasannejad and colleagues (2019). Briefly, neuroimaging studies have identified white matter hyperintensities, generalized brain atrophy, hippocampal atrophy, structural lesions, and damage to the white matter, including the corpus callosum and internal capsule, all suggestive of brain injury (Gunther et al., 2012; Hopkins et al., 2006; Jackson et al., 2015, 2018; Morandi et al., 2010, 2012; Wilson et al., 2018). Animal models have shown that breakdown of the blood–brain barrier and marked neural inflammation occur during critical illness and are associated with neuronal dysfunction and necrosis (Previgliano et al., 2015). A recent review found that neuroinflammation can occur, resulting in increased levels of circulating proinflammatory cytokines such as interleukin-10 and tumor necrosis factor and anti-inflammatory cytokines that damage the brain (Rengel et al., 2019). Damage to the blood–brain barrier also occurs from elevated peripheral cytokines that can bind to the endothelium, increasing its permeability to cytokines and thus further damaging the brain (Rengel et al., 2019). Both hypoxia and inflammation can lead to the development of oxygen radicals and subsequent neural apoptosis and necrosis (Hughes et al., 2016).

Risk factors

To understand or predict which patients may develop cognitive impairment after a critical illness, it is crucial to understand risk factors that have been identified. Predisposing risk factors include older age, apolipoprotein E4 allele, pre-ICU chronic disease (i.e., cardiovascular disease, pulmonary disorders), prior diagnosis of brain disease or injury (e.g., mild cognitive impairment, dementia, prior brain injury or stroke), and preexisting psychological and physical disorders

(Ely et al., 2007; Guerra et al., 2012; Pandharipande et al., 2013). Risk factors for cognitive impairment during and after critical illness include delirium, sepsis, hypoxia, glucose dysregulation, and readmission to the hospital or ICU (Sakusic et al., 2018).

A systematic review of 16,595 patients assessed delirium prevalence and its association with cognitive impairments in ICU survivors (Salluh et al., 2015). Delirium was an incident risk factor for cognitive impairment, and longer delirium duration was independently associated with cognitive impairment at 3- and 12-month follow-up (Salluh et al., 2015). Benzodiazepine use is also a risk factor for cognitive impairment, and higher benzodiazepine dosing during ICU treatment was associated with worse executive function at 3 but not 6 months after hospital discharge (Kok et al., 2018). Sakusic and colleagues (2018) found delirium, glucose dysregulation (hypoglycemia and hyperglycemia and glucose variability), and hypoxia to be associated with post-ICU cognitive impairment. Other risk factors include presence of sepsis, delirium, pre-sepsis depression, and higher Acute Physiologic Assessment and Chronic Health Evaluation-II (APACHE II) scores (Calsavara et al., 2018). Duration of mechanical ventilation and ICU length of stay were also identified as risk factors in a few studies, but most studies have not found such associations (Sakusic et al., 2018). Dissimilarities between studies are likely related to variations in research design, heterogeneity in study populations, variability in baseline risk factors, and differences in the timing of assessment and the measures used to assess cognitive function.

COVID-19 and cognitive outcomes

The novel coronavirus disease (COVID-19) is caused by severe acute respiratory coronavirus-2 (SARS-CoV-2), a beta-coronavirus that was initially reported in China in late 2019. COVID-19 presentation can be asymptomatic, can present with mild symptoms, or can be severe, resulting in hospitalization or admission to the ICU with severe respiratory distress or other organ failure. More severe illness is associated with a higher mortality rate (Richardson et al., 2020). COVID-19 has also been associated with neurologic symptoms and sequelae (Needham et al., 2020). Previously described coronaviruses such as severe acute respiratory syndrome coronavirus (SARS-CoV-1) and Middle Eastern Respiratory Syndrome coronavirus (MERS-CoV) can invade the brain and have direct neurologic effects (de Wit et al., 2016; Petrosillo et al., 2020).

We are only beginning to understand the morbidity of COVID-19. Early studies of individuals with COVID-19 identified neurologic symptoms such as dizziness, headache, loss of taste and smell, and loss of consciousness (Ellul et al., 2020). A study of 214 patients found that 36% had neurologic symptoms, the most common being headache and dizziness (Mao et al., 2020). A study of 509 hospitalized patients with COVID-19 found that 134 (26%) developed severe disease requiring mechanical ventilation along with neurologic symptoms, including headache, dizziness, and loss of taste; 31.8% developed encephalopathy (Liotta et al., 2020). Patients with neurologic symptoms were younger and had more severe COVID-19. Older patients were more likely to have encephalopathy (odds ratio [OR] 1.06; 95% CI 1.04–1.08). At discharge 28.9% of patients had poor functional outcome (assessed using the modified Rankin Scale); encephalopathy was associated with higher mortality and worse functional outcome (Liotta et al., 2020). The long-term neurologic consequences have also been associated with direct viral effects on the brain, including neuropathologic changes seen on neuroimaging and cognitive impairments; in turn, the neurologic changes may contribute to respiratory failure (Li et al., 2020; Montalvan et al., 2020).

Neuroimaging findings in COVID-19 patients with ARDS show a variety of neuropathologic changes, including microbleeds in subcortical brain regions such as the corpus callosum, cerebellar peduncles, and internal capsule (Fitsiori et al., 2020). A recent systematic review of neuroimaging findings in patients with COVID-19 found a variety of abnormalities, including stroke, temporal lobe atrophy, hippocampal atrophy, thalamic lesions, hemorrhage in the basal ganglia, hyperintensities and lesions in the temporal lobe, white matter hyperintensities, and loss of gray–white differentiation (Katal et al., 2021). Other neurologic disorders include encephalopathy, cerebrovascular events, psychosis, and dementia-like cognitive impairments (Ellul et al., 2020).

Studies find that ARDS is associated with the development of cognitive impairments in survivors of critical illness. Given that many COVID-19 patients who are treated in the ICU develop ARDS, they are also likely to develop cognitive impairments and additional sequelae similar to other ARDS survivors. A systematic review and meta-analysis of 72 studies that assessed survivors of SARS-CoV-1, MERS-CoV, and COVID-19 found that patients admitted to the hospital developed new depression, anxiety, PTSD, psychosis, confusion, and cognitive impairments, including impaired memory and executive function (Rogers et al., 2020). Data from a study from Toronto of 117 SARS-CoV-1-infected patients found that they had persistent physical impairments, including reduced distance walked in 6 minutes along with breathlessness and significant reduction in physical health as assessed using the Short-Form 36 (Tansey et al., 2007). In patients with SARS-CoV-1, 33% had significant reduction in mental health that was at least one standard deviation below normative data. During the first year after hospital discharge, visits to mental health providers accounted for most of the clinical care visits, suggesting that mental health was a significant problem for survivors. It is important to note that patients reported that the social stigma of the disease and acute stress due to isolation and quarantine were extremely difficult to cope with, and that these adversely affected their mental health (Tansey et al., 2007).

Cognitive impairments have also been reported in this population. A study of nine patients with COVID-19 found that one third had significant cognitive impairment on the Mini Mental State Examination (MMSE), with low scores in attention, memory, constructional apraxia, and written language at 30-day follow-up (Negrini et al., 2021). Only one person had impaired executive function. The cognitive impairments were associated with longer ICU length of stay. In addition, 66% had symptoms of anxiety and 22% had symptoms of depression (Negrini et al., 2021). A French study of 58 cases of COVID-19 found that 64% had abnormalities on their neurologic exam, and 33% of patients discharged home had dysexecutive problems, including impaired attention and disorganization of movements (Helms et al., 2020). A larger study assessed the relation between delirium and cognitive function at 1-month follow-up in survivors of COVID-19 (McLoughlin et al., 2020). Delirium was assessed in the hospital and cognitive function was assessed using the Modified Telephone Interview for Cognitive Status (TICS-m) at 4 weeks. Of the 71 patients enrolled in the study, only 36% underwent cognitive testing. The Mean TICS-m score of 34.5 was lower in the group with delirium compared to the mean score of 41.5 in the non-delirious group (p = .06). The authors concluded that cognitive function was not worse in the delirium group at 4 weeks (McLoughlin et al., 2020). However, the study was limited by the low rate of follow-up, likely resulting in insufficient power to determine the relation between cognitive impairments and delirium. In addition, TICS-m cutoff scores of 19 and 37 have been used to identify possible mild cognitive impairment (Lines et al., 2003). Taken together, these findings suggest that the delirium group, while not statistically different from the non-delirium group, scored in the range of mild cognitive impairment.

Critically ill COVID-19 survivors, both older and younger individuals, may develop significant physical, cognitive, and psychological morbidities. It remains to be determined if these patients recover and return to their pre-ICU functional abilities or if the impairments remain in the months to years after hospital discharge, which is typically what occurs in other critically ill populations. On October 20, 2020, a quick search of clinicaltrials.gov identified 24 studies assessing cognitive outcomes and/or interventions to improve outcomes in COVID-19 survivors. We eagerly await the results of these studies.

The following case studies illustrate the significant neurocognitive effects that can occur in patients with critical illness due to COVID-19.

CASE #1

A 51-year-old married man was admitted to the hospital with complaints of fatigue and shortness of breath. His medical history included diabetes, hypertension, and obesity. Prior to becoming ill, he was working full time as a high school English teacher. He tested positive for COVID-19, and shortly after admission he went into respiratory failure, requiring treatment in the ICU that included ventilator support and tracheostomy. His ICU clinical course was further complicated by deep vein thrombosis in all four extremities, which required aggressive anticoagulation. Three weeks into his critical illness, and while still on the ventilator, he sustained a cardiac arrest. He also developed acute kidney injury requiring hemodialysis as well as gastric ulcers with gastrointestinal bleeding. During his prolonged ICU course, he vacillated between being delirious and minimally responsive, even when sedation was lifted. Neuroimaging was negative for acute neuropathology.

After 35 days in the ICU, he was extubated and eventually transferred to the inpatient rehabilitation unit for treatment of critical illness myopathy, a decubitus ulcer, and cognitive impairments. He was initially somewhat disoriented, slow to process information, and easily fatigued. Due to pandemic restrictions, he was not allowed to have visitors physically present, but an iPad allowed him to visit with his wife and two teenage daughters. Secondary to cognitive and physical limitations, staff had to facilitate these interactions. He exhibited symptoms of depression and reported feeling lonely. Initially he had difficulty retaining new information and periodically forgot that he had spoken with his family. He had very little recollection of his ICU admission but did recall several vivid hallucinations and a delusional belief that the doctors were preparing to harvest his organs for donation while he was still alive. Over the course of rehabilitation, his endurance, mood, and cognition improved. A brief neuropsychological assessment before discharge found mild to moderate impairments in attention and memory as well as slow processing speed.

The critical care team members were concerned that this patient would not survive given the number of serious complications he experienced (e.g., delirium, respiratory failure, cardiac arrest, renal failure). After discharge he continued to display cognitive impairments and emotional adjustment issues. At the time of writing, the patient was living at home but had not returned to work due to persistent physical issues and cognitive impairments.

CASE #2

A 64-year-old woman was admitted to the hospital with cough and fever for 2 to 3 days. Prior to her hospital admission, she lived at home with her husband and functioned independently. Her medical history included chronic obstructive pulmonary disease, diabetes, hypertension, and stroke 5 years earlier. In the emergency department she was hypoxic and was placed on oxygen by nasal cannula. She tested positive for COVID-19. She was admitted to the ICU with septic shock and cytokine syndrome secondary to COVID-19. She required intubation, feeding tube placement, and intermittent dialysis. Prolonged mechanical ventilation was required, but she eventually was extubated.

She developed critical illness myopathy and was transferred to inpatient rehabilitation 1 month after her initial admission. The rehabilitation psychologist's evaluation revealed very slow mental processing speed. She could follow simple one-step commands but in delayed fashion. She was significantly lethargic with minimal initiation, requiring maximum cues for participation in therapy tasks. She could not read aloud and was largely nonverbal. She could not give her age or the date, nor could she talk about her symptoms or her plan of care. She was not agitated and had no evidence of emotional lability. The patient's family indicated that this was a significant regression from her baseline level of function, reporting that she had been independent in all ADLs after recovering from a "mild stroke" 5 years prior. Computed tomography (CT) scan of her brain showed an old left-sided lacunar infarct but no acute abnormalities. Severe cognitive impairments were thought to be related to multiple factors, including sepsis and ARDS complications from prolonged critical illness, in addition to preexisting declines in cognitive reserve due to cerebrovascular disease.

Unfortunately, as the patient could not tolerate more intense rehabilitation interventions, she was very slow to improve. She was eventually transferred to a long-term care facility, where she died 2 months later following a massive stroke.

Assessment in the critical care environment

In critical care settings the assessment and treatment of patients with neurocognitive disorders requires a multitiered, coordinated approach among a variety of clinicians on the interdisciplinary team. Although the role of the psychologist is emphasized in this chapter, the important and unique contributions made by physicians, nurses, speech and language pathologists (SLP), and other disciplines are also discussed.

The psychologist's assessment of an ICU patient with a known or suspected neurocognitive disorder typically serves three primary purposes: (1) differential diagnosis; (2) tracking and monitoring progression of cognitive and psychological symptoms or sequelae and/or response to treatment; and (3) determining decision-making capacity. A single assessment may serve all these purposes or just one, depending on the circumstances and the patient's unique needs.

COGNITIVE ASSESSMENT

Detailed discussion of the strengths and weaknesses of various assessment instruments is beyond the scope of this chapter, and it is assumed that readers are familiar with instruments commonly used to monitor delirium and orientation, such as the Confusion Assessment Method for the ICU (CAM-ICU) (Ely et al., 2001), the Richmond Agitation-Sedation Scale (RASS) (Sessler et al., 2002), and the Orientation Log (O-Log) (Novack et al., 2000), and cognitive assessment, including the Cognitive-Log (Cog-Log) (Alderson & Novack, 2003), the Montreal Cognitive Assessment (MoCA) (Nasreddine et al., 2005), the MMSE (Folstein et al., 1975; Kukull et al., 1994), and the TICS-m (Fong et al., 2009). In the sections that follow, cognitive assessment tools, questionnaires, and medical tests employed in the evaluation of neurocognitive disorders are briefly reviewed.

Before entering a discussion of cognitive assessment, it is important to clarify the differences among cognitive monitoring, cognitive screening, cognitive testing, and neuropsychological evaluation, given the inconsistent ways in which these terms are used in clinical settings. The definitions provided in what follows are largely based on commentary by Roebuck-Spencer and colleagues (2017) and Block and colleagues (2017).

Cognitive monitoring

In cognitive monitoring, (1) orientation to place, time, and circumstances and (2) confusion are assessed. In hospital settings cognitive monitoring is often conducted by nurses, as they can assess the patient's mental status throughout the day and several times during each shift. Cognitive monitoring can be used to track waxing and waning confusion, as occurs frequently in delirium. Measures such as the O-Log and CAM-ICU are commonly used measures in the ICU. These instruments can be repeated multiple times on the same day, generally without concern regarding practice effects.

Cognitive screening

Cognitive screening uses measures designed to assess basic aspects of cognitive function, such as orientation, memory, attention, and problem-solving (e.g., MMSE). Cognitive screening is more feasible and often preferred with patients who are severely cognitively compromised and cannot complete or tolerate more detailed assessment. Cognitive screening tests that assess multiple cognitive domains such as the MMSE, TICS-m, and MoCA can be administered by a variety of trained professionals.

When cognitive screening tests are used in isolation, they will frequently fail to identify patients with mild to moderate cognitive impairments and are almost always insufficient to inform differential diagnosis (Pfoh et al., 2015). In ICU populations the specificity of cognitive screening tests is very good, but sensitivity is poor, and the correlations of cognitive screening test scores and neuropsychological scores have been found to be weak to moderate (Pfoh et al., 2015). Further, cognitive screening test scores did not predict cognitive impairment at 6 months when compared to a comprehensive neuropsychological test battery (Woon et al., 2012). A systematic review of 46 cognitive outcome studies in ICU survivors found that the prevalence of cognitive impairment at 3 months was 35% in the 10 studies that used cognitive screening tests compared to 54% in the 26 studies that used neuropsychological test batteries (Honarmand et al., 2020). At 12 months the prevalence of cognitive impairment was 18% using cognitive screening tools and 43% using neuropsychological tests (Honarmand et al., 2020).

Cognitive screening tests also do not allow for in-depth investigation of higher-level cognitive abilities such as executive function, memory, or visuospatial skills. As with all neuropsychological tests, factors that can influence performance need to be accounted for in test interpretation (e.g., premorbid abilities and reading level, adequate attention and motivation, medication effects, pain, and psychiatric issues). The potential for harm due to false-positive or false-negative cognitive screening results cannot be overstated. A psychologist or physician may be able to use a screening instrument to determine that a patient has a neurocognitive disorder but will not likely be able to determine the cognitive domains impaired, severity of the impairments, and trajectory of the cognitive impairments without obtaining additional information, monitoring over time, and conducting more detailed studies or tests. For more in-depth discussion the reader is referred to the American Psychological Association's statement on cognitive screening (American Psychological Association Practice Organization, 2014).

Cognitive testing

Cognitive testing entails longer assessments typically conducted by clinicians with specific training backgrounds and roles. Cognitive testing provides more information regarding specific domains (e.g., attention, concentration, memory, visuospatial skills, language, and executive function). Short-test batteries typically require 30 to 60 minutes. They are administered for specific reasons such as determining current cognitive status, differential diagnosis, or outcome prediction. Brief focused batteries may be helpful in predicting outcomes in certain cases. For example, cognitive testing conducted in an inpatient rehabilitation setting can help predict functional outcome following moderate to severe TBI (Hanks et al., 2008). Similar studies in inpatient rehabilitation that predict functional outcomes in ICU survivors are still needed.

Neuropsychological assessment

Neuropsychological assessment is a specialized multidimensional procedure that can be particularly useful in identifying the nature and severity of cognitive impairments, exposing functional limitations, detecting change, and planning treatment. However, detailed neuropsychological assessment is rarely used in the ICU, being typically reserved for inpatient rehabilitation or outpatient settings. There are several reasons for this:

1. Neuropsychological assessment typically requires 2 or more hours, and most critically ill patients on the ICU are unable to participate in, or tolerate, such a lengthy assessment.
2. Cognitive function in patients on the ICU may wax and wane or improve once they are medically stable.
3. Patients fatigue easily, and testing is often interrupted for medical care and procedures.
4. The detailed information provided by neuropsychological assessment is typically aimed at informing long-term treatment planning, such as the patient's need for rehabilitation, school accommodations, work restrictions, and specific outpatient services.

In the ICU, psychologists are typically focused on urgent, short-term issues such as presence of delirium, cognitive screening, decision-making capacity, treatment selection, and level of supervision required. In critical care settings, lengthy neuropsychological examinations are not typically used to answer these questions. However, in outpatient ICU follow-up clinics for critical illness survivors, there is a growing appreciation for the importance of cognitive screening, which may lead to referral for more detailed neuropsychological testing and cognitive rehabilitation (Jackson et al., 2012). This is also discussed later in this chapter and in Chapter 13.

Questionnaires

Numerous questionnaires have been developed to assess cognitive, mental health, and behavioral symptoms. Although cognitive questionnaires have value in some settings, most studies of their utility in the critical care environment are limited or show little benefit (Jackson et al., 2003). A systematic review of studies that used cognitive questionnaires found the absence of cognitive impairment to be 40% using questionnaires compared to 15% using neuropsychological tests (Wolters et al., 2013). Generally, questionnaires designed to assess cognitive symptoms do not work very well in diverse populations (Polito et al., 2013; Sutter et al., 2015) for the following reasons:

1. Patients with severe cognitive impairments may also lack self-awareness and grossly underestimate or misrepresent their cognitive impairments.
2. Patients may not understand or accurately interpret questions about their cognitive status due to the presence of significant impairments in concentration, reading, and memory.
3. When family members fill out questionnaires about the patient's cognitive function, they sometimes report on cognitive abilities prior to the critical illness or have trouble recognizing impairment. For example, family members may not appreciate new memory impairments after the patient leaves the hospital and sometimes assume that their loved one's memory is "fine" because they can accurately recall remote information such as the names of family members, their address, and phone number, all of which represent highly overlearned information.

In addition, at discharge most people have not resumed their normal work and cognitive activities, so they have little basis on which to determine if their cognitive function has been affected by the critical illness.

Overall, it is inadvisable to use cognitive questionnaires to identify cognitive impairments in survivors of critical illness.

MEDICAL ASSESSMENT

In the sections that follow we briefly discuss medical assessment tools that should be familiar to the critical care psychologist who wishes to competently assess and evaluate neurocognitive disorders in the ICU.

Neuroimaging

For patients who present with or develop changes in mental status, a common practice is to obtain a magnetic resonance imaging (MRI) or CT scan of the brain. These tools are invaluable in identifying acute and chronic neuropathologic changes, including stroke, intraparenchymal hemorrhage, subdural hematoma, microhemorrhages, white matter changes, and other gray and white matter lesions. Studies of survivors of critical illness have found neuropathologic changes such as cortical and subcortical lesions, generalized and focal atrophy, and white matter lesions (Gunther et al., 2012; Hopkins et al., 2006; Morandi et al., 2012). It is important to recognize that initial scans may not identify lesions or atrophy in ICU survivors, but brain injury may manifest later in the illness or during recovery due to sepsis, hypoxia, and hypoglycemia or other factors that can damage the brain (Polito et al., 2013; Sutter et al., 2015). Even in the presence of persistent cognitive impairments, a sizable percentage of survivors of critical illness may have normal structural neuroimaging. Other neuroimaging modalities such as functional neuroimaging, diffusion tensor imaging, and perfusion imaging may identify other neuropathologic effects of critical illness on the brain (Hopkins et al., 2016).

Laboratory studies

To understand mental status changes, psychologists must understand how various metabolic derangements, organ failure, medications, infection, and other factors (e.g., abnormal thyroid, renal, and liver function; hypoxemia; complete blood count; electrolyte disorders; glucose dysregulation; abnormal toxicology tests) can adversely affect cognition. For example, hyponatremia and sepsis are common contributors to delirium and cognitive impairments.

Electroencephalography

Electroencephalography (EEG) is typically used to determine if patients are having seizures or if there are any focal abnormalities. In delirium the EEG can be abnormal and often shows nonfocal, generalized slowing or fast activity, especially in metabolic delirium. The EEG pattern will tell the clinician very little about the patient's cognition, behavior, or emotional status, but it is often used in combination with the clinical examination and other assessment instruments to reach diagnostic conclusions.

Differential diagnosis

In critical care settings there are often multiple predisposing and precipitating factors potentially contributing to a patient's cognitive function (e.g., metabolic instabilities, iatrogenic medication side effects, pain, preexisting cognitive impairment, new neurologic damage due to the critical illness). Patients in the ICU with delirium are more likely to die compared to non-delirious patients, which highlights the importance of prompt assessment, identification, and treatment of the underlying etiology (Ely et al., 2004; Shehabi et al., 2010). Unfortunately, despite advanced technology and increased clinician awareness, patients with cognitive impairments are often not assessed or are missed in the ICU (Barr et al., 2013; Gelinas et al., 2013; McCoy et al., 2017). The reasons for failure to diagnose cognitive impairment are multifactorial and include, but are not limited to, the following:

1. Important clinical care that takes precedence over delirium and cognitive assessment
2. Conflicting demands on staff time or lack of resources to assess and track cognitive function
3. Patient barriers to assessment such as mechanical ventilation, sedation, delirium, and coma

A competent and appropriately trained psychologist engaged in the care of patients in the ICU will be able to evaluate patients' abilities to engage in cognitive assessment and will assess at least some aspects of cognitive, psychological, and functional outcomes. The steps required in differential diagnosis are briefly described next.

MEDICAL HISTORY

The patient's history and current medical status can help the clinician develop a better sense of the patient's premorbid function and abilities and predisposing and precipitating factors while also finetuning the assessment plan. However, some homeless individuals or patients who are severely cognitively compromised may not be able to provide a history, and family may not be available.

INTERVIEW OF CLINICAL STAFF AND FAMILY

Input from clinical staff is essential in evaluating the patient. Some questions to address include:

Is the patient agitated, and if so, what specific behaviors are present and
    under what conditions?

Does the patient show any evidence of hallucinations or delusions?

What has the patient's orientation been like during the shift?

Have any neurobehavioral or cognitive changes been observed when the
    patient takes certain medications? Are these changes related to the
    timing of the medications?

How does pain affect behavior, cognition, mood, and participation?

Knowing the answers to these questions will help the psychologist identify which
behaviors are most problematic for staff and can also help generate targeted treatment recommendations. For example, the physician may express concern about
acute stress disorder, but staff members also report confusion and impulsive behaviors, raising the possibility of delirium.

To better understand the patient's preexisting issues, the clinician can also interview family. Learning that the patient has a history of dementia, substance use,
developmental disability, or other chronic conditions allows the clinician to generate estimates regarding premorbid abilities as well as vulnerability to new medical
complications and adverse long-term outcomes. For example, knowing that a patient
recovered from a stroke 2 years earlier will have implications for cognitive recovery
and function after this critical illness.

BEDSIDE ASSESSMENT

Assessment of cognitive function in the ICU and hospital may be quite brief for
some patients while requiring more time for others. When a neurocognitive disorder is under consideration, the clinician must be simultaneously attentive to behavioral changes, mood, cognitive abilities, motor and sensory function, and underlying
medical issues. Does the patient know where they are and why they are in the hospital? Are they able to sustain a conversation and follow commands consistently? Are
they able to understand and discuss their treatment options? Is the patient agitated,
physically aggressive, or hallucinating? When significant behavioral problems are
present, the clinician should not use comprehensive neuropsychological tests but
rather focus on identifying factors that contribute to agitation and investigate interventions at the bedside to determine tactics to manage these behaviors.

Face-to-face assessment in the ICU can be challenging. Many patients are on
mechanical ventilation, although alert and awake, cannot talk, and often are so
weak that they have difficulty using a pencil. Lethargy, somnolence, distractibility,

impulsivity, and/or irritability often preclude a more detailed evaluation. Individuals with hypoactive delirium may be unnoticed or mislabeled as unmotivated or depressed. Perceptual disturbances are also common, including misperceptions and hallucinations. Patients may not have their eyeglasses or hearing aids, which further contributes to confusion and difficulty communicating. By working with nurses, physical therapists, SLPs, and family members, the psychologist can address these barriers and/or conduct the assessment at a better time of the day.

Once the assessment is complete, by combining the known history with test findings and expert knowledge, conclusions based on a reasonable degree of scientific certainty can often be reached.

Tracking progression or response to treatment

One hallmark feature of neurocognitive disorders is that they are constantly evolving, and this necessitates frequent reassessment. All members of the clinical team, including physicians, psychologists, nurses, respiratory therapists, speech and language pathologists (SLPs), and physical and occupational therapy staff, are engaged in evaluation and care of patients with neurocognitive disorders. For example, at the second author's hospital, protocols have been created according to which nurses and/or SLPs administer cognitive screening assessments and share the findings with the team. In this model, trends and changes in mental status can be identified. The psychologist can use the data to focus on developing and monitoring behavioral management plans, ensuring that environmental management is coordinated, providing other interventions, and meeting with family members who may need additional support and education.

Determining decision-making capacity

Many patients admitted to the ICU lack the ability to participate in making decisions about their treatment (Cohen et al., 2005). Assessment of capacity to make informed health care decisions is a very important role fulfilled by physicians, psychologists, and psychiatrists in the ICU. The medicolegal and ethical concerns become quite apparent, especially considering that patients in critical care often require procedures and treatments that carry certain inherent risks. Even if the procedures or treatments go well, they may result in long-term problems. For example, patients who require prolonged ventilation are at increased risk for infection, delirium, debility, and decubitus ulcers. Nonetheless, many patients with cognitive impairments are still capable of making decisions about their medical care. For example, among patients with cognitive impairments who are aware of their diagnosis, symptoms, and prognosis, the majority are likely capable of making decisions regarding their medical treatment (Karlawish, 2008). Space does not permit detailed discussion of the complex clinical, ethical, legal, and practical issues at play or at odds in the assessment of decision-making capacity, and readers are encouraged to review some of the excellent books and articles on this topic (Grisso & Applebaum, 1998; Palmer & Harmell, 2016; please also see Chapter 15).

Treatment and interventions

Determining that a neurocognitive disorder is present is one step in what may be a long process of care and recovery. The treatment of neurocognitive disorders in the ICU can be broken down into component parts and should be part of a comprehensive treatment plan. The components briefly reviewed below are (1) environmental management, (2) sleep–wake schedules, (3) pharmacologic interventions, (4) staff training and support, (5) family education and support, and (6) rehabilitative interventions.

ENVIRONMENTAL MANAGEMENT

Patients in acute states of confusion require 24-hour supervision and monitoring in addition to standard medical care for the condition(s) that resulted in hospitalization. One-on-one safety observers are preferable to restraints whenever possible due to the risk of accidental injury, iatrogenic trauma, or unintended complications (e.g., skin breakdown). However, for patients who are a danger to self or others (e.g., physically aggressive, constantly trying to get out of bed, pulling at lines and tubes), restraints and medical safety devices (e.g., alarms, enclosure beds) may be needed.

After acute brain injury, the patient is unable to process information normally, is at risk for secondary injury (e.g., edema, catecholamine cascades, inflammation, apoptosis), and needs rest (Bechtold & Hosey, 2018; Sobbi & van den Boogaard, 2014). Some patients are placed in a medically induced coma to lower metabolic activity and reduce the risk of secondary injury. Low-stimulation protocols are also put in place to prevent excessive activation and potential exacerbation of factors that can delay or interfere with recovery. Examples include minimizing noise; keeping the lights low; frequent reorientation, cueing, and reassurance; use of large clocks and calendars; placing familiar objects in the room; having eyeglasses and hearing aids available; and removal of Foley catheters (Devlin et al., 2018; Geense et al., 2019). Critically ill patients can become easily agitated. Although they are not directly curative, various environmental and systematic interventions have been associated with lower fall risk, shorter lengths of stay, and reduced complication rates (Boutron et al., 2008; Stucky & Warren, 2019; Trzepacz & Meagher, 2009). A systematic review and meta-analysis of nonpharmacologic interventions found that they were effective in reducing the rates and duration of delirium but did not change the ICU length of stay or mortality rates (Kang et al., 2018).

SLEEP INTERVENTIONS

Patients frequently experience sleep–wake cycle disturbances in which the diurnal rhythm is reversed, with significant daytime lethargy and agitated hyperarousal in the evening. While medications are often required, behavioral and rehabilitative interventions designed to promote normal, proper, and uninterrupted sleep are a critical part of the structured routine. Ear plugs and eye shades are sometimes helpful, especially considering how busy ICU environments can be. Staff can endeavor to cluster nighttime care, thereby minimizing sleep interruptions. At night, the lights are kept off and stimulation is reduced, although some patients benefit from a night light, fan, or other soothing and reassuring interventions, or a white noise machine. For patients on mechanical ventilation, Devlin and colleagues (2018) endorsed assist–control ventilation (ventilator delivers the same tidal volume for each breath whether or not the breath is initiated by the patient or the ventilator) at night as helpful to improve sleep. During scheduled times throughout the day, the room lights should be kept on and the curtains open while paired with structured range-of-motion exercises, progressive mobility, and other out-of-bed activities.

PHARMACOLOGIC INTERVENTIONS

There is a large and increasing literature concerning medications to manage delirium, behavioral issues, and sleep–wake cycle disturbances in critically ill patients (Bienvenu et al., 2017; Rothberg et al., 2013; Shehabi et al., 2010). Ideal medications for use with patients experiencing or predisposed to delirium include those with low toxicity, minimal anticholinergic effects, short half-life, minimal effect on cardiovascular and respiratory systems, and no or negligible effect on seizure threshold (Clegg & Young, 2011; Kennedy & Ryan, 2009). Also, polypharmacy or idiosyncratic reactions to certain drugs can easily contribute to the development of delirium and subsequent cognitive impairments. A discussion of pharmacologic interventions is beyond the scope of this chapter. Additional relevant information can be found in Chapter 11.

STAFF TRAINING AND SUPPORT

The critical care team is a synergistic, mutually dependent group with expertise in identifying and managing neurocognitive disorders. In our view, psychologists should be part of critical care teams and be involved with patient care and in providing staff training and support. For example, the psychologist can not only administer cognitive tests and questionnaires but also can train nurses and SLPs to perform and document results of brief cognitive screening assessments (e.g., O-Log, CAM-ICU). Psychologists can also communicate with families and patients regarding cognitive and behavioral status and the treatment plan. Such teamwork can also help spread out the workload and potentially reduce overall stress for the team as a whole (Stucky & Warren, 2019).

FAMILY EDUCATION AND SUPPORT

A sizable percentage of family members or other support persons (anyone the patient wants involved with their care, related or unrelated) report symptoms of acute stress disorder, depression, and anxiety during and after a loved one's critical care admission (Warren et al., 2016). Visitors and relatives may not be aware of or understand the behavioral changes in their loved ones with neurocognitive disorders, which can place tremendous strain on the family. Family members are often grateful for practical tips on what they should and should not do to help the patient. Developing a working alliance with families is important, as they are often heavily relied on to provide medical care, reassurance, and social support for the patient when discharged home. For example, Partners in Healing involves care activities for family members while their loved one is in the hospital and helps to prepare the families for discharge and caring for the patient at home (Van De Graaff et al., 2018). Examples of care activities include use of an incentive spirometer, fluid intake and output measurement, activity support, and applying compression stockings. Of the families surveyed, 92% (n = 106) believed that the Partners in Healing improved their ability to care for their critically ill family member at home and would recommend the program to others (Van De Graaff et al., 2018). Helping families understand and use techniques that increase the patient's participation with various treatments, that improve recovery, and that may reduce hospital readmissions is essential to optimizing outcomes (Jackson & Jutte, 2016; Jutte et al., 2017). Educating the family about environmental interventions or introducing ICU diaries can also facilitate and improve the overall quality of life, reduce post-ICU psychological disorders, and increase consistency of treatments to improve patient recovery (Garrouste-Orgeas et al., 2012; Jones et al., 2012).

For many survivors of critical illness or injury who experienced neurocognitive changes in the ICU, cognitive impairment may persist for months to years after hospital discharge (Girard et al., 2018; Gunther et al., 2012; Jutte et al., 2015; Needham et al., 2012; Pandharipande et al., 2013). These individuals may not be able to return to independent living, work, or driving (Hopkins et al., 2017; Kamdar et al., 2017). However, unless the patient and family members are explicitly warned about this, some survivors may resume activities prematurely and then have to deal with the consequences (e.g., family strain and misunderstanding, fired or let go from work, traffic accidents or tickets). These activities may need to be restricted for some time after ICU discharge and until formal neuropsychological assessments or functional capacity evaluations are conducted. For this reason, outpatient ICU follow-up clinics for critical illness survivors have been established in Europe and are becoming more common in the United States (Iwashyna & Netzer, 2012; Sevin et al., 2018; van der Schaaf et al., 2009). ICU follow-up clinics can help coordinate and screen for post-ICU morbidities and may include rehabilitative, psychological, and medical interventions to help patients recover and return to ADLs in a measured stepwise fashion. In these recovery clinics, cognitive screening or testing can be carried out to identify patients with persistent neurocognitive and psychological impairments and pinpoint individuals who require more detailed neuropsychological assessment and referrals for cognitive and physical rehabilitation. See Chapter 13 for additional details regarding ICU follow-up clinics.

REHABILITATION INTERVENTIONS

Nurses, respiratory therapists, and physical and occupational therapists can work collaboratively to set up progressive mobility, physical therapy, occupational therapy, and other beneficial rehabilitative interventions (Banerjee et al., 2011; Brummel et al., 2012; Brummel, Jackson, et al., 2014). Chapter 3 provides more detail regarding the benefits of early mobility and range-of-motion exercises to reduce complications and facilitate discharge home (Desai et al., 2011; Ely, 2017; Jackson et al., 2012; Miller et al., 2015; Schweickert et al., 2009).

COGNITIVE REHABILITATION

Cognitive rehabilitation is becoming more of a focus in ICU research. However, currently only a handful of studies have assessed the effectiveness of cognitive rehabilitation in critical illness survivors (Jackson et al., 2003, 2012). Table 6.1 provides a summary of those studies.

To date, six studies have assessed the feasibility and/or effects of cognitive rehabilitation in ICU populations (Brummel, Girard, et al., 2014; Jackson et al., 2012; Khan et al., 2015; Turon et al., 2017; Wilson et al., 2018; Zhao et al., 2017). The studies used a variety of interventions and have relatively small sample sizes. Two studies used Goal Management Training (GMT) or modified GMT plus physical rehabilitation to improve executive function (Jackson et al., 2012; Brummel, Girard, et al., 2014). GMT is designed to improve organizational abilities and facilitate goal attainment, important aspects of executive function. The study by Jackson and colleagues (2012) compared GMT plus physical rehabilitation in 21 medical/surgical ICU survivors who were randomized to usual care or the intervention (Jackson et al., 2012). The intervention was provided for 12 weeks after hospital discharge with six in-person visits and six telehealth sessions. At 3-month follow-up the intervention was found to be feasible, and the cognitive intervention group had significant improvements in executive function compared to usual care (Jackson et al., 2012).

The Activity and Cognitive Therapy study randomized 87 ICU survivors to usual care (*n* = 22), once-daily early physical therapy (*n* = 22), or combined early physical therapy and cognitive rehabilitation (*n* = 43) (Brummel, Girard, et al., 2014). The cognitive and physical intervention was provided while patients were in the ICU and on the hospital wards. The cognitive intervention using GMT continued for 12 weeks (six sessions) after hospital discharge. The cognitive part of the intervention included exercises that focused on attention, memory, executive function, and orientation to person, place, and time. Of the 43 patients in the cognitive and physical intervention group, most had cognitive therapy every day in the ICU and hospital. The researchers found that cognitive plus physical rehabilitation was feasible and safe in ICU survivors (Brummel, Girard, et al., 2014). However, there was no difference in cognitive function among the three groups at 3-month follow-up, which may be due to the sample size or loss to follow-up of patients who withdrew in the cognitive and physical rehabilitation group (Brummel, Girard, et al., 2014).

Other studies of cognitive rehabilitation in ICU survivors have used different cognitive interventions. Zhao and colleagues (2017) used a novel cognitive intervention that included learning to play an electronic keyboard, learning and speaking simple Spanish, memory for the time set on a clock face, and talking to a psychiatrist to improve psychological function 4 days per week for 3 months (see Table 6.1).

TABLE 6.1.

Studies of cognitive rehabilitation in the survivors of critical illness

Study	ICU population	Study type	N	Intervention	Major findings
Jackson et al., 2012	Medical/surgical	RCT with intervention and control groups	N = 21 (8 usual care; 13 physical and cognitive rehabilitation)	GMT and physical therapy	Significant improvement in executive function in the intervention group at 3-month follow-up
Brummel et al., 2014	Medical/surgical	RCT with intervention and control group	N = 87 (22 usual care; 22 physical therapy; 43 physical and cognitive rehabilitation)	Modified GMT and physical therapy	The study was feasible as nearly all patients were able to participate in cognitive and physical therapy. Physical therapy occurred on a majority of study days. The study was safe. There was no difference between intervention and control groups at 3 months.
Zhao et al., 2017	Mixed ICU population	RCT with intervention and control groups	N = 332 (165 controls; 167 intervention)	Cognitive intervention (including play a musical keyboard, learn simple Spanish, view a clock, and draw from memory 10 minutes later) and talk to psychiatrist for mental health	The cognitive intervention reduced worsening of cognitive function. Cognitive intervention improved memory, attention, and language. Younger patients were more likely to have improved cognitive function than were older patients.

Study	Population	Design	Sample	Intervention	Findings
Khan et al., 2015	Mixed ICU population	Prospective cohort study	$N = 52$; 24 were evaluated on their first clinic visit and at least one additional visit	The Critical Care Recovery Center developed standardized minimal care components including assessment and cognitive management. Each patient received an individualized management plan.	The cognitive score declined from the initial assessment, improving from 19.21 to 14.75 (lower scores suggest better cognitive function). The Critical Care Recovery Center is using an innovative approach to interventions to improve cognitive outcome.
Turon et al., 2017	Medical/ surgical	Prospective cohort study	$N = 20$	Daily cognitive stimulation sessions for 20 minutes using Early Neurocognitive Rehabilitation in Intensive Care (ENRIC) platform	Virtual reality for cognitive rehabilitation was safe and feasible and patients were able to tolerate the training. Patients completed 87% of possible neurocognitive stimulation sessions. Critically ill patients reported that the virtual reality sessions were enjoyable and relaxing.
Wilson et al., 2018	Medical/ surgical	Prospective cohort study	$N =33$; comparison of baseline scores with post-training scores	Computerized cognitive rehabilitation with training in memory, auditory and verbal processing, attention, executive control, and response speed, 5 days a week for 12 weeks	Cognitive function improved across the cognitive domains from baseline performance. The amount of improvement was associated with the number of training hours. In addition, neuropsychological tests showed significant improvement in digit span, spatial span, and Trail Making Test parts A and B compared to these same measures at baseline.

GMT = Goal Management Training; RCT = randomized controlled trial

The intervention improved memory, attention, and language and reduced worsening cognitive function in the intervention group (Zhao et al., 2017). Khan and colleagues (2015) assessed and developed an individual management plan to improve cognitive impairments for patients seen in an ICU follow-up clinic. ICU survivors' cognitive function improved in the group that received an individualized management plan (Khan et al., 2015). Turon and colleagues (2017) used virtual reality for cognitive rehabilitation and found it to be safe and feasible, and patients were able to tolerate the intervention. Finally, Wilson and colleagues (2018) used computerized cognitive rehabilitation focused on improving memory, attention, executive control, and response time. They found that cognitive function improved across cognitive domains when comparing baseline performance to post-intervention scores (Wilson et al., 2018).

While the number of studies is limited and sample sizes are small, these studies suggest that cognitive rehabilitation with critical illness survivors may be a promising strategy. Research is needed to determine (1) which interventions provide benefit; (2) the optimal timing, duration, and intensity of the intervention; (3) what ICU populations will benefit from cognitive rehabilitation; (4) whether the effect of cognitive rehabilitation generalizes beyond the specific tasks used; and (5) whether combined cognitive and physical rehabilitation provides greater benefit than cognitive rehabilitation alone.

REHABILITATION DURING COVID-19

Physical and cognitive rehabilitation of survivors of critical illness is an important part of care following ICU discharge to address the physical, cognitive, and psychological morbidities. Patients who survive COVID-19 after admission to the ICU will likely require inpatient and outpatient rehabilitation. However, implementation of rehabilitation is challenging in patients with COVID-19 and other highly infectious diseases, as personal protective equipment (PPE) must be worn by staff and rehabilitation units need to adopt restrictive procedures to minimize spread of the disease (Simpson & Robinson, 2020). In both inpatient and outpatient settings, telemedicine sessions may be essential to provide rehabilitation services, prevent spread of the disease, protect clinicians, and preserve PPE (Simpson & Robinson, 2020). Several physical and cognitive rehabilitation studies in ICU patients that used a combination of acute in-person rehabilitation and telerehabilitation interventions were shown to be safe and feasible and to improve cognitive function at 3-month follow-up (Brummel, Girard, et al., 2014; Jackson et al., 2012). However, it should be noted that telerehabilitation has limitations, including lack of rehabilitation equipment in the homes, limited abilities to conduct physical examination, and lack of rehabilitation personnel to help with activities and ensure safety (Simpson & Robinson, 2020).

There is a need to adapt quickly to provide rehabilitation services to the large and growing group of survivors of COVID-19. In the future, patients with highly infectious conditions like COVID-19 will have rehabilitation needs that require an evidence-based approach (Ceravolo et al., 2020). A systematic review of rehabilitation in patients with COVID-19 (Ceravolo et al., 2020) provided several recommendations, including:

1. Early rehabilitation and progressive mobility should be carried out whenever safe and possible on the ICU.
2. For patients in quarantine or lockdown, rehabilitation should focus on mobility while also addressing cognitive decline and emotional adjustment issues.
3. Telerehabilitation may be the first option for patients discharged home.
4. Protection of rehabilitation professionals is essential for rehabilitation to occur.

Physical and cognitive rehabilitation is essential to facilitate recovery after hospital discharge in patients with COVID-19. Development and use of telerehabilitation and telecognitive rehabilitation along with other novel interventions are essential to provide the care that COVID-19 survivors need.

Conclusion

Critical illness and injury survivors often incur or develop major neurocognitive disorders that can persist months to years after leaving the hospital. The neurocognitive impairments have profound long-term effects on ability to return to work, instrumental ADLs, and quality of life. Caring for these survivors requires a comprehensive interdisciplinary team approach because they often present with a complex array of medical, behavioral, emotional, and cognitive sequelae. Specialty psychologists, particularly those with expertise in rehabilitation psychology, are uniquely qualified and can be a tremendous asset to the critical care team.

References

Alderson, A. L., & Novack, T. A. (2003). Reliable serial measurement of cognitive processes in rehabilitation: The Cognitive Log. *Archives of Physical Medicine and Rehabilitation, 84*(5), 668–672. doi:10.1016/s0003-9993(02)04842-6

American Psychological Association Practice Organization. (2014, December). Distinguishing between screening and assessment for mental and behavioral health problems: A statement from an American Psychological Association Practice Organization work group on screening and psychological assessment. http://www.apapracticecentral.org/reimbursement/billing/assessment-screening.aspx

Banerjee, A., Girard, T. D., & Pandharipande, P. (2011). The complex interplay between delirium, sedation, and early mobility during critical illness: Applications in the trauma unit. *Current Opinion in Anaesthesiology, 24*(2), 195–201. doi:10.1097/ACO.0b013e3283445382

Barr, J., Fraser, G. L., Puntillo, K., Ely, E. W., Gelinas, C., Dasta, J. F., . . . American College of Critical Care Medicine. (2013). Clinical practice guidelines for the management of pain, agitation, and delirium in adult patients in the intensive care unit. *Critical Care Medicine, 41*(1), 263–306. doi:10.1097/CCM.0b013e3182783b72

Bechtold, K. T., & Hosey, M. M. (2018). Consciousness: Disorders, assessment, and intervention. In J. E. Morgan & J. H. Ricker (Eds.), *Textbook of clinical neuropsychology* (2nd ed., pp. 332–350). Taylor and Francis.

Bienvenu, O. J., Jones, C., & Hopkins, R. O. (2017). *Psychological and cognitive impact of critical illness*. Oxford University Press.

Block, C. K., Johnson-Greene, D., Pliskin, N., & Boake, C. (2017). Discriminating cognitive screening and cognitive testing from neuropsychological assessment: Implications for professional practice. *Clinical Neuropsychologist, 31*(3), 487–500. doi:10.1080/13854046.2016.1267803

Boutron, I., Moher, D., Altman, D. G., Schulz, K. F., Ravaud, P., & Group, C. (2008). Extending the CONSORT statement to randomized trials of nonpharmacologic treatment: Explanation and elaboration. *Annals of Internal Medicine, 148*(4), 295–309. doi:10.7326/0003-4819-148-4-200802190-00008

Bruck, E., Schandl, A., Bottai, M., & Sackey, P. (2018). The impact of sepsis, delirium, and psychological distress on self-rated cognitive function in ICU survivors: A prospective cohort study. *Journal of Intensive Care, 6*, 2. doi:10.1186/s40560-017-0272-6

Brummel, N. E., Girard, T. D., Ely, E. W., Pandharipande, P. P., Morandi, A., Hughes, C. G., . . . Jackson, J. C. (2014). Feasibility and safety of early combined cognitive and physical therapy for critically ill medical and surgical patients: The Activity and Cognitive Therapy in ICU (ACT-ICU) trial. *Intensive Care Medicine, 40*(3), 370–379. doi:10.1007/s00134-013-3136-0

Brummel, N. E., Jackson, J. C., Girard, T. D., Pandharipande, P. P., Schiro, E., Work, B., . . . Ely, E. W. (2012). A combined early cognitive and physical rehabilitation program for people who are critically ill: The Activity and Cognitive Therapy in the Intensive Care Unit (ACT-ICU) trial. *Physical Therapy, 92*(12), 1580–1592. doi:10.2522/ptj.20110414

Brummel, N. E., Jackson, J. C., Pandharipande, P. P., Thompson, J. L., Shintani, A. K., Dittus, R. S., . . . Girard, T. D. (2014). Delirium in the ICU and subsequent long-term disability among survivors of mechanical ventilation. *Critical Care Medicine, 42*(2), 369–377. doi:10.1097/CCM.0b013e3182a645bd

Calsavara, A. J. C., Costa, P. A., Nobre, V., & Teixeira, A. L. (2018). Factors associated with short- and long-term cognitive changes in patients with sepsis. *Scientific Reports, 8*(1), 4509. doi:10.1038/s41598-018-22754-3

Ceravolo, M. G., de Sire, A., Andrenelli, E., Negrini, F., & Negrini, S. (2020). Systematic rapid "living" review on rehabilitation needs due to COVID-19: Update to March 31st,

2020. *European Journal of Physical Rehabilitation Medicine, 56*(3), 347–353. doi:10.23736/S1973-9087.20.06329-7

Clegg, A., & Young, J. B. (2011). Which medications to avoid in people at risk of delirium: A systematic review. *Age Ageing, 40*(1), 23–29. doi:10.1093/ageing/afq140

Cohen, S., Sprung, C., Sjokvist P., Lippert, A., Ricou, B., Baras, M., . . . Woodcock, T. (2005), Communication of end-of-life decisions in European intensive care units. *Intensive Care Medicine, 31*(9), 1215–1221.

Desai, S. V., Law, T. J., & Needham, D. M. (2011). Long-term complications of critical care. *Critical Care Medicine, 39*(2), 371–379. doi:10.1097/CCM.0b013e3181fd66e5

Devlin, J. W., Skrobik, Y., Gelinas, C., Needham, D. M., Slooter, A. J. C., Pandharipande, P. P., . . . Alhazzani, W. (2018). Clinical practice guidelines for the prevention and management of pain, agitation/sedation, delirium, immobility, and sleep disruption in adult patients in the ICU. *Critical Care Medicine, 46*(9), e825–e873. doi:10.1097/CCM.0000000000003299

de Wit, E., van Doremalen, N., Falzarano, D., & Munster, V. J. (2016). SARS and MERS: Recent insights into emerging coronaviruses. *Nature Reviews Microbiology, 14*(8), 523–534. doi:10.1038/nrmicro.2016.81

Elliott, D., Davidson, J. E., Harvey, M. A., Bemis-Dougherty, A., Hopkins, R. O., Iwashyna, T. J., . . . Needham, D. M. (2014). Exploring the scope of post-intensive care syndrome therapy and care: Engagement of non-critical care providers and survivors in a second stakeholders meeting. *Critical Care Medicine, 42*(12), 2518–2526. doi:10.1097/CCM.0000000000000525

Ellul, M. A., Benjamin, L., Singh, B., Lant, S., Michael, B. D., Easton, A., . . . Solomon, T. (2020). Neurological associations of COVID-19. *Lancet Neurology, 19*(9), P767–P783. doi:10.1016/S1474-4422(20)30221-0

Ely, E. W. (2017). The ABCDEF bundle: Science and philosophy of how ICU liberation serves patients and families. *Critical Care Medicine, 45*(2), 321–330. doi:10.1097/CCM.0000000000002175

Ely, E. W., Girard, T. D., Shintani, A. K., Jackson, J. C., Gordon, S. M., Thomason, J. W., . . . Laskowitz, D. T. (2007). Apolipoprotein E4 polymorphism as a genetic predisposition to delirium in critically ill patients. *Critical Care Medicine, 35*(1), 112–117.

Ely, E. W., Margolin, R., Francis, J., May, L., Truman, B., Ditus, R., Speroff, T., Gautam, S., Bernard, G. R., & Inouye, S. K. (2001). Evaluation of delirium in critically ill patients: Validation of the Confusion Assessment Method for the Intensive Care Unit (CAM-ICU). *Critical Care Medicine, 29*(7), 1370–1379. doi:10.1097/00003246-200107000-00012

Ely, E. W., Shintani, A., Truman, B., Speroff, T., Gordon, S. M., Harrell, F. E., Jr., . . . Dittus, R. S. (2004). Delirium as a predictor of mortality in mechanically ventilated patients in the intensive care unit. *Journal of the American Medical Association, 291*(14), 1753–1762.

Fitsiori, A., Pugin, D., Thieffry, C., Lalive, P., & Vargas, M. I. (2020). Unusual microbleeds in brain MRI of Covid-19 patients. *Journal of Neuroimaging, 30*(5), 593–597. doi:10.1111/jon.12755

Folstein, M. F., Folstein, S. E., & Mchugh, P. R. (1975). "Mini-Mental State": A practical method for grading cognitive state of patients for the clinician. *Journal of Psychiatric Research, 12*, 189–198.

Fong, T. G., Fearing, M. A., Jones, R. N., Pellin, S., Marcantonio, E. R., Rudolph, J. L., Yang, F. M., Kiely, D. K., & Inouye, S. K. (2009). The Telephone Interview for Cognitive Status: Creating a crosswalk with the Mini-Mental State Exam. *Alzheimer's & Dementia, 5*(6), 492–497. doi:10.1016/j.jalz.2009.02.007

Garrouste-Orgeas, M., Coquet, I., Perier, A., Timsit, J. F., Pochard, F., Lancrin, F., . . . Misset, B. (2012). Impact of an intensive care unit diary on psychological distress in patients and relatives. *Critical Care Medicine, 40*(7), 2033–2040. doi:10.1097/CCM.0b013e31824e1b43

Geense, W. W., van den Boogaard, M., van der Hoeven, J. G., Vermeulen, H., Hannink, G., & Zegers, M. (2019). Nonpharmacologic interventions to prevent or mitigate adverse long-term outcomes among ICU survivors: A systematic review and meta-analysis. *Critical Care Medicine, 47*(11), 1607–1618. doi:10.1097/CCM.0000000000003974

Gelinas, C., Klein, K., Naidech, A. M., & Skrobik, Y. (2013). Pain, sedation, and delirium management in the neurocritically ill: Lessons learned from recent research. *Seminars in Respiratory and Critical Care Medicine, 34*(2), 236–243. doi:10.1055/s-0033-1342986

Girard, T. D., Thompson, J. L., Pandharipande, P. P., Brummel, N. E., Jackson, J. C., Patel, M. B., . . . Ely, E. W. (2018). Clinical phenotypes of delirium during critical illness and severity of subsequent long-term cognitive impairment: A prospective cohort study. *Lancet Respiratory Medicine, 6*(3), 213–222. doi:10.1016/S2213-2600(18)30062-6

Grisso, T., & Applebaum, P. S. (1998). *Assessing competence to consent to treatment: A guide for physicians and other health professionals.* Oxford University Press.

Guerra, C., Linde-Zwirble, W. T., & Wunsch, H. (2012). Risk factors for dementia after critical illness in elderly Medicare beneficiaries. *Critical Care, 16*(6), R233. doi:10.1186/cc11901

Gunther, M. L., Morandi, A., Krauskopf, E., Pandharipande, P., Girard, T. D., Jackson, J. C., Thompson, J., Shintani, A. K., Geevarghese, S., Miller, R. R. III, Canonico, A., Merkle, K., Cannistraci, C. J., Rogers, B. P., Gatenby, J. C., Heckers, S., Gore, J. C., Hopkins, R. O., Ely, E. W., for the VISIONS Investigation (VISualizing Icu SurvivOrs Neuroradiological Sequelae). (2012). The association between brain volumes, delirium duration, and cognitive outcomes in intensive care unit survivors: The VISIONS cohort magnetic resonance imaging study. *Critical Care Medicine, 40*(7), 2022–2032. doi:10.1097/CCM.0b013e318250acc0

Hanks, R. A., Millis, S. R., Ricker, J. H., Giacino, J. T., Nakese-Richardson, R., Frol, A. B., . . . Gordon, W. A. (2008). The predictive validity of a brief inpatient neuropsychologic battery for persons with traumatic brain injury. *Archives of Physical Medicine and Rehabilitation, 89*(5), 950–957. doi:10.1016/j.apmr.2008.01.011

Hauschildt, K. E., Seigworth, C., Kamphuis, L. A., Hough, C. L., Moss, M., McPeake, J. M., Iwashyna, T. J., & National Heart, Lung, and Blood Institute Prevention and Early Treatment of Acute Lung Injury (PETAL) Network. (2020). Financial toxicity after acute respiratory distress syndrome: A national qualitative cohort study. *Critical Care Medicine, 48*(8), 1103–1110. doi:10.1097/CCM.0000000000004378

Helms, J., Kremer, S., Merdji, H., Clere-Jehl, R., Schenck, M., Kummerlen, C., . . . Meziani, F. (2020). Neurologic features in severe SARS-CoV-2 infection. *New England Journal of Medicine, 382*(23), 2268–2270. doi:10.1056/NEJMc2008597

Honarmand, K., Lalli, R. S., Priestap, F., Chen, J. L., McIntyre, C. W., Owen, A. M., & Slessarev, M. (2020). Natural history of cognitive impairment in critical illness survivors: A systematic review. *American Journal of Respiratory and Critical Care Medicine, 202*(2), 193–201. doi:10.1164/rccm.201904-0816CI

Hopkins, R. O., Gale, S. D., & Weaver, L. K. (2006). Brain atrophy and cognitive impairment in survivors of acute respiratory distress syndrome. *Brain Injury, 20*(3), 263–271. doi:10.1080/02699050500488199

Hopkins, R. O., Suchyta, M. R., Beene, K., & Jackson, J. C. (2016). Critical illness acquired brain injury: Neuroimaging and implications for rehabilitation. *Rehabilitation Psychology, 61*(2), 151–164. doi:10.1037/rep0000088

Hopkins, R. O., Suchyta, M. R., Kamdar, B. B., Darowski, E., Jackson, J. C., & Needham, D. M. (2017). Instrumental activities of daily living after critical illness: A systematic review. *Annals of the American Thoracic Society, 14*(8), 1332–1343.:10.1513/AnnalsATS.201701-059SR

Hopkins, R. O., Weaver, L. K., Collingridge, D., Parkinson, R. B., Chan, K. J., & Orme, J. F., Jr. (2005). Two-year cognitive, emotional, and quality-of-life outcomes in acute respiratory distress syndrome. *American Journal of Respiratory and Critical Care Medicine, 171*(4), 340–347. http://www.atsjournals.org/doi/pdf/10.1164/rccm.200406-763OC.

Hopkins, R. O., Weaver, L. K., Pope, D., Orme, J. F., Jr., Bigler, E. D., & Larson-Lohr, V. (1999). Neuropsychological sequelae and impaired health status in survivors of severe acute respiratory distress syndrome. *American Journal of Respiratory and Critical Care Medicine, 160*(1), 50–56.

Hughes, C. G., Pandharipande, P. P., Thompson, J. L., Chandrasekhar, R., Ware, L. B., Ely, E. W., & Girard, T. D. (2016). Endothelial activation and blood-brain barrier injury as risk factors for delirium in critically ill patients. *Critical Care Medicine, 44*(9), e809–e817. doi:10.1097/CCM.0000000000001739

Iwashyna, T. J., Ely, E. W., Smith, D. M., & Langa, K. M. (2010). Long-term cognitive impairment and functional disability among survivors of severe sepsis. *Journal of the American Medical Association, 304*(16), 1787–1794.

Iwashyna, T. J., & Netzer, G. (2012). The burdens of survivorship: An approach to thinking about long-term outcomes after critical illness. *Seminars in Respiratory and Critical Care Medicine, 33*(4), 327–338. doi:10.1055/s-0032-1321982

Jackson, J. C., Ely, E. W., Morey, M. C., Anderson, V. M., Denne, L. B., Clune, J., . . . Hoenig, H. (2012). Cognitive and physical rehabilitation of intensive care unit survivors: Results of the RETURN randomized controlled pilot investigation. *Critical Care Medicine, 40*(4), 1088–1097. doi:10.1097/CCM.0b013e3182373115

Jackson, J. C., Hart, R. P., Gordon, S. M., Shintani, A., Truman, B., May, L., & Ely, E. W. (2003). Six-month neuropsychological outcome of medical intensive care unit patients. *Critical Care Medicine, 31*(4), 1226–1234.

Jackson, J. C., & Jutte, J. E. (2016). Rehabilitating a missed opportunity: Integration of rehabilitation psychology into the care of critically ill patients, survivors, and caregivers. *Rehabilitation Psychology, 61*(2), 115–119. doi:10.1037/rep0000091

Jackson, J. C., Morandi, A., Girard, T. D., Merkle, K., Graves, A. J., Thompson, J. L., Shintani, A. K., Gunther, M. L., Cannistraci, C. J., Rogers, B. P., Gore, J. C., Warrington, H. J., Ely, E. W., Hopkins, R. O., & VISualizing Icu SurvivOrs Neuroradiological Sequelae (VISIONS) Investigation. (2015). Functional brain imaging in survivors of critical illness: A prospective feasibility study and exploration of the association between delirium and brain activation patterns. *Journal of Critical Care, 30*(3), 653 e651–657. doi:10.1016/j.jcrc.2015.01.017

Jackson, J. C., Warrington, H. J., Kessler, R., Kiehl, A. L., & Ely, W. E. (2018). Florbetapir-PET beta-amyloid imaging and associated neuropsychological trajectories in survivors of critical illness: A case series. *Journal of Critical Care, 44*, 331–336. doi:10.1016/j.jcrc.2017.10.016

Jones, C., Bäckman, C., & Griffiths, R. D. (2012). Intensive care diaries and relatives' symptoms of posttraumatic stress disorder after critical illness: A pilot study. *American Journal of Critical Care, 21*(3), 172–176. doi:10.4037/ajcc2012569

Jutte, J. E., Erb, C. T., & Jackson, J. C. (2015). Physical, cognitive, and psychological disability following critical illness: What is the risk? *Seminars in Respiratory and Critical Care Medicine, 36*(6), 943–958. doi:10.1055/s-0035-1566002

Jutte, J. E., Jackson, J. C., & Hopkins, R. O. (2017). Rehabilitation psychology insights for treatments of critical illness. In O. J. Bienvenu, C. Jones, & R. O. Hopkins (Eds.), *Psychological and cognitive impact of critical illness* (pp. 105–139). Oxford University Press.

Kamdar, B. B., Huang, M., Dinglas, V. D., Colantuoni, E., von Wachter, T. M., Hopkins, R. O., Needham, D. M., & National Heart, Lung, and Blood Institute Acute Respiratory Distress Syndrome Network. (2017). Joblessness and lost earnings after acute respiratory distress syndrome in a 1-year national multicenter study. *American Journal of Respiratory and Critical Care Medicine, 196*(8), 1012–1020. doi:10.1164/rccm.201611-2327OC

Kamdar, B. B., Suri, R., Suchyta, M. R., Digrande, K. F., Sherwood, K. D., Colantuoni, E., . . . Hopkins, R. O. (2020). Return to work after critical illness: A systematic review and meta-analysis. *Thorax, 75*(1), 17–27. doi:10.1136/thoraxjnl-2019-213803

Kang, J., Lee, M., Ko, H., Kim, S., Yun, S., Jeong, Y., & Cho, Y. (2018). Effect of nonpharmacological interventions for the prevention of delirium in the intensive care unit: A systematic review and meta-analysis. *Journal of Critical Care, 48*, 372–384. doi:10.1016/j.jcrc.2018.09.032

Karlawish, J. (2008). Measuring decision-making capacity in cognitively impaired individuals. *Neurosignals, 16*(1), 91–98.

Katal, S., Balakrishnan, S., & Gholamrezanezhad, A. (2021). Neuroimaging and neurologic findings in COVID-19 and other coronavirus infections: A systematic review in 116 patients. *Journal of Neuroradiology, 48*(1), 43–50. doi:10.1016/j.neurad.2020.06.007

Kennedy, K. A., & Ryan, M. (2009). Neurotoxic effects of pharmaceutical agents III: Neurological agents. In M. R. Dobbs (Ed.), *Clinical neurotoxicology: Syndromes, substances, environments* (pp. 358–371). Saunders and Elsevier.

Khan, B. A., Lasiter, S., & Boustani, M. A. (2015). CE: Critical care recovery center: An innovative collaborative care model for ICU survivors. *American Journal of Nursing, 115*(3), 24–31; quiz 34, 46. doi:10.1097/01.NAJ.0000461807.42226.3e

Kok, L., Slooter, A. J., Hillegers, M. H., van Dijk, D., & Veldhuijzen, D. S. (2018). Benzodiazepine use and neuropsychiatric outcomes in the ICU: A systematic review. *Critical Care Medicine, 46*(10), 1673–1680. doi:10.1097/CCM.0000000000003300

Kukull, W. A., Larson, E. G., Teri, L., Bowen, J., McCormick, W., & Pfanschmidt, M. G. (1994). The Mini-Mental State Examination score and the clinical diagnosis of dementia. *Clinical Epidemiology, 47*, 1061–1067.

Li, Y. C., Bai, W. Z., & Hashikawa, T. (2020). The neuroinvasive potential of SARS-CoV2 may play a role in the respiratory failure of COVID-19 patients. *Journal of Medical Virology, 92*(6), 552–555. doi:10.1002/jmv.25728

Lines, C. R., McCarroll, K. A., Lipton, R. B., & Block, G. A. (2003). Telephone screening for amnestic mild cognitive impairment. *Neurology, 60*(2), 261–266. doi:10.1212/01.wnl.0000042481.34899.13

Liotta, E. M., Batra, A., Clark, J. R., Shlobin, N. A., Hoffman, S. C., Orban, Z. S., & Koralnik, I. J. (2020). Frequent neurologic manifestations and encephalopathy-associated morbidity in Covid-19 patients. *Annals of Clinical and Translational Neurology, 7*(11), 2221–2230. doi:10.1002/acn3.51210

Mao, L., Jin, H., Wang, M., Hu, Y., Chen, S., He, Q., Chang, J., Hong, C., Zhou, Y., Wang, D., Miao, X., Li, Y., &. Hu, B. (2020). Neurologic manifestations of hospitalized patients with coronavirus disease 2019 in Wuhan, China. *JAMA Neurology, 77*(6), 683–690. doi:10.1001/jamaneurol.2020.1127

Marra, A., Pandharipande, P. P., Girard, T. D., Patel, M. B., Hughes, C. G., Jackson, J. C., . . . Brummel, N. E. (2018). Co-occurrence of post-intensive care syndrome problems among 406 survivors of critical illness. *Critical Care Medicine, 46*(9), 1393–1401. doi:10.1097/CCM.0000000000003218

McCoy, T. H., Jr., Hart, K. L., & Perlis, R. H. (2017). Characterizing and predicting rates of delirium across general hospital settings. *General Hospital Psychiatry, 46*, 1–6. doi:10.1016/j.genhosppsych.2017.01.006

McLoughlin, B. C., Miles, A., Webb, T. E., Knopp, P., Eyres, C., Fabbri, A., Humphries, F., & Davis, D. (2020). Functional and cognitive outcomes after COVID-19 delirium. *European Geriatric Medicine, 11*(6), 857–862. doi:10.1007/s41999-020-00353-8

Mikkelsen, M. E., Christie, J. D., Lanken, P. N., Biester, R. C., Thompson, B. T., Bellamy, S. L., . . . Angus, D. C. (2012). The adult respiratory distress syndrome cognitive outcomes study: Long-term neuropsychological function in survivors of acute lung injury. *America Journal of Respiratory and Critical Care Medicine, 185*(12), 1307–1315. doi:10.1164/rccm.201111-2025OC

Miller, M. A., Govindan, S., Watson, S. R., Hyzy, R. C., & Iwashyna, T. J. (2015). ABCDE, but in that order? A cross-sectional survey of Michigan intensive care unit sedation, delirium, and early mobility practices. *Annals of the American Thoracic Society, 12*(7), 1066–1071.

Montalvan, V., Lee, J., Bueso, T., De Toledo, J., & Rivas, K. (2020). Neurological manifestations of COVID-19 and other coronavirus infections: A systematic review. *Clinical Neurology and Neurosurgery, 194*, 105921. doi:10.1016/j.clineuro.2020.105921

Morandi, A., Gunther, M. L., Vasilevskis, E. E., Girard, T. D., Hopkins, R. O., Jackson, J. C., . . . Ely, E. W. (2010). Neuroimaging in delirious intensive care unit patients: A preliminary case series report. *Psychiatry, 7*(9), 28–33.

Morandi, A., Rogers, B. P., Gunther, M. L., Merkle, K., Pandharipande, P., Girard, T. D., Jackson, J. C., Thompson, J., Shintani, A. K., Geevarghese, S., Miller, R. R. 3rd, Canonico, A., Cannistraci, C. J., Gore, J. C., Ely, E. W., Hopkins, R. O., &. . . Visions Investigation, VISualizing Icu SurvivOrs Neuroradiological Sequelae. (2012). The relationship between delirium duration, white matter integrity, and cognitive impairment in intensive care unit survivors as determined by diffusion tensor imaging: The VISIONS prospective cohort magnetic resonance imaging study. *Critical Care Medicine, 40*(7), 2182–2189. doi:10.1097/CCM.0b013e318250acdc

Nasreddine, A. S., Phillips, N. A., Vedirian, V., Charbonneau S., Whitehead, V., Collin I., Cummings, J. L., & Chertkow, H., (2005). The Montreal Cognitive Assessment, MoCA: A brief screening tool for mild cognitive impairment. *Journal of the American Geriatrics Society, 53*(4), 695–699. doi:10.1111/j.1532-5415.2005.53221.x

Needham, D. M., Colantuoni, E., Dinglas, V. D., Hough, C. L., Wozniak, A. W., Jackson, J. C., . . . Hopkins, R. O. (2016). Rosuvastatin versus placebo for delirium in intensive care and subsequent cognitive impairment in patients with sepsis-associated acute respiratory distress syndrome: An ancillary study to a randomised controlled trial. *Lancet Respiratory Medicine, 4*(3), 203–212. doi:10.1016/S2213-2600(16)00005-9

Needham, D. M., Davidson, J., Cohen, H., Hopkins, R. O., Weinert, C., Wunsch, H., . . . Harvey, M. A. (2012). Improving long-term outcomes after discharge from intensive care unit: Report from a stakeholders' conference. *Critical Care Medicine, 40*(2), 502–509. doi:10.1097/CCM.0b013e318232da75

Needham, D. M., Dinglas, V. D., Bienvenu, O. J., Colantuoni, E., Wozniak, A. W., Rice, T. W., Hopkins, R. O., & NIH NHLBI ARDS Network. (2013). One year outcomes in patients with acute lung injury randomised to initial trophic or full enteral feeding: Prospective follow-up of EDEN randomised trial. *British Medical Journal, 346,* f1532. doi:10.1136/bmj.f1532

Needham, D. M., Dinglas, V. D., Morris, P. E., Jackson, J. C., Hough, C. L., Mendez-Tellez, P. A., Wozniak, A. W., Colantuoni, E., Ely, E. W., Rice, T. W., Hopkins, R. O, & NIH NHLBI ARDS Network. (2013). Physical and cognitive performance of patients with acute lung injury 1 year after initial trophic versus full enteral feeding. EDEN trial follow-up. *American Journal of Respiratory and Critical Care Medicine, 188*(5), 567–576. doi:10.1164/rccm.201304-0651OC

Needham, E. J., Chou, S. H., Coles, A. J., & Menon, D. K. (2020). Neurological implications of COVID-19 infections. *Neurocritical Care, 32*(3), 667–671. doi:10.1007/s12028-020-00978-4

Negrini, F., Ferrario, I., Mazziotti, D., Berchicci, M., Bonazzi, M., de Sire, A., Negrini, S., & Zapparoli, L. (2021). Neuropsychological features of severe hospitalized COVID-19 patients at clinical stability and clues for post-acute rehabilitation. *Archives of Physical Medicine and Rehabilitation, 102*(1), 155–158. doi:10.1016/j.apmr.2020.09.376

Novak, T. A., Dowler, R. N., Bush, B. A., Glen, T, & Schneider, J. J., (2000). Validity of the Orientation log, relative to the Galveston Orientation and Amnesia Test. *Journal of Head Trauma Rehabilitation, 15*(3), 957–961. doi: 10.1097/00001199-200006000-00008

Palmer, B.W. & Harmell, A.L. (2016). Assessment of healthcare decision-making capacity. *Archives of Clinical Neuropsychology, 31*, 530–540.

Pandharipande, P. P., Girard, T. D., Jackson, J. C., Morandi, A., Thompson, J. L., Pun, B. T., . . . Ely, E. W. (2013). Long-term cognitive impairment after critical illness. *New England Journal of Medicine, 369*(14), 1306–1316. doi:10.1056/NEJMoa1301372

Petrosillo, N., Viceconte, G., Ergonul, O., Ippolito, G., & Petersen, E. (2020). COVID-19, SARS and MERS: Are they closely related? *Clinical Microbiology Infection, 26*(6), 729–734. doi:10.1016/j.cmi.2020.03.026

Pfoh, E. R., Chan, K. S., Dinglas, V. D., Girard, T. D., Jackson, J. C., Morris, P. E., . . . Hopkins, R. O. (2015). Cognitive screening among acute respiratory failure survivors: A cross-sectional evaluation of the Mini-Mental State Examination. *Critical Care, 19*, 220. doi:10.1186/s13054-015-0934-5

Polito, A., Eischwald, F., Maho, A. L., Polito, A., Azabou, E., Annane, D., . . . Sharshar, T. (2013). Pattern of brain injury in the acute setting of human septic shock. *Critical Care, 17*(5), R204. doi:10.1186/cc12899

Previgliano, I. J., Andres, B., & Ciesiclczyk, P. J. (2015). Long-term cognitive impairment after critical illness: Definition, incidence, pathophysiology and hypothesis of neurotrophic treatment. *European Neurological Review, 10*(2), 195–203. http://doi.org/10.17925/ENR.2015.10.02.195

Rawal, G., Yadav, S., & Kumar, R. (2017). Post-intensive care syndrome: An overview. *Journal of Translational Internal Medicine, 5*(2), 90–92.

Rengel, K. F., Hayhurst, C. J., Pandharipande, P. P., & Hughes, C. G. (2019). Long-term cognitive and functional impairments after critical illness. *Anesthesia and Analgesia, 128*(4), 772–780. doi:10.1213/ANE.0000000000004066

Richardson, S., Hirsch, J. S., Narasimhan, M., Crawford, J. M., McGinn, T., Davidson, K. W., . . . Zanos, T. P. (2020). Presenting characteristics, comorbidities, and outcomes among 5700 patients hospitalized with COVID-19 in the New York City area. *Journal of the American Medical Association, 323*(20), 2052–2059. doi:10.1001/jama.2020.6775

Roebuck-Spencer, T. M., Glen, T., Puente, A. E., Denney, R. L., Ruff, R. M., Hostetter, G., & Bianchini, K. J. (2017). Cognitive screening tests versus comprehensive neuropsychological test batteries: A National Academy of Neuropsychology education paper *Archives of Clinical Neuropsychology, 32*(4), 491–498. doi:10.1093/arclin/acx021

Rogers, J. P., Chesney, E., Oliver, D., Pollak, T. A., McGuire, P., Fusar-Poli, P., . . . David, A. S. (2020). Psychiatric and neuropsychiatric presentations associated with severe coronavirus infections: A systematic review and meta-analysis with comparison to the COVID-19 pandemic. *Lancet Psychiatry, 7*(7), 611–627. doi:10.1016/S2215-0366(20)30203-0

Rothberg, M. B., Herzig, S. J., Pekow, P. S., Avrunin, J., Lagu, T., & Lindenauer, P. K. (2013). Association between sedating medications and delirium in older inpatients. *Journal of the American Geriatric Society, 61*(6), 923–930. doi:10.1111/jgs.12253

Sakusic, A., O'Horo, J. C., Dziadzko, M., Volha, D., Ali, R., Singh, T. D., . . . Rabinstein, A. A. (2018). Potentially modifiable risk factors for long-term cognitive impairment after critical illness: A systematic review. *Mayo Clinic Proceedings, 93*(1), 68–82. doi:10.1016/j.mayocp.2017.11.005

Salluh, J. I., Wang, H., Schneider, E. B., Nagaraja, N., Yenokyan, G., Damluji, A., . . . Stevens, R. D. (2015). Outcome of delirium in critically ill patients: Systematic review and meta-analysis. *British Medical Journal, 350*, h2538. doi:10.1136/bmj.h2538

Sasannejad, C., Ely, E. W., & Lahiri, S. (2019). Long-term cognitive impairment after acute respiratory distress syndrome: A review of clinical impact and pathophysiological mechanisms. *Critical Care, 23*(1), 352. doi:10.1186/s13054-019-2626-z

Schweickert, W. D., Pohlman, M. C., Pohlman, A. S., Nigos, C., Pawlik, A. J., Esbrook, C. L., . . . Kress, J. P. (2009). Early physical and occupational therapy in mechanically ventilated, critically ill patients: A randomised controlled trial. *Lancet, 373*(9678), 1874–1882. doi:S0140-6736(09)60658-9

Sessler, C. N., Gosnell, M. S., Grap, M. J., Brophy, G. M., O'Neal, P. V., Keane, K. A., . . . Elswick, R. K. (2002). The Richmond Agitation-Sedation Scale: Validity and reliability in adult intensive care unit patients. *American Journal of Respiratory and Critical Care Medicine, 166*(10), 1338–1344. doi:10.1164/rccm.2107138

Sevin, C. M., Bloom, S. L., Jackson, J. C., Wang, L., Ely, E. W., & Stollings, J. L. (2018). Comprehensive care of ICU survivors: Development and implementation of an ICU recovery center. *Journal of Critical Care, 46*, 141–148. doi:10.1016/j.jcrc.2018.02.011

Shehabi, Y., Riker, R. R., Bokesch, P. M., Wisemandle, W., Shintani, A., & Ely, E. W. (2010). Delirium duration and mortality in lightly sedated, mechanically ventilated intensive care patients. *Critical Care Medicine, 38*(12), 2311–2318. doi:10.1097/CCM.0b013e3181f85759

Simpson, R., & Robinson, L. (2020). Rehabilitation after critical illness in people with COVID-19 infection. *American Journal of Physical Medicine and Rehabilitation, 99*(6), 470–474. doi:10.1097/PHM.0000000000001443

Smith, G., & Nielsen, M. (1999). ABC of intensive care. Criteria for admission. *British Medical Journal, 318*(7197), 1544–1547.:10.1136/bmj.318.7197.1544

Sobbi, S. C., & van den Boogaard, M. (2014). Inflammation biomarkers and delirium in critically ill patients: New insights? *Critical Care, 18*(3), 153. doi:10.1186/cc13930

Stucky, K. J., & Warren, A. M. (2019). Rehabilitation psychologists in critical care settings. In L. A. Brenner, S. Reid-Arndt, T. R. Elliot, R. G. Frank, & B. Caplan (Eds.), *The rehabilitation psychology handbook* (3rd ed., pp. 483–496). American Psychological Association.

Sutter, R., Chalela, J. A., Leigh, R., Kaplan, P. W., Yenokyan, G., Sharshar, T., & Stevens, R. D. (2015). Significance of parenchymal brain damage in patients with critical illness. *Neurocritical Care, 23*(2), 243–252. doi:10.1007/s12028-015-0110-4

Tansey, C. M., Louie, M., Loeb, M., Gold, W. L., Muller, M. P., de Jager, J., . . . Herridge, M. S. (2007). One-year outcomes and health care utilization in survivors of severe acute respiratory syndrome. *Archives of Internal Medicine, 167*(12), 1312–1320. doi:10.1001/archinte.167.12.1312

Trzepacz, P. T., & Meagher, D. J. (2009). Neuropsychiatric aspects of delirium. In S. C. Ydofsky & R. E. Hales (Eds.), *Textbook of neuropsychiatry and behavioral neurosciences* (pp. 455–518). American Psychiatric Publishing, Inc.

Turon, M., Fernandez-Gonzalo, S., Jodar, M., Goma, G., Montanya, J., Hernando, D., . . . Blanch, L. (2017). Feasibility and safety of virtual-reality-based early neurocognitive stimulation in critically ill patients. *Annals of Intensive Care, 7*(1), 81. doi:10.1186/s13613-017-0303-4

Van De Graaff, M., Beesley, S. J., Butler, J., Benuzillo, J., Poll, J. B., Oniki, T., . . . Brown, S. M. (2018). Partners in healing: Postsurgical outcomes after family involvement in nursing care. *Chest, 153*(2), 572–574. doi:10.1016/j.chest.2017.09.046

van der Schaaf, M., Beelen, A., Dongelmans, D. A., Vroom, M. B., & Nollet, F. (2009). Functional status after intensive care: A challenge for rehabilitation professionals to improve outcome. *Journal of Rehabilitation Medicine, 41*(5), 360–366. doi:10.2340/16501977-0333

Warren, A. M., Rainey, E. E., Weddle, R. J., Bennett, M., Roden-Foreman, K., & Foreman, M. L. (2016). The intensive care unit experience: Psychological impact on family members of patients with and without traumatic brain injury. *Rehabilitation Psychology, 61*(2), 179–185. doi:10.1037/rep0000080

Wilson, J. E., Collar, E. M., Kiehl, A. L., Lee, H., Merzenich, M., Ely, E. W., & Jackson, J. (2018). Computerized cognitive rehabilitation in intensive care unit survivors: Returning to everyday tasks using rehabilitation networks-computerized cognitive rehabilitation pilot investigation. *Annals of the American Thoracic Society, 15*(7), 887–891. doi:10.1513/AnnalsATS.201709-744RL

Wolters, A. E., Slooter, A. J., van der Kooi, A. W., & van Dijk, D. (2013). Cognitive impairment after intensive care unit admission: A systematic review. *Intensive Care Medicine, 39*(3), 376–386. doi:10.1007/s00134-012-2784-9

Woon, F. L., Dunn, C. B., & Hopkins, R. O. (2012). Predicting cognitive sequelae in survivors of critical illness with cognitive screening tests. *American Journal of Respiratory and Critical Care Medicine, 186*(4), 333–340. doi:10.1164/rccm.201112-2261OC

Zhao, J., Yao, L., Wang, C., Sun, Y., & Sun, Z. (2017). The effects of cognitive intervention on cognitive impairments after intensive care unit admission. *Neuropsychological Rehabilitation, 27*(3), 301–317. doi:10.1080/09602011.2015.1078246

7 The Psychologist's Role in Pain Management in the Intensive Care Unit

Christina J. Hayhurst and Mina Nordness

Introduction

Being critically ill is often a painful experience, and the demands and complexities of care in the intensive care unit (ICU) can make managing—or even assessing—patients' pain a formidable challenge. In recent years, the importance of adequate pain relief in the critical care setting has only increased for patients and clinicians, as ICU mortality rates have declined in the United States to new lows of 10% to 29% (Zimmerman et al., 2013). Many critical care patients have pain at baseline from a variety of causes, and many must also contend with pain related to necessary medical procedures. Furthermore, undertreated or unrecognized pain in the ICU can lead to acute alterations in physiology and psychological stress that can worsen short- and long-term outcomes. Recent research has borne out that significant psychosocial factors undeniably influence pain (Frischenschlager & Pucher, 2002), suggesting that a greater role for psychologists may be emerging in the critical care setting. This chapter explores the prevalence, causes, and consequences of pain in the ICU, discussing not only possible pharmacologic treatment strategies but also opportunities for improved assessment and psychological treatment strategies. Areas of interest for future research are also addressed.

Christina J. Hayhurst and Mina Nordness, *The Psychologist's Role in Pain Management in the Intensive Care Unit* In: *Critical Care Psychology and Rehabilitation*. Edited by: Kirk J. Stucky and Jennifer E. Jutte, Oxford University Press. © Oxford University Press 2022. DOI: 10.1093/oso/9780190077013.003.0007

Etiology of pain

The etiology of pain is often complex, a reality that is particularly relevant in the ICU. At the most basic level, a patient's pain can be somatic or visceral, including acute postoperative pain and acute pain from injury or trauma. Many patients entering the ICU also experience chronic pain related to inflammatory or neuropathic processes. Furthermore, in critically ill patients, secondary inflammatory processes such as urosepsis, abdominal sepsis, or physiologic response to surgery have been linked to pain, likely due to mediation of nociception and alteration of sensation (Baumbach et al., 2016; Bruehl, 2015). Factors within the ICU can also cause or exacerbate pain. For example, many critically ill patients, especially those who are on mechanical ventilation, receive opioid-based sedatives, and these have been linked to physiologic dependence that for many produces a degree of hyperalgesia when tapered (Brown et al., 2000; Martyn et al., 2019; Puntillo & Naidu, 2016). Nonsurgical invasive procedures in the ICU also have been associated with pain, with chest tube removal, drain removal, arterial line insertion, and endotracheal suctioning among the most painful (Puntillo et al., 2014).

To fully understand the etiology of pain in critically ill patients, it is instructive to consider the definition of pain established by the International Association for the Study of Pain: "an unpleasant sensory and emotional experience associated with, or resembling that associated with, actual or potential tissue damage" (Raja et al., 2020). This definition, which allows that the experience of pain is multidimensional and not a purely physical entity, helps to illuminate the experience of pain in the ICU. In the critical care setting, pain may often be augmented by the psychological distress of being hospitalized and the loss of a sense of control. In addition to the sudden dependence on others for survival that is inherent in the ICU, many patients must contend with pain while experiencing a limited ability to communicate or, in some cases, a near-total loss of the ability to communicate (e.g., while receiving mechanical ventilation). Evidence also suggests that "pain distress," an emotional component of pain, may be experienced by patients undergoing certain procedures (Barr et al., 2013).

Prevalence of pain in the ICU

Given these realities, it is not surprising that moderate to severe pain is highly prevalent among critically ill patients. Rates of pain in the ICU have been reported as high as 50% of patients at rest, and as high as 80% during procedures (Barr et al., 2013; Chanques et al., 2006, 2007; Devlin et al., 2018; Payen et al., 2007; Puntillo et al.,

2014). This contrasts with the 28% of patients admitted to a general medicine ward who reported severe pain (Whelan et al., 2004). Interestingly, pain prevalence is the same across surgical/trauma and medical ICUs (Chanques et al., 2007). Chanques and colleagues (2007) demonstrated that rates of moderate to severe pain at rest were no different between medical and surgical patients, although their etiologies differed. Medical patients had more back and limb pain, while surgical and trauma patients reported more pain associated with their surgical or injury site (Chanques et al., 2007). One possible explanation for the similar pain rates across these two groups is that the degree of somatic pain in trauma and surgical patients is matched by the visceral and inflammatory pain in medical patients, the latter experiencing higher rates of sepsis and severity of illness on admission compared with their surgical counterparts (Chanques et al., 2007).

Complexity of pain in the ICU

Many factors can influence how a critically ill patient experiences and responds to pain. To elucidate these, it is helpful first to consider pain from a general view. Pain is a protective mechanism to encourage avoidance of tissue injury or damage; typically, when a person encounters a painful stimulus, the protective reflex encourages a quick withdrawal and avoidance of that stimulus to protect from or prevent further tissue injury. This signal is relayed through a complex nociceptive pathway regulated by various neurotransmitters. Because the nociceptive pathway is closely related to the sympathetic nervous system, nociceptive stimuli can increase sympathetic or adrenergic stimulation (Janig, 1985). Sustained painful stimuli and activation of the nociceptive pathway can induce elevated sympathetic nervous system responses that can have an impact on the cardiovascular system (Burton et al., 2016; Liu et al., 1995). Given this increase of sympathetic nervous system activity, critically ill patients with untreated pain have higher levels of energy expenditure (Reade & Finfer, 2014; Swinamer et al., 1988), and in the long term this may have immuno-modulatory effects (Colacchio et al., 1994; Page et al., 2001). Life-sustaining interventions such as mechanical ventilation, arterial lines, and patient repositioning have been reported by ICU survivors to be some of the most noxious stimuli (Puntillo et al., 2014, 1997), making the potential impact of acute pain on the physiologic state of critically ill patients even more complex. Furthermore, patients in the ICU are limited in their ability to independently avoid noxious stimuli to protect against tissue injury, hampered by pharmacologic sedation, restraints, lines, tubes, and frequently a limited ability to communicate effectively.

Pain among the critically ill is also intricately interwoven with a concern paramount in the ICU: delirium. Delirium is highly prevalent among critically ill patients, affecting up to 70% to 80% of adults admitted to ICUs (Girard et al., 2008). Although the causes of delirium are complex and not fully understood, it is essential to recognize that delirium and pain are often intertwined in the ICU. This will be discussed in more detail later in this chapter.

Assessing pain in the ICU

The need to assess pain consistently in the ICU is "paramount," according to the Society of Critical Care Medicine (SCCM)'s 2018 Pain, Agitation/Sedation, Delirium, Immobility, and Sleep Disruption (PADIS) clinical practice guidelines (Devlin et al., 2018). One of its key recommendations states that "the management of pain for adult ICU patients should be guided by routine pain assessment" (Devlin et al., 2018).

Although the notion of assessing pain before treating it makes logical sense, studies suggest that this ordering is not always practiced in adult ICUs. In the multicenter DOLOREA trial, Payen and colleagues (2009) found that of 1,144 mechanically ventilated patients, only 45% had a pain assessment by day 2 of admission. Furthermore, the authors report that in spite of the relatively low rate of assessment, 90% of the patients received concomitant opioids, a finding that runs counter to current opioid-sparing recommendations. In a prospective multicenter cohort observational study of Canadian ICUs, more than 50% of units had a pain assessment tool and standardized treatment protocol available, but the tool was used to guide therapy in just 19% of patients and the protocol for pain was used in only 25% of patients (Burry et al., 2014).

Failing to properly assess pain in critically ill patients has a multitude of negative physiologic and psychological effects, in both the short and long term.

SHORT-TERM OUTCOMES

In the short term, studies generally support the idea that appropriate assessment and subsequent treatment of pain improves outcomes, decreasing the number of days on mechanical ventilation, ICU length of stay (LOS), and rates of delirium and even mortality (Barr et al., 2013; Devlin et al., 2018; Kastrup et al., 2009; Payen et al., 2009). Adequate pain assessment has also been shown to reduce sedative use, including benzodiazepines (Payen et al., 2009), as recommended in the 2018 PADIS clinical practice guidelines (Devlin et al., 2018). Gélinas and colleagues (2011) found that the number of propofol boluses and the overall dose of propofol were significantly reduced when pain was assessed.

There are mixed results regarding improved pain assessment and management on the duration of mechanical ventilation. In an observational study, Payen and colleagues (2009) found median duration of mechanical ventilation to be 11 days among patients not assessed for pain versus 8 days for those who were assessed. Similarly, Arbour and Gélinas (2011) found the mean duration of mechanical ventilation in trauma ICU patients to be reduced from approximately 7 to 4 days after initiating pain assessment with the Care Pain Observation Tool (CPOT). Several other studies, however, did not find an association with improved pain assessment and the duration of mechanical ventilation (Radtke et al., 2012; Rose et al., 2013; Williams et al., 2008).

Studies are also mixed regarding the impact of pain assessment on ICU LOS. Payen and colleagues (2009) found ICU LOS to be reduced by 5 days, while a trend toward decreased LOS was observed by Rose and colleagues (2013) and Arbour and Gélinas (2011). In several other studies, however, LOS was increased or not affected by pain assessment. This likely indicates that pain is not often the major driver of admission to the ICU or a primary contributor to LOS.

LONG-TERM OUTCOMES

Inadequate pain assessment has been shown to have a negative impact on long-term outcomes. Postintensive care syndrome (PICS) (Needham et al., 2012), for example, is a syndrome characterized by new or worsened physical, cognitive, and/or psychological functioning related to critical illness. Pain is considered an aspect of PICS, and, indeed, 33% to 77% of patients report persistent pain after discharge from the ICU (Baumbach et al., 2016; Hayhurst et al., 2018). Such chronic pain can persist for years. In a retrospective review of 196 mixed medical and surgical patients, 44% were still reporting chronic pain 1 year after their discharge from the ICU (Battle et al., 2013). Hayhurst and colleagues (2018) found even higher rates of persistent pain at 12 months after discharge, with 74% of patients reporting any pain; 31% had moderate to severe pain at 3 months, and 35% had moderate to severe pain at 12 months, consistent with the findings of others. Baumbach and colleagues (2016) found similar rates, with 33% of patients reporting chronic pain at 6 months after discharge. Half of those patients, or 16% total, reported new chronic pain specific to their ICU stay, not simply worsening of their prior chronic pain syndrome. A smaller study found that 66% of mixed medical and surgical patients had "new" pain associated with their critical illness (Devine et al., 2019). Several other studies have found similar rates of chronic pain within the first year after a critical illness (Battle et al., 2013;

Langerud et al., 2018). At least one study suggested that post-ICU chronic pain is persistent in the long term, with 57% of patients reporting pain at 6 to 11 years after discharge (Timmers et al., 2011).

The impact on daily life of this increased rate of chronic pain is significant. Several studies focusing on PICS have demonstrated the impact of the syndrome on patients' ability to return to their normal daily life. In the few studies specifically examining it, pain interfered with patients' ability to enjoy life, sleep, spend time with their families, or return to work (Baumbach et al., 2016; Devine et al., 2019; Hayhurst et al., 2018). Cuthbertson and colleagues (2010) showed that at least 75% of the physical component scores of a quality-of-life assessment tool were below the population mean during the 5 years after ICU discharge, possibly reflecting a component of pain. In addition, in the study by Timmers and colleagues (2011), 29% of patients experienced anxiety or depression, conditions closely intertwined with the negative experience of physical pain.

ASSESSMENT TOOLS

The use of validated assessment tools for sedation, pain, and delirium, therefore, is essential to the appropriate management of the critically ill patient. In general patient populations, the most common method of pain assessment is a numeric scale, but how best to assess pain among ICU patients depends on their level of consciousness and ability to communicate verbally and/or physically. The 2018 PADIS clinical practice guidelines (Devlin et al., 2018) offer an in-depth review of pain assessment tools in the ICU, which will be summarized here.

Vital sign assessment

Vital sign changes are unreliably associated with pain in critically ill patients (Arbour & Gélinas, 2010; Devlin et al., 2018; Gélinas & Arbour, 2009). Given the physiologic variability across critically ill patients, vital sign changes have not been shown to be a valid measure of pain in these patients. Furthermore, vital sign changes have been associated with both painful and nonpainful experiences in the ICU and can be overinterpreted as pain by clinical personnel (Arbour & Gélinas, 2010; Devlin et al., 2018; Gélinas & Arbour, 2009).

Patient-reported scales

Patient-reported numeric rating scales are commonly used to assess pain. Several scales are available, but those with the best psychometric properties for ICU patients who are able to self-report pain include the numeric pain rating scale with visual component (NRS-V), in which patients report their pain on a scale from 0 to 10, with 0 indicating no pain. The visual component shows the scale in large font, with "no pain" next to the number 0 on the left side of the scale and "extreme pain" next to the number 10 on the right side. The NRS-V can be used with patients who are verbal and those who are nonverbal but alert enough to communicate. Intubated patients can point to their corresponding pain level with the use of a large communication board including the NRS-V scale.

The verbal descriptor scale (VDS) (Chanques et al., 2010; Devlin et al., 2018) rates pain more qualitatively from "no pain" to "severe pain." Though it is not the preferred method of assessment, the VDS can be useful in patients who have difficulties with numbers.

Validated behavioral assessment tools

There are two widely accepted behavioral-based assessment tools for nonverbal patients who are unable to self-report pain: the Behavioral Pain Scale (BPS) (Payen et al., 2001) and the Critical-Care Pain Observation Tool (CPOT) (Gélinas et al., 2006). These tools are designed, and have been validated, for the assessment of behavioral symptoms of pain.

The BPS is a scoring system that ranges from 3 to 12 and includes three domains: facial expression, upper limbs, and compliance with ventilation. A BPS score of 6 or more signifies pain that should be addressed with treatment (Payen et al., 2001).

The CPOT scoring system is similar to the BPS, including facial expression; body movements; compliance with the ventilator or, for extubated patients, vocalization; and muscle tension. This scoring system uses a scale from 0 to 8, with scores greater than 2 signifying an unacceptable level of pain (Gélinas et al., 2006).

Treatment of pain in the ICU

The treatment of pain in an ICU should involve a multimodal approach including pharmacologic and non-pharmacologic modalities.

PHARMACOLOGIC INTERVENTIONS

The standard pharmacologic approach can be taken from the current PADIS guidelines (Devlin et al., 2018), which recommend regularly assessing pain, as previously discussed, and standardized pain management protocols. SCCM guidelines recommend opioids as the first-line treatment for non-neuropathic pain (Table 7.1), while urging carefully titrated, analgesic dosing.

TABLE 7.1.

Opioids recommended by SCCM for the ICU

Opiate	IV potency ratio (relative to morphine)	Onset (IV)	Half-life (h)	Active metabolite	Metabolism	Clinical considerations
Fentanyl	100:1	1–2 min	2–4	No	Demethylation, CYP3A4 substrate	Accumulation with hepatic impairment
Hydromorphone	5:1	5–15 min	2–3	No	Glucuronidation	Accumulation with hepatic/renal impairment
Morphine	1:1	5–10 min	1.5–5	Yes	Demethylation, glucuronidation	Accumulation with hepatic/renal impairment; histamine release; active metabolite
Remifentanil	20:1	1–3 min	0.05	No	Hydrolysis by plasma esterases	Use ideal body weight for obese patients; cost; glycine neurotoxicity

IV = intravenous
Devlin et al., 2018

Adjuncts such as ketamine infusions, gabapentinoids, acetaminophen, and nefopam are recommended. In select patient populations nonsteroidal anti-inflammatories (NSAIDs), lidocaine infusions, and regional anesthesia can be used as well (Table 7.2). Analgosedation, a method of treating a patient's pain first, and subsequently providing sedation only if needed, is also emphasized in the guidelines (Devlin et al., 2018).

The implementation of standardized pain assessment protocols appears to correlate with a more efficient use of analgesics. In several studies, administered doses of opioid analgesics decreased while patient-reported numeric rating scale pain scores improved (Gélinas et al., 2011; Radtke et al., 2012). Interestingly, in a study with a cardiac and mixed ICU population, implementing a standardized pain assessment protocol changed the median dose of morphine from 5 mg to 4 mg in the cardiac ICU but increased it significantly from 27 mg to 75 mg in the mixed ICU group (Rose et al., 2013). The reason for the difference in dosing was unclear, but it could be that morphine was previously being used as a sedative in the cardiac ICU, where almost all patients are intubated for the initial part of their admission. In patients assessed for pain, versus those who were not, the use of multimodal adjuvants increased, including the use of ketamine, paracetamol, and nefopam (Payen et al., 2009), as was the use of dedicated pain treatment during procedural pain (Payen et al., 2009; Williams et al., 2008).

Particular care must be taken in ascertaining the best pharmacologic approach as it relates to the prevention of delirium, as delirium, pain, and sedation are closely interwoven (Barr et al., 2013; Chanques et al., 2006; Devlin et al., 2018; Ely & Barr, 2013; Ely & Pisani, 2006; Gélinas et al., 2013; Reade & Finfer, 2014). Untreated pain has been associated with delirium in several patient populations (Agnoletti et al., 2005; Chrispal et al., 2010; Maldonado et al., 2003; Mckoy, 2004; Santos et al., 2004). In addition, in critically ill patients, the balance among pain, delirium, and sedation can be complex. Some common sedatives, particularly benzodiazepines, have been associated with increased delirium (Pandharipande et al., 2010; Pisani et al., 2009). One takeaway recommendation from the PADIS guidelines (Devlin et al., 2018) is that the use of benzodiazepines is a modifiable risk factor associated with increased risk for delirium in critically ill adults (strong evidence).

The long-term impact of delirium is significant. Many patients who experience delirium in the ICU will develop long-term cognitive impairment, lasting even up to a year after hospital discharge (Gunther et al., 2012; Hopkins & Jackson, 2006; Jackson et al., 2010, 2003; James C Jackson et al., 2007; Jutte et al., 2015; Karnatovskaia et al., 2015; Pandharipande et al., 2013). Delirium is also associated with the development of posttraumatic stress disorder (PTSD) after hospitalization, which is closely related to pain and uncomfortable experiences during critical

TABLE 7.2.

Nonopioid analgesics for the ICU

Drug	Dose	Metabolism/Clearance	Considerations
Acetaminophen	<4 g/d	Hepatic	Adjust dose for cirrhosis: up to 2 g/d
Gabapentinoids:		Renal	Adjust dose for GFR; can commonly cause somnolence, blurry vision
Gabapentin	100–1,200 mg TID		
Pregabalin	50–300 mg TID		
Ketamine infusion	2–5 mcg/kg/min	Hepatic	Avoid if history of PTSD/psychosis due to risk of hallucinations
Lidocaine infusion*	1–2 mg/min	Hepatic	Avoid if history of seizure disorder, on anti-arrhythmics
NSAIDs	Varies	Renal	Caution with reduced GFR, peptic ulcers, age >65
SNRIs*	Varies	Hepatic	Analgesic effect has faster onset than antidepressant effect; helps with anxiety component

* Not recommended for routine use by SCCM (Devlin et al., 2018)

TID = three times daily, GFR = glomerular filtration rate, SNRIs = serotonin/norepinephrine reuptake inhibitors illness (Jackson et al., 2011, 2014, 2016; Jackson, Hart et al., 2007; Parker et al., 2015; Patel et al., 2016). Patients with delirium are more likely to die compared with ICU patients without delirium (Ely et al., 2004; Shehabi et al., 2010; van den Boogaard et al., 2010); thus, prompt assessment, identification, and treatment of the underlying etiology of delirium are essential.

In the postoperative patient population, untreated pain or lack of appropriate analgesia can also incite delirium. Institution of a validated care bundle targeted at decreasing ICU delirium titled the ABCDEF bundle has been shown to decrease ICU delirium but interestingly did not improve pain scores (Morandi et al., 2011; Pun et al., 2019):

Assess, Prevent and Manage Pain

Both Spontaneous Awakening Trial (SAT) and Spontaneous Breathing Trials (SBT)

Choice of Analgesia or Sedation

Delirium: Assess, Prevent, Manage

Early Mobility and Exercise

Family Engagement and Empowerment.

This is likely due to patients being less sedated and better able to communicate their pain.

Pain management surrounding procedures in the ICU can have a significant impact on the pain experiences of critically ill patients (Chanques et al., 2006; Puntillo et al., 2014, 2018). In particular, although ICU procedures are necessary and lifesaving, caution should be taken in how these procedures are implemented and what strategies are taken for pain management periprocedurally. Procedural pain, depending on the invasiveness, can be managed with local or regional anesthesia, opioid analgesics, procedural sedation, and, as discussed later in this chapter, nonpharmacologic techniques.

There is a suspected interplay among analgesia, anxiety, and the long-term impact of ICU-related pain on quality of life. A post hoc analysis of a large prospective cohort study by Puntillo and colleagues (2018) investigated pain distress, the emotional component of pain experienced by patients in the ICU. Pain distress and intensity were assessed immediately before and after undergoing ICU procedures. Pain distress was positively correlated with pain intensity. Having preprocedural pain, having pre-hospital anxiety, and receiving pethidine/meperidine or haloperidol before the procedure all significantly increased the odds of having higher procedural pain distress (Puntillo et al., 2018). Further work is needed to understand the best approach to address the psychological and physical components of pain in the ICU.

NONPHARMACOLOGIC INTERVENTIONS

In the ICU, the treatment of pain must focus on the entire experience of pain, including physical, psychological, cultural, and emotional components. One model of the multiple dimensions of the pain experience outlines the following components:

- Sensory/discriminative: underlying physical pathology and nervous system pathways
- Affective-motivational: emotional responses to pain
- Cognitive-evaluative: individual beliefs and assignment of meaning to the pain experience.

The treatment of pain should focus on all components, as possible. This is often difficult in critically ill patients, with limits in cognition from such things as medications, delirium, ischemia, and, often, barriers to communication. However, as noted, treatment of acute pain can improve both short- and long-term outcomes, and every effort should be made to use nonpharmacologic means to help reduce pain in the critically ill.

In its newest guidelines, the SCCM recommends several nonpharmacologic pain therapies (Devlin et al., 2018), including massage therapy, cold therapy (applying ice packs prior to painful procedures), music therapy, and relaxation techniques. They do not recommend virtual reality or hypnosis as methods for acute pain control in the general critically ill population, based on the current low quality of evidence. Further study is needed in these areas.

In a study of relaxation techniques administered by a bedside nurse, cardiac surgery patients had significantly lower pain scores when combining deep-breathing exercises with opioids than with opioids alone at the time of chest tube removal (Friesner et al., 2006). Guided-imagery therapy in the form of prerecorded tapes decreased pain scores, opioid use, and LOS in several studies (Deisch et al., 2000; Halpin et al., 2002). A Cochrane review found little high-quality evidence to suggest that psychological interventions (multiple methodologies) helped reduce pain after cardiac surgery, but they did note that it reduced mental stress (Ziehm et al., 2017). This indicates the need for further high-quality studies to examine these relations. The risk of using techniques such as music therapy or calm breathing exercises is exceedingly low, however, which makes them attractive modalities to supplement other forms of analgesia while further study is ongoing.

THE PSYCHOLOGIST'S EVOLVING ROLE

To date, very little research has examined the effect of in-ICU psychologist intervention on the outcomes of patients with acute or chronic pain after critical illness, but there is increased interest and need for such studies. In a recent study, 47% of hospital-based psychologists reported working in a critical care setting, but only 17% did so on a daily basis (Stucky et al., 2016). That same survey found that neuropsychologists and rehabilitation psychologists were most often used in an ICU, mainly in medical/surgical ICUs in level 1 trauma centers (Stucky et al., 2016). In a 2019 study of psychology consultations for critically ill patients in a medical ICU, there were 79 consultations in 10 months (Hosey et al., 2019). This was in an academic center with an attending psychologist on staff in the unit once a week. The majority (56%) of referrals were for emotional distress, while only 4% were for pain.

Increased PTSD scores after critical illness have been associated with higher baseline pain scores after discharge and recall of frightening experiences in the ICU (Elliott et al., 2016). Having a mental health comorbidity has been linked to prolonged worsened mental health and reduced quality of life following a critical illness hospitalization (Bienvenu et al., 2018; Nikayin et al., 2016; Rabiee et al., 2016). As discussed, chronic pain after critical illness also contributes to a decreased quality of life. It is likely that these two factors are interconnected, as coping strategies, ability to adjust to new cognitive and physical disabilities, and mood disorders all contribute to the experience of pain. Increased levels of anxiety, depression, and catastrophizing have been shown to portend worse postoperative acute and chronic pain (Dunn et al., 2018; Theunissen et al., 2012). Therefore, the ability of the clinical psychologist to help patients with acute anxiety, depression, and feelings of loss of control will likely positively influence their experience of pain (e.g., through reframing, thought stopping). Specific interventions are discussed in the following section.

PSYCHOLOGICAL INTERVENTIONS

Patients' ability to cope with pain and the overwhelming experience of critical illness depends on multiple cognitive and psychological functions as well as the level and quality of emotional and social support available. Stress and negative emotions affect patients' psychological and physical well-being in both the acute phase and long term (Deja et al., 2006) and have been linked to delayed physical recovery (Sukantarat et al., 2007). As stated, anxiety and depression can exacerbate the impact of pain, and unfortunately critically ill patients have higher rates of anxiety, depression, and PTSD than the general population. In a United Kingdom survey of 4,943 patients following critical illness, 46% met criteria for anxiety, 40% for depression, and 22% for PTSD up to 2 years after discharge (Hatch et al., 2018). When one psychological disorder was present, there was a 65% chance that it would co-occur with one of the other disorders. Strikingly, those with depression had a 47% greater likelihood of death within the first 2 years after their critical illness. While it is known that depression and anxiety exacerbate pain, it is unclear how much these disorders affect acute and long-term outcomes. Still, addressing these disorders should go hand in hand with addressing pain. For example, patients who are cognitively intact may have difficulty discriminating or understanding the difference between normal or desirable pain (e.g., stretching during therapy or soreness after exercise) versus pain that is potentially harmful or requires cessation of activity. Psychologists are specifically trained in helping patients reframe their thoughts and experience in the service of improving overall coping, reducing distress, and lowering preoccupation with pain.

The psychological strategies most often used for acute pain management include information provision, relaxation, and cognitive techniques (Table 7.3). Unfortunately, there is a paucity of guidance and data on how to implement these interventions, the ideal dose and timing, and the effect of these techniques in the ICU with the critically ill population. Peris and colleagues (2011) conducted a

TABLE 7.3.

Possible psychological interventions for acute pain in the critically ill

Categories	Intervention types
Relaxation	Progressive muscle relaxation
	Abdominal breathing
	Paced breathing
	Hypnosis
Information	Preemptive truthful information regarding sensations or process of a medical procedure; 1:1, video or audio recording
	Psychoeducation about the mind–body connection and its impact on pain
	Education regarding the benefits of exercise and mobility versus consequences of activity avoidance
Cognitive	Distraction
	Cognitive-behavioral therapy to reduce catastrophizing and maladaptive thoughts
	Self-reflection
	Mindfulness
	Positive thinking styles

before/after observational cohort study of 209 trauma patients to assess the impact of psychological intervention on these mental health disorders in the critically ill (Peris et al., 2011). In-ICU psychologist intervention helped reduce rates of anxiety, depression (statistically insignificant), and scoring as high risk for PTSD (Peris et al., 2011). In addition, fewer patients in the intervention group required psychiatric medications 1 year after discharge. The interventions included counseling on stress management, educational interventions, psychological support, and teaching coping strategies. The last of these were designed to address anxiety, depression, fear, and a sense of hopelessness and helplessness and to reduce the discomfort of medical procedures and general health conditions. Caregivers led by the in-ICU psychologist were also taught cognitive and emotional restructuring to help with stress management. Psychologists also provided interventions with the patient's family while the patient was still unconscious to promote family-centered decision-making and provide support. Of note, not all interventions were performed by the psychologist; in several instances, the nurses and intensivists were taught to deliver the psychological interventions as well. Unfortunately, while mental health did seem to improve with these interventions, there was no difference in pain scores at 1 year. It is unclear how pain scores were affected in the acute setting, and this should be explored in further studies.

Some evidence for the effectiveness of these techniques can be found in patients with acute pain, although there are few large-scale randomized controlled trials (RCTs) and data are mixed. Pain from burns has been successfully treated with psychological interventions, including music distraction and controlled breathing during debridement (Fratianne et al., 2001). Hypnosis with relaxation and guided imagery also reduced pain scores during burn debridements (Wright & Drummond, 2000). During coronary angiography, a recorded relaxation intervention lead to reduced pain scores and fewer requests for medication when compared with a music distraction group or no-intervention group (Mandle et al., 1990). However, in a relatively large RCT, a combined intervention of information provision, positive self-statements, relaxation, and guided imagery during autologous bone-marrow transplantation did not affect pain scores or distress (Gaston-Johansson et al., 2000).

In a novel case series, a psychologist was added to the rounding team on the acute pain service (Childs et al., 2014). The authors' aim was to see if early psychological intervention could reduce the impact of adverse psychological comorbidities on pain, and also help the physicians and staff create a healing environment, even when the patients' behavioral phenotypes were incongruent with the biopsychosocial models of the health care professionals. The authors presented three postsurgical patients, all of whom had high pain scores that were minimally responsive to standard analgesics. They found that fear, anxiety, low mood, and anger were present in most cases as well as significant communication barriers with the medical team in some cases. Using a combination of cognitive-behavioral therapy to reduce maladaptive thoughts, mindfulness, relaxation, and positive-thinking styles, the clinical psychologists were able to help the patients interact with their medical team in a more productive manner, be discharged home with adequate pain control, and, in two cases, continue mindfulness and cognitive-behavioral therapy as outpatients. This case series presents what is likely a valuable role of psychological intervention in acute pain: an integral player on an interdisciplinary team designed to promote a patient- and family-centered healing environment.

Another role of the clinical psychologist in the ICU is to help address not only patient pain conditions and concomitant psychological pathology but also to offer insight into patient and family relationships and communication with the medical team. The interaction between patients and all members of their medical team can have an impact on recovery, but interactions are not always harmonious. Due to the highly acute nature of the critical care environment, significant conflicts often emerge between nurses and physicians, nurses and families, and between nurses, often due to mistrust and communication gaps (Azoulay et al., 2009). In addition, patients in pain are often considered challenging. If nurses perceive the patient or family interactions as negative, they can engage in avoidance behavior, which might impair good care and pain control. Similarly, if patients are not responding to analgesics as expected, physicians might label them as "drug seeking" or "difficult." Anger and aggression can frequently be caused by pain, yet these undesirable behaviors in the patient elicit avoidance by the team (Fishbain et al., 2011). There is very little education in medical or nursing school about how psychological comorbidities affect the experience of pain; thus, these comorbidities are often not addressed. Guidance from an in-ICU psychologist can help mitigate related risks. Indeed, an article accompanying the PADIS guidelines includes psychologists on a list of potential "implementation leaders" (Balas et al., 2018). Furthermore, psychologists can help members of the ICU team improve their own coping and communication skills, which are necessary in the high-stress environment of the ICU. There are no studies of this more holistic model on pain outcomes in the ICU, but this should provide impetus for further study.

Conclusions

Pain is a complex sensation affected by a variety of physical, emotional, cognitive, and psychosocial inputs. Unfortunately, it is exceedingly common in the critically ill, both medical and surgical patients. Undertreated pain can lead to worsened short- and long-term outcomes. Pain related to a critical illness can persist well past the time of recovery, and recent data show that patients may still experience pain up to 11 years after discharge. This pain affects patients' ability to return to their life before hospitalization. Many do not return to work, have difficulty spending time with family, and have trouble enjoying life due to pain. Unfortunately, the experience of chronic pain is linked with and exacerbated by psychological disorders, including depression and anxiety, which are found at high rates in the critically ill population.

The inclusion of clinical psychologists in the care of critically ill patients is increasing, but currently consultations to psychologists for pain control, specifically, appear to occur less often than for other indications. There is a paucity of data in critically ill patients on the impact of psychological interventions on pain and there are mixed data in the general medical population with acute pain. Psychological interventions to help alleviate pain are designed to target not only patients' perception of pain but also their cognitive and emotional responses to pain. The interventions also focus on the treatment of depression and anxiety, as these can exacerbate pain. Psychological interventions could include facilitation of medical team communication with patients and families by addressing barriers to communication such as anger, aggression, and avoidance. Further study is needed, but particularly in the midst of the current opioid crisis, focus on nonpharmacologic interventions for pain is paramount, and clinical psychologists are perfectly positioned to implement and teach these interventions.

References

Agnoletti, V., Ansaloni, L., Catena, F., Chattat, R., De Cataldis, A., Di Nino, G., . . . Taffurelli, M. (2005). Postoperative delirium after elective and emergency surgery: Analysis and checking of risk factors. A study protocol. *BMC Surgery, 5*, 12. doi:10.1186/1471-2482-5-12

Arbour, C., & Gélinas, C. (2010). Are vital signs valid indicators for the assessment of pain in postoperative cardiac surgery ICU adults? *Intensive and Critical Care Nursing, 26*(2), 83–90.

Azoulay, E., Timsit, J. F., Sprung, C. L., Soares, M., Rusinova, K., Lafabrie, A., . . . for the Ethics Section of the European Society of Intensive Care Medicine. (2009). Prevalence and factors of intensive care unit conflicts: The Conflicus study. *American Journal of Respiratory and Critical Care Medicine, 180*(9), 853–860. doi:10.1164/rccm.200810-1614OC

Balas, M. C., Weinhouse, G. L., Denehy, L., Chanques, G., Rochwerg, B., Misak, C. J., . . . Fraser, G. L. (2018). Interpreting and implementing the 2018 pain, agitation/sedation, delirium, immobility, and sleep disruption clinical practice guideline. *Critical Care Medicine, 46*(9), 1464–1470. doi:10.1097/CCM.0000000000003307

Barr, J., Fraser, G. L., Puntillo, K., Ely, E. W., Gélinas, C., Dasta, J. F., . . . Jaeschke, R. (2013). Clinical practice guidelines for the management of pain, agitation, and delirium in adult patients in the intensive care unit. *Critical Care Medicine, 41*(1), 263–306. doi:10.1097/CCM.0b013e3182783b72

Battle, C. E., Lovett, S., & Hutchings, H. (2013). Chronic pain in survivors of critical illness: A retrospective analysis of incidence and risk factors. *Critical Care, 17*(3), R101. doi:10.1186/cc12746

Baumbach, P., Gotz, T., Gunther, A., Weiss, T., & Meissner, W. (2016). Prevalence and characteristics of chronic intensive care-related pain: The role of severe sepsis and septic shock. *Critical Care Medicine, 44*(6), 1129–1137. doi:10.1097/CCM.0000000000001635

Bienvenu, O. J., Friedman, L. A., Colantuoni, E., Dinglas, V. D., Sepulveda, K. A., Mendez-Tellez, P., . . . Needham, D. M. (2018). Psychiatric symptoms after acute respiratory distress syndrome: A 5-year longitudinal study. *Intensive Care Medicine, 44*(1), 38–47. doi:10.1007/s00134-017-5009-4

Brown, C., Albrecht, R., Pettit, H., McFadden, T., & Schermer, C. (2000). Opioid and benzodiazepine withdrawal syndrome in adult burn patients. *American Surgeon, 66*(4), 367–370.

Bruehl, S. (2015). Complex regional pain syndrome. *British Medical Journal, 351,* h2730. doi:10.1136/bmj.h2730

Burry, L. D., Williamson, D. R., Perreault, M. M., Rose, L., Cook, D. J., Ferguson, N. D., . . . Mehta, S. (2014). Analgesic, sedative, antipsychotic, and neuromuscular blocker use in Canadian intensive care units: A prospective, multicentre, observational study. *Canadian Journal of Anaesthesia, 61*(7), 619–630. doi:10.1007/s12630-014-0174-1

Burton, A. R., Fazalbhoy, A., & Macefield, V. G. (2016). Sympathetic responses to noxious stimulation of muscle and skin. *Frontiers in Neurology, 7,* 109. doi:10.3389/fneur.2016.00109

Chanques, G., Jaber, S., Barbotte, E., Violet, S., Sebbane, M., Perrigault, P. F., . . . Eledjam, J. J. (2006). Impact of systematic evaluation of pain and agitation in an intensive care unit. *Critical Care Medicine, 34*(6), 1691–1699. doi:10.1097/01.CCM.0000218416.62457.56

Chanques, G., Sebbane, M., Barbotte, E., Viel, E., Eledjam, J. J., & Jaber, S. (2007). A prospective study of pain at rest: Incidence and characteristics symptom in surgical and trauma versus intensive care patients. *Anesthesiology, 107*(5), 858–860.

Chanques, G., Viel, E., Constantin, J. M., Jung, B., de Lattre, S., Carr, J., . . . Jaber, S. (2010). The measurement of pain in intensive care unit: Comparison of 5 self-report intensity scales. *Pain, 151*(3), 711–721. doi:10.1016/j.pain.2010.08.039

Childs, S. R., Casely, E. M., Kuehler, B. M., Ward, S., Halmshaw, C. L., Thomas, S. E., . . . Bantel, C. (2014). The clinical psychologist and the management of inpatient pain: A small case series. *Neuropsychiatric Disease and Treatment, 10,* 2291–2297. doi:10.2147/NDT.S70555

Chrispal, A., Mathews, K. P., & Surekha, V. (2010). The clinical profile and association of delirium in geriatric patients with hip fractures in a tertiary care hospital in India. *Journal of the Association of Physicians of India, 58,* 15–19.

Colacchio, T. A., Yeager, M. P., & Hildebrandt, L. W. (1994). Perioperative immunomodulation in cancer surgery. *American Journal of Surgery, 167*(1), 174–179. doi:10.1016/0002-9610(94)90070-1

Cuthbertson, B. H., Roughton, S., Jenkinson, D., Maclennan, G., & Vale, L. (2010). Quality of life in the five years after intensive care: A cohort study. *Critical Care, 14*(1), R6. doi:10.1186/cc8848

Deisch, P., Soukup, S. M., Adams, P., & Wild, M. C. (2000). Guided imagery: Replication study using coronary artery bypass graft patients. *Nursing Clinics of North America, 35*(2), 417–425.

Deja, M., Denke, C., Weber-Carstens, S., Schroder, J., Pille, C. E., Hokema, F., . . . Kaisers, U. (2006). Social support during intensive care unit stay might improve mental impairment and consequently health-related quality of life in survivors of severe acute respiratory distress syndrome. *Critical Care, 10*(5), R147. doi:10.1186/cc5070

Devine, H., Quasim, T., McPeake, J., Shaw, M., McCallum, L., & Mactavish, P. (2019). Chronic pain in intensive care unit survivors: Incidence, characteristics and side-effects up to one-year post-discharge. *Journal of Rehabilitation Medicine, 51*(6), 451–455. doi:10.2340/16501977-2558

Devlin, J. W., Skrobik, Y., Gélinas, C., Needham, D. M., Slooter, A. J. C., Pandharipande, P. P., . . . Alhazzani, W. (2018). Clinical practice guidelines for the prevention and management of pain, agitation/sedation, delirium, immobility, and sleep disruption in adult patients in the ICU. *Critical Care Medicine, 46*(9), e825–e873. doi:10.1097/CCM.0000000000003299

Dunn, L. K., Durieux, M. E., Fernandez, L. G., Tsang, S., Smith-Straesser, E. E., Jhaveri, H. F., . . . Naik, B. I. (2018). Influence of catastrophizing, anxiety, and depression on in-hospital opioid consumption, pain, and quality of recovery after adult spine surgery. *Journal of Neurosurgery: Spine, 28*(1), 119–126. doi:10.3171/2017.5.SPINE1734

Elliott, R., McKinley, S., Fien, M., & Elliott, D. (2016). Posttraumatic stress symptoms in intensive care patients: An exploration of associated factors. *Rehabilitation Psychology, 61*(2), 141–150. doi:10.1037/rep0000074

Ely, E. W., & Barr, J. (2013). Pain/agitation/delirium. *Seminars in Respiratory and Critical Care Medicine, 34*(2), 151–152. doi:10.1055/s-0033-1342974

Ely, E. W., & Pisani, M. A. (2006). Monitoring and treatment of pain, anxiety, and delirium in the ICU. In R. K. Albert, A. Slutsky, M. Ranieri, J. Takala, & A. Torres (Eds.), *Clinical critical care medicine* (pp. 51–59). Mosby Elsevier.

Ely, E. W., Shintani, A., Truman, B., Speroff, T., Gordon, S. M., Harrell, F. E., Jr., . . . Dittus, R. S. (2004). Delirium as a predictor of mortality in mechanically ventilated patients in the intensive care unit. *Journal of the American Medical Association, 291*(14), 1753–1762. doi:10.1001/jama.291.14.1753

Fishbain, D. A., Lewis, J. E., Bruns, D., Disorbio, J. M., Gao, J., & Meyer, L. J. (2011). Exploration of anger constructs in acute and chronic pain patients vs. community patients. *Pain Practice, 11*(3), 240–251. doi:10.1111/j.1533-2500.2010.00410.x

Fratianne, R. B., Prensner, J. D., Huston, M. J., Super, D. M., Yowler, C. J., & Standley, J. M. (2001). The effect of music-based imagery and musical alternate engagement on the burn debridement process. *Journal of Burn Care and Rehabilitation, 22*(1), 47–53. doi:10.1097/00004630-200101000-00010

Friesner, S. A., Curry, D. M., & Moddeman, G. R. (2006). Comparison of two pain-management strategies during chest tube removal: Relaxation exercise with opioids and opioids alone. *Heart Lung, 35*(4), 269–276. doi:10.1016/j.hrtlng.2005.10.005

Frischenschlager, O., & Pucher, I. (2002). Psychological management of pain. *Disability and Rehabilitation, 24*(8), 416–422. doi:10.1080/09638280110108841

Gaston-Johansson, F., Fall-Dickson, J. M., Nanda, J., Ohly, K. V., Stillman, S., Krumm, S., & Kennedy, M. J. (2000). The effectiveness of the comprehensive coping strategy program on clinical outcomes in breast cancer autologous bone marrow transplantation. *Cancer Nursing, 23*(4), 277–285. doi:10.1097/00002820-200008000-00004

Gélinas, C., & Arbour, C. (2009). Behavioral and physiologic indicators during a nociceptive procedure in conscious and unconscious mechanically ventilated adults: Similar or different? *Journal of Critical Care, 24*(4), 628.e7–17.

Gélinas, C., Arbour, C., Michaud, C., Vaillant, F., & Desjardins, S. (2011). Implementation of the critical-care pain observation tool on pain assessment/management nursing practices in an intensive care unit with nonverbal critically ill adults: A before and after study. *International Journal of Nursing Studies, 48*(12), 1495–1504. doi:10.1016/j.ijnurstu.2011.03.012

Gélinas, C., Fillion, L., Puntillo, K. A., Viens, C., & Fortier, M. (2006). Validation of the critical-care pain observation tool in adult patients. *American Journal of Critical Care, 15*(4), 420–427.

Gélinas, C., Klein, K., Naidech, A., & Skrobik, Y. (2013). Pain, sedation, and delirium management in the neurocritically ill: Lessons learned from recent research. *Seminars in Respiratory and Critical Care Medicine, 34*(02), 236–243.

Girard, T. D., Pandharipande, P. P., & Ely, E. W. (2008). Delirium in the intensive care unit. *Critical Care, 12*(Suppl 3), S3. doi:10.1186/cc6149

Gunther, M. L., Morandi, A., Krauskopf, E., Pandharipande, P., Girard, T. D., Jackson, J. C., . . . Ely, E. W. (2012). The association between brain volumes, delirium duration, and cognitive outcomes in intensive care unit survivors: The VISIONS cohort magnetic resonance imaging study. *Critical Care Medicine, 40*(7), 2022–2032. doi:10.1097/CCM.0b013e318250acco

Halpin, L. S., Speir, A. M., CapoBianco, P., & Barnett, S. D. (2002). Guided imagery in cardiac surgery. *Journal of Clinical Outcomes Management, 6*(3), 132–137.

Hatch, R., Young, D., Barber, V., Griffiths, J., Harrison, D. A., & Watkinson, P. (2018). Anxiety, depression and post-traumatic stress disorder after critical illness: A UK-wide prospective cohort study. *Critical Care, 22*(1), 310. doi:10.1186/s13054-018-2223-6

Hayhurst, C. J., Jackson, J. C., Archer, K. R., Thompson, J. L., Chandrasekhar, R., & Hughes, C. G. (2018). Pain and its long-term interference of daily life after critical illness. *Anesthesia and Analgesia, 127*(3), 690–697. doi:10.1213/ANE.0000000000003358

Hopkins, R. O., & Jackson, J. C. (2006). Long-term neurocognitive function after critical illness. *Chest, 130*(3), 869–878.

Hosey, M. M., Ali, M. K., Mantheiy, E. C., Albert, K., Wegener, S. T., & Needham, D. M. (2019). Psychology consultation patterns in a medical intensive care unit: A brief report. *Rehabilitation Psychology, 64*(3), 360–365. doi:10.1037/rep0000264

Jackson, J. C., Archer, K. R., Bauer, R., Abraham, C. M., Song, Y., Greevey, R., . . . Obremskey, W. (2011). A prospective investigation of long-term cognitive impairment and psychological distress in moderately versus severely injured trauma intensive care unit survivors without intracranial hemorrhage. *Journal of Trauma and Acute Care Surgery, 71*(4), 860–866. doi:10.1097/TA.0b013e318215161

Jackson, J. C., Girard, T. D., Gordon, S. M., Thompson, J. L., Shintani, A. K., Thomason, J. W., . . . Ely, E. W. (2010). Long-term cognitive and psychological outcomes in the awakening and breathing controlled trial. *American Journal of Respiratory and Critical Care Medicine, 182*(2), 183–191. doi:10.1164/rccm.200903-0442OC

Jackson, J. C., Hart, R. P., Gordon, S. M., Hopkins, R. O., Girard, T. D., & Ely, E. W. (2007). Post-traumatic stress disorder and post-traumatic stress symptoms following critical illness in medical intensive care unit patients: Assessing the magnitude of the problem. *Critical Care, 11*(1), R27. doi:10.1186/cc5707

Jackson, J. C., Hart, R. P., Gordon, S. M., Shintani, A., Truman, B., May, L., & Ely, E. W. (2003). Six-month neuropsychological outcome of medical intensive care unit patients. *Critical Care Medicine*, *31*(4), 1226–1234.

Jackson, J. C., Jutte, J. E., Hunter, C. H., Ciccolella, N., Warrington, H., Sevin, C., & Bienvenu, O. J. (2016). Posttraumatic stress disorder (PTSD) after critical illness: A conceptual review of distinct clinical issues and their implications. *Rehabilitation Psychology*, *61*(2), 132–140. doi:10.1037/rep0000085

Jackson, J. C., Obremskey, W., Bauer, R., Greevy, R., Cotton, B., Anderson, V., . . . Ely, W. (2007). Long-term cognitive, emotional, and functional outcomes in trauma intensive care unit survivors without intracranial hemorrhage. *Journal of Trauma and Acute Care Surgery*, *62*(1), 80–88.

Jackson, J. C., Pandharipande, P. P., Girard, T. D., Brummel, N. E., Thompson, J. L., Hughes, C. G., . . . Incidence of Neuropsychological Dysfunction in ICU Survivors (BRAIN-ICU) Study Investigators (2014). Depression, post-traumatic stress disorder, and functional disability in survivors of critical illness in the BRAIN-ICU study: A longitudinal cohort study. *Lancet Respiratory Medicine*, *2*(5), 369–379. doi:10.1016/S2213-2600(14)70051-7

Janig, W. (1985). Systemic and specific autonomic reactions in pain: Efferent, afferent and endocrine components. *European Journal of Anaesthesiology*, *2*(4), 319–346.

Jutte, J. E., Erb, C. T., & Jackson, J. C. (2015). Physical, cognitive, and psychological disability following critical illness: What is the risk? *Seminars in Respiratory and Critical Care Medicine*, *36*(6), 943–958. doi:10.1055/s-0035-1566002

Karnatovskaia, L. V., Johnson, M. M., Benzo, R. P., & Gajic, O. (2015). The spectrum of psychocognitive morbidity in the critically ill: A review of the literature and call for improvement. *Journal of Critical Care*, *30*(1), 130–137. doi:10.1016/j.jcrc.2014.09.024

Kastrup, M., von Dossow, V., Seeling, M., Ahlborn, R., Tamarkin, A., Conroy, P., . . . Spies, C. (2009). Key performance indicators in intensive care medicine: A retrospective matched cohort study. *Journal of International Medical Research*, *37*(5), 1267–1284. doi:10.1177/147323000903700502

Langerud, A. K., Rustoen, T., Brunborg, C., Kongsgaard, U., & Stubhaug, A. (2018). Prevalence, location, and characteristics of chronic pain in intensive care survivors. *Pain Management Nursing*, *19*(4), 366–376. doi:10.1016/j.pmn.2017.11.005

Liu, S., Carpenter, R. L., & Neal, J. M. (1995). Epidural anesthesia and analgesia: Their role in postoperative outcome. *Anesthesiology*, *82*(6), 1474–1506. doi:10.1097/00000542-199506000-00019

Maldonado, J. R., van der Starre, P. J., & Wysong, A. (2003). Post-operative sedation and the incidence of ICU delirium in cardiac surgery patients. *Anesthesiology*, *99*, A465.

Mandle, C. L., Domar, A. D., Harrington, D. P., Leserman, J., Bozadjian, E. M., Friedman, R., & Benson, H. (1990). Relaxation response in femoral angiography. *Radiology*, *174*(3 Pt 1), 737–739. doi:10.1148/radiology.174.3.2406782

Martyn, J. A. J., Mao, J., & Bittner, E. A. (2019). Opioid tolerance in critical illness. *New England Journal of Medicine*, *380*(4), 365–378. doi:10.1056/NEJMra1800222

Mckoy, J. M. (2004). Effect of delirium on length of stay for post-operative surgical patients. *Journal of the American Geriatrics Society*, *52*(4), S167–S167.

Morandi, A., Brummel, N. E., & Ely, E. W. (2011). Sedation, delirium and mechanical ventilation: The "ABCDE" approach. *Current Opinion in Critical Care*, *17*(1), 43–49. doi:10.1097/MCC.0b013e3283427243

Needham, D. M., Davidson, J., Cohen, H., Hopkins, R. O., Weinert, C., Wunsch, H., . . . Harvey, M. A. (2012). Improving long-term outcomes after discharge from intensive care unit: Report from a stakeholders' conference. *Critical Care Medicine, 40*(2), 502–509. doi:10.1097/CCM.0b013e318232da75

Nikayin, S., Rabiee, A., Hashem, M. D., Huang, M., Bienvenu, O. J., Turnbull, A. E., & Needham, D. M. (2016). Anxiety symptoms in survivors of critical illness: A systematic review and meta-analysis. *General Hospital Psychiatry, 43*, 23–29. doi:10.1016/j.genhosppsych.2016.08.005

Page, G. G., Blakely, W. P., & Ben-Eliyahu, S. (2001). Evidence that postoperative pain is a mediator of the tumor-promoting effects of surgery in rats. *Pain, 90*(1–2), 191–199. doi:10.1016/s0304-3959(00)00403-6

Pandharipande, P. P., Girard, T. D., Jackson, J. C., Morandi, A., Thompson, J. L., Pun, B. T., . . . BRAIN-ICU Study Investigators. (2013). Long-term cognitive impairment after critical illness. *New England Journal of Medicine, 369*(14), 1306–1316. doi:10.1056/NEJMoa1301372

Pandharipande, P. P., Sanders, R. D., Girard, T. D., McGrane, S., Thompson, J. L., Shintani, A. K., . . . Ely, E. W. (2010). Effect of dexmedetomidine versus lorazepam on outcome in patients with sepsis: An a priori-designed analysis of the MENDS randomized controlled trial. *Critical Care, 14*(2), R38. doi:10.1186/cc8916

Parker, A. M., Sricharoenchai, T., Raparla, S., Schneck, K. W., Bienvenu, O. J., & Needham, D. M. (2015). Posttraumatic stress disorder in critical illness survivors: A meta-analysis. *Critical Care Medicine, 43*(5), 1121–1129. doi:10.1097/CCM.0000000000000882

Patel, M. B., Jackson, J. C., Morandi, A., Girard, T. D., Hughes, C. G., Thompson, J. L., . . . Pandharipande, P. P. (2016). Incidence and risk factors for intensive care unit-related post-traumatic stress disorder in veterans and civilians. *American Journal of Respiratory and Critical Care Medicine, 193*(12), 1373–1381. doi:10.1164/rccm.201506-1158OC

Payen, J. F., Bosson, J. L., Chanques, G., Mantz, J., & Labarere, J. (2009). Pain assessment is associated with decreased duration of mechanical ventilation in the intensive care unit: A post hoc analysis of the DOLOREA study. *Anesthesiology, 111*(6), 1308–1316. doi:10.1097/ALN.0b013e3181c0d4f0

Payen, J. F., Bru, O., Bosson, J. L., Lagrasta, A., Novel, E., Deschaux, I., . . . Jacquot, C. (2001). Assessing pain in critically ill sedated patients by using a behavioral pain scale. *Critical Care Medicine, 29*(12), 2258–2263. doi:10.1097/00003246-200112000-00004

Payen, J. F., Chanques, G., Mantz, J., Hercule, C., Auriant, I., Leguillou, J. L., . . . Bosson, J. L. (2007). Current practices in sedation and analgesia for mechanically ventilated critically ill patients: A prospective multicenter patient-based study. *Anesthesiology, 106*(4), 687–695. doi:10.1097/01.anes.0000264747.09017.da

Peris, A., Bonizzoli, M., Iozzelli, D., Migliaccio, M. L., Zagli, G., Bacchereti, A., . . . Belloni, L. (2011). Early intra-intensive care unit psychological intervention promotes recovery from post-traumatic stress disorders, anxiety and depression symptoms in critically ill patients. *Critical Care, 15*(1), R41. doi:10.1186/cc10003

Pisani, M. A., Murphy, T. E., Araujo, K. L. B., Slattum, P., Van Ness, P. H., & Inouye, S. K. (2009). Benzodiazepine and opioid use and the duration of intensive care unit delirium in an older population. *Critical Care Medicine, 37*(1), 177–183. doi:10.1097/Ccm.0b013e318192fcf9

Pun, B. T., Balas, M. C., Barnes-Daly, M. A., Thompson, J. L., Aldrich, J. M., Barr, J., . . . Ely, E. W. (2019). Caring for critically ill patients with the ABCDEF Bundle: Results of the ICU liberation collaborative in over 15,000 adults. *Critical Care Medicine, 47*(1), 3–14. doi:10.1097/CCM.0000000000003482

Puntillo, K. A., Max, A., Timsit, J. F., Ruckly, S., Chanques, G., Robleda, G., . . . Azoulay, E. (2018). Pain distress: The negative emotion associated with procedures in ICU patients. *Intensive Care Medicine, 44*(9), 1493–1501. doi:10.1007/s00134-018-5344-0

Puntillo, K. A., Max, A., Timsit, J. F., Vignoud, L., Chanques, G., Robleda, G., . . . Azoulay, E. (2014). Determinants of procedural pain intensity in the intensive care unit. The Europain(R) study. *American Journal of Respiratory and Critical Care Medicine, 189*(1), 39–47. doi:10.1164/rccm.201306-1174OC

Puntillo, K. A., Miaskowski, C., Kehrle, K., Stannard, D., Gleeson, S., & Nye, P. (1997). Relationship between behavioral and physiological indicators of pain, critical care patients' self-reports of pain, and opioid administration. *Critical Care Medicine, 25*(7), 1159–1166. doi:10.1097/00003246-199707000-00017

Puntillo, K. A., & Naidu, R. (2016). Chronic pain disorders after critical illness and ICU-acquired opioid dependence: Two clinical conundra. *Current Opinion in Critical Care, 22*(5), 506–512. doi:10.1097/mcc.0000000000000343

Rabiee, A., Nikayin, S., Hashem, M. D., Huang, M., Dinglas, V. D., Bienvenu, O. J., . . . Needham, D. M. (2016). Depressive symptoms after critical illness: A systematic review and meta-analysis. *Critical Care Medicine, 44*(9), 1744–1753. doi:10.1097/CCM.0000000000001811

Radtke, F. M., Heymann, A., Franck, M., Maechler, F., Drews, T., Luetz, A., . . . Spies, C. D. (2012). How to implement monitoring tools for sedation, pain and delirium in the intensive care unit: An experimental cohort study. *Intensive Care Medicine, 38*(12), 1974–1981. doi:10.1007/s00134-012-2658-1

Raja, S. N., Daniel, D. B., Cohen, M., Finnerup, N. B., Flor, H., Gibson, S., . . . Vader, K. (2020). The revised International Association for the Study of Pain definition of pain: Concepts, challenges, and compromises. *Pain, 161*(9), 1976–1982.

Reade, M. C., & Finfer, S. (2014). Sedation and delirium in the intensive care unit. *New England Journal of Medicine, 370*(5), 444–454.

Rose, L., Haslam, L., Dale, C., Knechtel, L., & McGillion, M. (2013). Behavioral pain assessment tool for critically ill adults unable to self-report pain. *American Journal of Critical Care, 22*(3), 246–255. doi:10.4037/ajcc2013200

Santos, F. S., Velasco, I. T., & Fraguas, R., Jr. (2004). Risk factors for delirium in the elderly after coronary artery bypass graft surgery. *International Psychogeriatrics, 16*(2), 175–193.

Shehabi, Y., Riker, R. R., Bokesch, P. M., Wisemandle, W., Shintani, A., & Ely, E. W. (2010). Delirium duration and mortality in lightly sedated, mechanically ventilated intensive care patients. *Critical Care Medicine, 38*(12), 2311–2318. doi:10.1097/CCM.0b013e3181f85759

Stucky, K., Jutte, J. E., Warren, A. M., Jackson, J. C., & Merbitz, N. (2016). A survey of psychology practice in critical-care settings. *Rehabilitation Psychology, 61*(2), 201–209. doi:10.1037/rep0000071

Sukantarat, K., Greer, S., Brett, S., & Williamson, R. (2007). Physical and psychological sequelae of critical illness. *British Journal of Health Psychology, 12*(Pt 1), 65–74. doi:10.1348/135910706X94096

Swinamer, D. L., Phang, P. T., Jones, R. L., Grace, M., & King, E. G. (1988). Effect of routine administration of analgesia on energy expenditure in critically ill patients. *Chest, 93*(1), 4–10. doi:10.1378/chest.93.1.4

Theunissen, M., Peters, M. L., Bruce, J., Gramke, H. F., & Marcus, M. A. (2012). Preoperative anxiety and catastrophizing: A systematic review and meta-analysis of the association with chronic postsurgical pain. *Clinical Journal of Pain, 28*(9), 819–841. doi:10.1097/AJP.0b013e31824549d6

Timmers, T. K., Verhofstad, M. H., Moons, K. G., van Beeck, E. F., & Leenen, L. P. (2011). Long-term quality of life after surgical intensive care admission. *Archives of Surgery, 146*(4), 412–418. doi:10.1001/archsurg.2010.279

van den Boogaard, M., Peters, S. A., van der Hoeven, J. G., Dagnelie, P. C., Leffers, P., Pickkers, P., & Schoonhoven, L. (2010). The impact of delirium on the prediction of in-hospital mortality in intensive care patients. *Critical Care, 14*(4), R146.

Whelan, C. T., Jin, L., & Meltzer, D. (2004). Pain and satisfaction with pain control in hospitalized medical patients: No such thing as low risk. *Archives of Internal Medicine, 164*(2), 175–180. doi:10.1001/archinte.164.2.175

Williams, T. A., Martin, S., Leslie, G., Thomas, L., Leen, T., Tamaliunas, S., . . . Dobb, G. (2008). Duration of mechanical ventilation in an adult intensive care unit after introduction of sedation and pain scales. *American Journal of Critical Care, 17*(4), 349–356.

Wright, B. R., & Drummond, P. D. (2000). Rapid induction analgesia for the alleviation of procedural pain during burn care. *Burns, 26*(3), 275–282. doi:10.1016/s0305-4179(99)00134-5

Ziehm, S., Rosendahl, J., Barth, J., Strauss, B. M., Mehnert, A., & Koranyi, S. (2017). Psychological interventions for acute pain after open heart surgery. *Cochrane Database of Systematic Reviews, 7*, CD009984. doi:10.1002/14651858.CD009984.pub3

Zimmerman, J. E., Kramer, A. A., & Knaus, W. A. (2013). Changes in hospital mortality for United States intensive care unit admissions from 1988 to 2012. *Critical Care, 17*(2), R81. doi:10.1186/cc12695

8 Psychological Considerations in the Intersection of Infectious Disease with Critical Care Medicine

Julie Highfield, Matt Morgan, and Paul Twose

Introduction

While preparing this chapter, the world is plagued by the novel coronavirus pandemic. Coronaviruses are a family of viruses that cause illnesses. In humans, several coronaviruses are known to cause respiratory infections, including the common cold and more severe diseases such as Middle East respiratory syndrome (MERS) and severe acute respiratory syndrome (SARS). The most recently discovered coronavirus (SARS-CoV-2) causes coronavirus disease (COVID-19).

Most people infected with COVID-19 develop a mild to moderate influenza-like illness. Figures from the United Kingdom suggest that 20% of patients are unwell enough to require hospitalization, with 5% needing admission to an intensive care unit (ICU). Early data from the United States suggest a different picture, with 12% of patients hospitalized and approximately one quarter admitted to the ICU (Centers for Disease Control and Prevention, 2020). In China, of the 55% of patients experiencing respiratory distress, approximately half needed ICU admission, and half of those required invasive ventilation (Wang et al., 2020).

An intersection between infectious disease and critical care has affected critical care medicine as well as the ability to provide rehabilitation and psychological intervention. Working with an infectious disease brings challenges but also innovation.

Julie Highfield, Matt Morgan, and Paul Twose, *Psychological Considerations in the Intersection of Infectious Disease with Critical Care Medicine* In: *Critical Care Psychology and Rehabilitation* Edited by: Kirk J. Stucky and Jennifer E. Jutte, Oxford University Press. © Oxford University Press 2022. DOI: 10.1093/oso/9780190077013.003.0008

It has created a distance and barriers between clinicians and patients but also global connections within the critical care community.

Preparation for pandemic capacity

Preparation of the whole hospital system, and especially critical care, is key: monitoring patterns of infectious disease, predicting demand, and creating surge capacity. Consensus suggests that planning should be systemic, involving all levels from hospital to government, with clear communication and regional coordination (Dichter et al., 2014). In most developed countries critical care is close to capacity during usual times, and the 2003 SARS coronavirus (SARS-CoV) outbreak indicated how quickly critical care capacity was stretched to the limit in countries such as Canada (Low, 2004). Following the 2009 H1N1 influenza pandemic, the International Health Regulations committee concluded that "the world is ill-prepared to respond to a severe influenza pandemic or to any similarly global, sustained, and threatening public-health emergency" (World Health Organization [WHO], 2011, p. 128). Given that this publication is 9 years old, there is potential for resentment among the health care community that further preparation had not taken place sooner.

Preparation for patient-related care

SARS, MERS, and COVID-19 are three major coronavirus outbreaks that have occurred in the last century, with SARS in 2002, MERS in 2012, and now COVID-19 in 2019–2020. There is a lack of long-term research into COVID-19; however, one may extrapolate evidence from SARS and MERS in order to develop hypotheses regarding postintensive care outcomes from COVID-19. SARS and MERS survivors have long-term physical and psychological effects requiring high health care utilization: A meta-analysis of 28 pooled studies of SARS and MERS survivors 6 months after hospitalization found lung function abnormalities in 27%, reduced exercise capacity, a 39% prevalence of posttraumatic stress disorder (PTSD), 33% with depression, and 30% with anxiety (Ahmed et al., 2020).

We also now know that even without contracting the virus, there are substantial mental health consequences of living during a pandemic. Given these figures for patients with COVID-19 and the wider population, psychologists have needed to prepare and respond accordingly but have been greatly hampered by the requirement to provide input while using personal protective equipment (PPE) or via telemedicine. For licensed psychologists in wider settings, issues include the effects of COVID-19 (e.g., personal exposure, exposure of a loved one, bereavement), the secondary impacts of the pandemic (e.g., self-isolation, physical distancing and quarantine, economic loss), and psychological impacts (e.g., depression, anxiety disorders, generalized stress, insomnia, increased substance use and domestic violence) (Pfefferbaum & North, 2020).

Preparation for hospital staff support

Pandemics are known to provoke significant psychological stressors affecting hospital staff and health care workers (Maunder et al., 2006). Hospital-based transmission of the virus to other patients and transmission to health care workers, with resulting severe infection and even death, was a feature of both outbreaks of SARS and MERS and now COVID-19. This places great importance on the use of PPE. At the start of the COVID-19 pandemic, the WHO (2020) indicated a global shortage of PPE of 40%.

High exposure to infection exerts significant levels of psychological stress on the staff. During the SARS and MERS outbreaks, health care workers reported concerns for their own or their family's health as well as experiences of fear and even stigmatization. In a meta-analysis of 19 studies investigating the psychological effects of the SARS pandemic on hospital-based health care workers, clinically significant PTSD symptoms were found in 23% of staff during the acute phase; although there was some spontaneous recovery, prevalence remained at 12% beyond 12 months. For other psychologically significant concerns (e.g., anxiety or depressive symptoms), the prevalence was 34% in the early stages and 29% beyond 12 months (Allan et al., 2020). The authors of this review suggested that COVID-19 may represent a more serious psychological threat than previous pandemics due to factors such as concerns about the availability of PPE, lockdown, and physical distancing requirements. The prolonged and uncertain nature of the pandemic and the likelihood of further waves of increased cases are likely to present a significant continuing emotional and physical threat to many clinical personnel. Staff may be required to work at a more intense pace for a prolonged period of time; they may not have adequate time to rest and recover; they may experience uncertainty about the adequacy of hospital resources. Allan and colleagues (2020) therefore argue that prevalence rates from previous pandemics may provide underestimates of likely prevalence rates for the current pandemic. Undetected and untreated mental health problems such as PTSD and depression are likely to have significant long-term effects on workplace functioning (e.g., as a result of sleeping problems, reduced concentration, workplace avoidance, reduced motivation and loss of interest, increased alcohol and substance use) and increased sickness-related absences, therefore creating a strain on the health care system.

Reflections on the impact of COVID-19 on the critical care setting so far

CREATING CAPACITY

Indications from an April 2020 national survey of 4,875 U.S. ICU clinicians suggested that although hospitals were preparing early for additional bed capacity, clinicians had concerns about preparedness, staffing, and resource allocation (Kaplan et al., 2020). In early February 2020, when it became clear that COVID-19 had arrived in the United States with the first confirmed case in Washington State on January 20, 2020, along with news and images of the impact on hospitals in China and then Italy, a wave of anticipatory anxiety began as clinicians realized the fate that awaited them. Others within hospital and personal communities seemed less concerned; anecdotally, some colleagues thought critical care professionals might be overreacting.

Critical care teams began anticipating the requirement to create surge capacity. This entailed canceling elective surgeries, creating bed capacity from surgical recovery and neurologic high-care areas, and redeploying staff to critical care. There was also consideration of strategies for wider containment and revising and updating protocols, especially for PPE.

IMPACT ON THE TEAM

The authors of this chapter have reflected on the impact on our team of both a sense of coming together to rise to the challenge and experiencing a sense of anxiety and chaos. As the first COVID-19 patients arrived, many units needed to create a "suspected" COVID-19 patient area in addition to a confirmed area, while also treating patients who required critical care but had no indication of infection. With variable sizes and layouts of units, this posed a great challenge, and many critical care units needed to take over other areas within their hospital. We found that this quickly diminished team communication, as team members were dispersed over different areas. Our teams became less integrated geographically, but with time, core staffing was increased to cover the larger number of patients and surge areas, so staff were less likely to see each other and more likely to work with redeployed individuals. To deal with increasing demand, many former critical care personnel and other staff were redeployed; while this brought greater staff support, it also diluted the core ICU staff team.

To create more physical distancing, staff took fewer breaks together, losing their time to connect informally. With the much-needed introduction of lockdown, the opportunities for staff to come together outside work were greatly reduced as well. Staff found that their ability to communicate with patients and each other was hampered by wearing PPE; therefore, communication within the "PPE zone" became more basic and functional, with the use of shorter sentences, less social conversation, and more practical focus. The emphasis on efficiency and preservation of PPE meant that entry into critical care from physicians was less frequent and more functional and could be perceived as less supportive. The once-cohesive interdisciplinary team fractured into transient visits from individual specialties whose practitioners were often unfamiliar with critical care. The social fabric of the critical care environment started to fray.

POSTINTENSIVE CARE SYNDROME AND COVID-19 RECOVERY

It is too early to produce robust outcome data on the impact of COVID-19 in the longer term, but many, anticipating a wave of patients with postintensive care syndrome (PICS), have called for a focus on longer-term rehabilitation needs, given what we know from outcomes of SARS survivors (Stam et al., 2020). Despite the low-level evidence, many societies and organizations have attempted to rapidly produce guidance on the treatment and rehabilitation of patients during and after COVID-19. Guidelines from multiple organizations and collaboratives have highlighted the need for ongoing rehabilitation (e.g., Chartered Society of Physiotherapy, 2020). Patients recovering from COVID-19 will require a range of rehabilitation services and staff, including but not limited to physiotherapy, occupational therapy, speech and language therapy, and psychologists. This requirement is not new, having been required for survivors of critical illnesses in the United Kingdom and elsewhere for decades. However, there is now a surge in patient numbers combined with greater expectations from the wider public.

Early reports are now emerging about the longer-term effects of COVID-19 in those who develop critical illness and require hospitalization and also for a small percentage of those who did not require such treatment. Some are referring to this as "long COVID" (Boseley, 2020), which is characterized by respiratory effects, physical weakness and fatigue, psychological impacts, and neurologic and cognitive consequences. Early anecdotal evidence suggests that 50% of survivors of hospitalized COVID-19, in addition to a minority of non-hospitalized patients, will experience significant problems such as those associated with PICS.

Patients discharged from critical care for other reasons are known to experience ongoing physical limitations for up to 5 years after hospital discharge (Herridge et al., 2011). Patients frequently report ongoing physical weakness, reduced exercise tolerance, and challenges in independently completing activities of daily living. With COVID-19, all of these are apparent, with the addition of severe viral fatigue further inhibiting natural recovery.

Postviral fatigue seems to be prevalent in patients who are hospitalized generally (i.e., not in the ICU), and evidence from SARS suggests this should be a consideration (Perrin et al., 2020). We know little about the specific critical illness neuromuscular pathology in COVID-19, let alone the longer-term patient-centered outcomes. A large funded study, the Post-Hospitalisation COVID-19 Study (PHOSP-COVID) led by the Leicester Biomedical Research Centre, may provide much-needed data in this area. Anecdotal evidence from local colleagues suggests that fatigue is prevalent in longer-stay critical care patients, and it is hard to differentiate that which may be due to their prolonged hospital stay from that due to postviral fatigue.

Early anecdotal reports also suggest a high incidence of laryngeal dysfunction, because of both prolonged intubation and the occurrence of viral laryngitis (Royal College of Speech and Language Therapists, 2020). Patients requiring a tracheostomy may experience ongoing difficulties with both speech and swallowing. Furthermore, it is anticipated that those severely affected by COVID-19 will also experience ongoing respiratory symptoms, including shortness of breath, altered gas exchange, and dysfunctional breathing patterns (George et al., 2020).

There are known psychological effects of an admission to the ICU, with studies indicating that more than 50% of ICU survivors develop symptoms of severe anxiety, depression, or PTSD in the months or years after leaving critical care (Needham et al., 2012; Wade et al., 2012). Although it is early, research seems to suggest that similar outcomes are experienced by COVID-19 survivors, with an added complication of the global fear and awareness of a high-mortality virus. A systematic review of COVID-19 survivors found indications of depression (14.9%), anxiety (14.8%), and PTSD (32.2%) as well as rarer conditions such as hypoxic encephalopathy (Rogers et al., 2020). The British Psychological Society (2020) has produced extensive guidance across a number of areas of COVID-19–related outcomes.

Increasing evidence shows that effects of coronaviruses are not always confined to the respiratory tract; they may also invade the central nervous system, inducing neurologic diseases and/or complications. Patients are likely to experience cognitive impairments related to the direct and indirect effects of the virus and iatrogenic effects of an ICU stay. The combination of prolonged ventilation, sedation, and immobilization has been described as "the perfect storm" leading to increased delirium and post-ICU cognitive and psychological difficulties (Belluck, 2020). The incidence of delirium in patients in the ICU with COVID has been high, many reporting some level of delirium prior to ICU admission that is often missed (McLoughlin et al., 2020). In some cases, brain inflammation and early evidence indicate that a significant proportion of patients hospitalized with COVID-19 will experience neurologic impairments, including impairments in cognitive functioning. In a study of 214 patients, 78 (36.4%) patients had neurologic manifestations. More severely affected patients were likely to have neurologic symptoms such as acute cerebrovascular diseases (5.7%) (Mao et al., 2020).

Impacts on treatment and rehabilitation

A CHANGING ROLE IN PSYCHOLOGY PRACTICE: PATIENTS AND STAFF

Across the world, the role of the psychologist in critical care varies. It includes advising teams in early stages and working directly with patients when de-sedated, especially with regard to delirium management, mood management, and engagement in rehabilitation. Some psychologists work directly in supporting the emotional well-being of critical care staff. Many psychologists will follow a patient into an outpatient setting.

During the current pandemic, the focus of psychological assessment and intervention for patients has shifted away from the ICU to the wards for many shorter-stay patients. Wards have been set up to receive patients who continued to shed virus. Staff were focused on preventing spread of infection, with patients reporting that staff would remain out of the patient environment as much as possible, adding to their increased feelings of isolation and perpetuating delirium.

For the psychology team, our experience has been that ward staff, who had not commonly witnessed delirium, were now baffled by the high rates of confusion and at a loss at what to do. Thus, one primary focus of psychological intervention has been to educate ward staff on managing delirium. What had previously taken many years of educating staff had to be repeated in a rapid timeframe with new teams.

In addition, many recovering patients experience high levels of fatigue and breathlessness—a significant cause of anxiety, therefore requiring an additional role for the critical care or ward psychologist in helping patients and staff manage this more effectively through education about the impact of anxiety on breathlessness, and the role of pacing and patient expectations in physical energy management.

In follow-up clinics, psychologists are now seeing patients who have been home for 8 to 12 weeks. There are similarities in the expression of PICS as found in other post-ICU patients, including stress and anxiety, psychological adjustment difficulties, and PTSD. However, perhaps due to the extensive press coverage of COVID-19 and critical care and increased public awareness in the United Kingdom following this, our experience is that patients attending clinic are already aware of the consequences of delirium. The impact of fatigue and breathlessness on psychological adjustment and recovery is also clear.

There have also been increased referrals of distressed relatives for critical care psychology support. During the ICU stay, relatives' problems include high levels of worry, feeling unable to comprehend what their loved one is facing, and feelings of helplessness. After discharge home, relatives report concerns and anxieties dealing with the distress and trauma in their loved one. Many staff report a level of personal distress at not being able to talk directly with relatives while the patient is in hospital due to restrictions on visitors. This deprives them of an opportunity to hear much of a background story of the patient they are treating.

Many critical care psychologists who previously focused on patient interventions have found their role shifting more to supporting the emotional impact of the pandemic on staff. There has been a temporary increase in the number of team members seeking critical care psychologists for help with personal and work-related stressors in some units, but not in all areas. For instance, in Wuhan an extensive psychological service that was offered to all hospital staff was underused (Chen et al., 2020).

Many staff have found the pace of the experience to cause stress and exhaustion, provoking psychological distress in some and exacerbating mental health issues for those who have underlying mental health vulnerabilities such as clinical depression and anxiety disorders. Psychologists in occupational health have worked in conjunction with psychologists in critical care to teach staff skills to manage stress while also offering reflective group sessions such as Schwartz Center Rounds (Taylor et al., 2018) to help the team members discuss their experiences. This is an evidence-based forum where hospital staff from all backgrounds can come together to talk about the emotional and social challenges of caring for patients. The aim is to offer staff a safe environment in which to share their stories and offer support to one another. This has proven tricky due to physical distancing requirements, and many sessions are conducted via group or individual video call. As the first wave of the pandemic has settled, in some units staff are now being offered group video call sessions to allow time to reflect and consider the psychological impacts of their experiences, but much of the early discussion has focused on the impact of the uncertain and changing supply of PPE; many team members are not yet ready to process what they have witnessed. Offering services via video call introduces new challenges to a psychologist. On the one hand, it enables both patients and staff to connect without the need for travel and allows for more people within a room. On the other hand, video can be experienced as distancing, and in group work this may diminish the feeling of safety to share personal information and be honest. Psychological societies have produced guidelines to help psychologists with these new technologies (American Psychological Association, 2020).

It is important to note that in helping staff make sense of the trauma they have witnessed, the psychologists shared this lived experience and needed to access clinical supervision and their own formal and informal support structures to make sense of their experience.

MEDICAL TREATMENT

The ability to deliver treatment to patients is also changed by the nature of a pandemic. In the first instance, COVID-19 has not responded as a typical pneumonia, so, for the first patients, staff were rapidly learning from other units to formulate effective responses. Like MERS and SARS, there are no distinguishing clinical features of COVID-19, and symptoms overlap substantially with other severe acute respiratory infections, creating a challenge for the intensive care consultant; however, many anecdotal reports indicate that clinicians found the new learning positive and exhilarating. The pathophysiology of COVID-19, involving complex respiratory physics and physiology, is often what attracted many critical care physicians to the specialty in the first place. They are now faced with understanding, treating, and (hopefully) overcoming a new entity using these concepts.

For our medical colleagues, dealing with high numbers of patients with a single disease type has led to more formulaic medicine. Although this may have brought advantages of consistency, at the same time it has diluted the humanity of care. Working with new teams, often brought together at short notice, has made trust difficult to build and even harder to keep. Even familiar faces often become unrecognizable through the fog of PPE. Drug and equipment shortages have made once-familiar tasks more complex. Along with high patient sedation requirements, emergence following de-sedation has been difficult, and delirium has become more common. Interventions such as proning patients are known to be physically demanding and have required the coordination of multiple teams. It is possible that physicians have also had a psychological barrier to suggest these treatments, despite their efficiency, knowing the additional burden it would place on an already stretched workforce.

REHABILITATION

Rehabilitation staff have been limited in their ability to work effectively in full PPE within the "red" zone (as the acute COVID-19 zone has been described in many ICUs). Also, critical care stays have often been longer than was previously typical in ICUs, with an average length of stay for those with COVID-19 of 12 days in ICU and 20 days in the hospital, although experience between units has varied (Docherty et al., 2020). The majority of patients in critical care have remained intubated and deeply sedated for prolonged periods, immobilized and isolated from family members due to visitor restrictions. Delirium has been seen in as many as 70% in some cohorts (Khan, 2020). Staff report on critical care rounds has returned to the ways of over 10 years ago, with patients fully sedated and immobilized; as a result, the opportunity for ICU-based early rehabilitation has rapidly diminished. With wariness around the use of PPE, both in terms of risk to self but also in maintaining adequate supply, rehabilitation staff cluster their working days around time in PPE zones. Although this does not alter the nursing approach, in our experience as clinicians, this has meant that during the height of the first wave of the COVID-19 pandemic, patients' rehabilitation has been harder to coordinate.

Rehabilitation works best when delivered by a fully integrated interdisciplinary team with input from nursing, medical, and allied health care professions. The restrictions of PPE have challenged the status quo. Interaction between professions has become harder, frequently resulting in a return to "silo" working. This was compounded by the increase in patient numbers and the understandable drive to discharge patients to ward environments as soon as possible to release critical care capacity.

As with nursing, rehabilitation staff have relied on redeployment of therapists from non–critical care areas who likely have little experience in hyperacute rehabilitation within critical care. This has required considerable upskilling, supervision, and training, which further reduced the capacity of specialist staff to provide specialized rehabilitation to those in need.

Rehabilitation staff have had to learn from each other's experience and the experiences of those who worked during previous pandemics, seeking information from other hospitals and critical care units that gained early experience in managing those admitted with COVID-19. Viral fatigue has been a predominant feature, with patients able to complete only very short bursts of treatment, and frequently unable to manage both physical rehabilitation and ventilatory weaning at the same time. This has resulted in the need to provide input in shorter sessions and more frequently; however, this has not always been possible due to concerns about PPE availability.

As time has progressed, a significant number of patients have been slow to wean from mechanical ventilation. Even when the amount of respiratory support is low, removal from a ventilator often fails for reasons that are unclear. This, combined with weakness, means that a longer duration of weaning is often required, with longer times needing higher levels of respiratory support and frequent use of tracheostomy. This requires full multidisciplinary team (MDT) rehabilitation within the critical care context, which feels more familiar, although in practice it is far from this. An element of PPE is still required, and MDT staff are challenged to reduce delirium and encourage engagement while wearing surgical masks. In fact, some patients have reported delusional thinking in relation to the PPE itself (e.g., "That is not your face").

For those providing rehabilitation, a new "normal" has been required. Using everything we know about the impact of critical illness and the requirement for early rehabilitation, balanced against ongoing PPE requirements, concerns about using aerosol-generating procedures have reduced staff–patient interaction. Prolonged ventilation, sedation type and use, and neuromuscular blockades all had, and still have, significant impacts. The combination of profound intensive care–acquired weakness, severe postviral fatigue, and significant delirium has resulted in significant rehabilitation requirements. Rehabilitation staff have had to revert to a coordinated approach, timing interventions to ensure maximum benefit without overload. We have continuously had to balance the importance of weaning from mechanical ventilation while ensuring physical and emotional recovery. However, this was a modified "normal," not a completely new way of working. The format of rehabilitation remains the same as for those admitted for reasons other than COVID-19. Rehabilitation has continued to consist of physical rehabilitation such as sitting on the edge of the bed, transfers to the chair, strengthening exercises, and, when possible, walking. Patient communication has been key: The incidence of tracheostomy insertion has been higher than initially anticipated, but this has provided the opportunity for early communication with inline speaking valves, and this has been essential for reducing delirium, assessing orientation, and improving patient–health care professional interaction (Vallès Fructuoso et al., 2015).

Visitor restrictions have meant that family involvement in rehabilitation has all but disappeared. Many units have opted to create a system of telephone updates to family and the use of video calling with the awake and alert patient. However, this is a poor substitute for being at the bedside. The use of speaking valves has provided the opportunity for patients to talk to relatives and loved ones via telephone or video calls; however, because of aerosolization concerns, not all units use them, or they will do so only where staff remain in full PPE.

Due to stretched medical rosters and high demand on nursing staff, rehabilitation staff have often become the most consistent presence for patients, providing holistic patient management that includes creation of integrated rehabilitation and ventilatory weaning plans, tracheostomy weaning, and discharge planning. All of these will have an ongoing positive impact beyond COVID-19 and have only served to increase the need for allied health professionals within critical care.

THE FUTURE OF CRITICAL CARE IN A CONTINUED CONTEXT
OF INFECTIOUS DISEASES

Even before the last patient has recovered from COVID-19, medicine will have changed forever. Technologies that struggled for decades to enter clinical practice will remain as essential tools. Video consultations, distant follow-up, and telemedicine will continue to be used, even after visiting restrictions have been lifted. A knowledge of what intensive care staff can, and importantly cannot, do will remain in the minds of the public and professionals alike. The advantages of a public health care system to respond to global challenges will remind us that private medicine has disadvantages. Reemergence of faith in science and experts will hopefully dilute exploitative and fake medical news. But there may be disadvantages too. When the experience of lockdown for those remaining at home for months was so radically different compared with health care workers, some may reflect on the injustice of low pay and difficult working conditions for the latter. The psychological burden may also remain, with staff carrying the distress felt by families and patients with them into a post-COVID world.

There are challenges, too, in the administration and business of health care. Separation of "clean" work, often the province of private medicine, such as joint replacements, is simple. However, complex major surgery, cancer care (such as chemotherapy and radiotherapy), and health care where patients are critically unwell must become safely integrated into the risk environment where COVID-19 may be ever-present. This requires not only the physical goods such as PPE but also developed governance systems to allow risk prediction, patient flow, paperwork, and people to flow smoothly.

Patients admitted to critical care with COVID-19 or any other pathology will continue to require specialist rehabilitation from a range of professions. Similarly, the challenges of PPE, grouping patients into areas depending on infection status, and unpredictable patient numbers are not going to change anytime soon. Rehabilitation will need to continue to adapt both within critical care and along the recovery continuum to reflect patient and service demands. As "usual" services resume, staff redeployment will diminish, and the core cohort of rehabilitation staff will remain. On the one hand, this will allow a return to familiar ways of working, a more interdisciplinary approach, and greater specialist input. However, it will also result in a reduction of staffing, a return to previous models of working (e.g., 5-day working patterns rather than 7-day ones), and the risk of those core staff continuing to face the burden of viral exposure, lack of PPE, and high patient numbers.

Luckily, as yet in the United Kingdom, we have not had to limit the range of treatments available to patients, and careful planning and communication have meant that those who benefit most from a critical care stay have been admitted. However, there was significant early anticipation of a point of setting additional treatment limitations and a fear of the moral distress that would induce, with some reports of rationing at the peak of the pandemic in parts of Italy. Time will tell if we are to reach that point.

Conclusion

The response to the coronavirus pandemic has resulted in many positive outcomes. Rehabilitation services have shown their ability to adapt to suit patients' needs. Furthermore, the requirement for post–critical care rehabilitation has never been more apparent, with significant media coverage and the publication of multiple guidance documents. For many who have worked tirelessly to promote the field of critical care rehabilitation, this has come as a mixed blessing; on the one hand, it has shined a positive spotlight on an undersupported area, while on the other, despite good intentions, it has led to some misinformation and confusion. There is potential for conflict between different groups as is often seen in the context of a disaster; we must encourage cooperation via shared interests and the collective sense of what is the morally right thing to do (for a good overview, see Van Bavel et al., 2020). These gains must not be lost, and rehabilitation services must continue to develop to provide for all patients requiring critical care, due to COVID-19 or other reasons. Furthermore, the mental health impact of pandemics on patients, families, and staff alike cannot be underestimated, and for all the pressure and burden that it brings, the role of the psychologist within critical care and beyond has become more clearly recognized.

References

Ahmed, H., Patel, K., Greenwood, D. C., Halpin, S., Lewthwaite, P., Salawu, A., . . . Sivan, M. (2020). Long-term clinical outcomes in survivors of severe acute respiratory syndrome (SARS) and Middle East respiratory syndrome (MERS) coronavirus outbreaks after hospitalisation or ICU admission: A systematic review and meta-analysis. *Journal of Rehabilitation Medicine*, *52*(5), jrm00063.

Allan, S. M., Bealey, R., Birch, J., Cushing, T., Parke, S., Sergi, G., . . . Meiser-Stedman, R. (2020). The prevalence of common and stress-related mental health disorders in healthcare workers based in pandemic-affected hospitals: A rapid systematic review and meta-analysis. *European Journal of Psychotraumatology*, *11*, 1810903. https://doi.org/10.1080/20008198.2020.1810903

American Psychological Association. (2020). Five tips for transitioning your practice to tele-health. https://www.apaservices.org/practice/business/management/transitioning-telehealth

Belluck, P. (2020, June 28). "They want to kill me:" Many COVID patients have terrifying delirium. *New York Times.* https://www.nytimes.com/2020/06/28/health/coronavirus-delirium-hallucinations.html

Boseley, S. (2020, September 8). Coronavirus: 60,000 may have "long Covid" for more than three months—UK study. *The Guardian.* https://www.theguardian.com/society/2020/sep/08/60000-may-have-long-covid-for-more-than-three-months-uk-study

British Psychological Society. (2020, July 23). Coronavirus resources and guidance. https://www.bps.org.uk/coronavirus-resources

Centers for Disease Control and Prevention. (2020). Severe outcomes among patients with coronavirus disease 2019 (COVID-19). https://www.cdc.gov/mmwr/volumes/69/wr/mm6912e2.htm

Chartered Society of Physiotherapy. (2020, July 23). Coronavirus guidelines. https://www.csp.org.uk/news/coronavirus/clinical-guidance/rehabilitation-coronavirus/covid-19-rehabilitation-standards

Chen, Q., Liang, M., Li, Y., Guo, J., Fei, D., Wang, L., . . . Zhang, Z. (2020). Mental health care for medical staff in China during the COVID-19 outbreak. *Lancet Psychiatry, 7,* e15–e16.

Dichter, J. R., Kanter, R. K., Dries, D., Luyckx, V., Lim, M. L., Wilgis, J., . . . Kissoon, N. (2014). System-level planning, coordination, and communication: Care of the critically ill and injured during pandemics and disasters: CHEST consensus statement. *Chest, 146*(4 suppl), e87S–e102S.

Docherty, A. B., Harrison, E. M., Green, C. A., Hardwick, H., Pius, R., Norman, L., . . . Semple, M. G. (2020). Features of 16,749 hospitalised UK patients with COVID-19 using the ISARIC WHO Clinical Characterisation Protocol. medRxiv. https://doi.org/10.1101/2020.04.23.20076042

George, P. M., Barratt, S. L., Condliffe, R., Desai, S. R., Devaraj, A., Forrest, I., . . . Spencer, L. G. (2020). Respiratory follow-up of patients with COVID-19 pneumonia. *Thorax, 75,* 1009–1016.

Herridge, M. S., Tansey, C. M., Matte, A., Tomlinson, G., Diaz-Granados, N., Cooper, A., . . . Cheung, A. M. (2011). Functional disability 5 years after acute respiratory distress syndrome. *New England Journal of Medicine, 364,* 1293–1304.

Kaplan, L. J., Kleinpell, R., Maves, R. C., Doersam, J. K., Raman, R., & Ferraro, D. M. (2020). Critical care clinician reports on coronavirus disease 2019: Results from a national survey of 4,875 ICU providers. *Critical Care Explorations, 2,* e0125. doi:10.1097/CCE.0000000000000125

Khan, S. H., Lindroth, H., Perkins, A. J., Jamil, Y., Wang, S., Roberts, S., . . . Khan, B. A. (2020). Delirium incidence, duration and severity in critically ill patients with COVID-19. medRxiv. https://doi.org/10.1101/2020.05.31.20118679

Li, Y. C., Bai, W. Z., & Hashikawa, T. (2020). The neuroinvasive potential of SARS-CoV2 may play a role in the respiratory failure of COVID-19 patients. *Journal of Medical Virology, 92*(6), 552–555.

Lodigiani, C., Iapichino, G., Carenzo, L., Cecconi, M., Ferrazzi, P., Sebastian, T., . . . Barco, S. (2020). Venous and arterial thromboembolic complications in COVID-19 patients admitted to an academic hospital in Milan, Italy. *Thrombosis Research, 191,* 9–14.

Low, D. E. (2004). SARS: Lessons from Toronto. In S. Knobler, A. Mahmoud, S. Lemon, A. Mack, L. Sivitz, & K. Oberholtzer (Eds.), *Learning from SARS: Preparing for the next disease outbreak.* Institute of Medicine (US) Forum on Microbial Threats. National Academies Press. https://www.ncbi.nlm.nih.gov/books/NBK92467/

Mao, L., Jin, H., Wang, M., Hu, Y., Chen, S., He, Q., Chang, J., . . . Hu, B. (2020). Neurologic manifestations of hospitalized patients with coronavirus disease 2019 in Wuhan, China. *JAMA Neurology, 77*(6), 683–690.

Maunder, R. G., Lancee, W. J., Balderson, K. E., Bennett, J. P., Borgundvaag, B., Evans, S., . . . Wasylenki, D. A. (2006). Long-term psychological and occupational effects of providing hospital healthcare during SARS outbreak. *Emerging Infectious Diseases, 12*(12), 1924–1932.

McLoughlin, B. C., Miles, A., Webb, T. E., Knopp, P., Eyres, C., Fabbri, A., . . . Davis, D. (2020). Functional and cognitive outcomes after COVID-19 delirium. *European Geriatric Medicine, 11*, 857–862.

Needham, D. M., Davidson, J., Cohen, H., Hopkins, R. O., Weinert, C., Wunsch, H., . . . Harvey, M. A. (2012). Improving long-term outcomes after discharge from intensive care unit: Report from a stakeholders' conference. *Critical Care Medicine, 40*(2), 502–509.

Perrin, R., Riste, L., & Hann, M. (2020). Into the looking glass: Post-viral syndrome post COVID-19. *Medical Hypotheses, 144*, 110055. doi: 10.1016/j.mehy.2020.110055

Pfefferbaum, B., & North, C. S. (2020). Mental health and the Covid-19 pandemic. *New England Journal of Medicine, 383*, 510–512.

Rogers, J. P., Chesney, E., Oliver, D., Pollack, T. A., McGuire, P., Fusar-Poli, P., . . . David, A. S. (2020). Psychiatric and neuropsychiatric presentations associated with severe coronavirus infections: A systematic review and meta-analysis with comparison to the COVID-19 pandemic. *Lancet Psychiatry, 7*(7), 611–627.

Royal College of Speech and Language Therapists. (2020). COVID-19 speech and language therapy rehabilitation pathway. https://www.rcslt.org/wp-content/uploads/media/docs/Covid/RCSLT-COVID-19-SLT-rehab-pathway_15-July-2020_FINAL.pdf?la=en&hash=29A7914A98103BDDF61ECAA072A70C80FBF50551

Stam, H. J., Stucki, G., Bickenbach, J., & European Academy of Rehabilitation Medicine. (2020). Covid-19 and post-intensive care syndrome: A call for action. *Journal of Rehabilitation Medicine, 52*(4), jrm00044. doi:10.2340/16501977-2677

Taylor, C., Xyrichis, A., Leamy, M. C., Reynolds, E., & Maben, J. (2018). Can Schwartz Center Rounds support healthcare staff with emotional challenges at work, and how do they compare with other interventions aimed at providing similar support? A systematic review and scoping reviews. *BMJ Open, 8*, e024254. doi:10.1136/bmjopen-2018-024254

Vallès Fructuoso, O., Ruiz de Pablo, B., Fernández Plaza, M., Fernández Olgoso, M. J., & Martínez Estalella, G. (2015). Does the speaking valve improve tracheostomized ICU patients communication and emotional security? *Intensive Care Medicine Experimental, 3*(Suppl 1), A557.

Van Bavel, J. J., Baicker, K., Boggio, P. S., Capraro, V., Cichocka, A., Cikara, M., . . . Willer, R. (2020). Using social and behavioural science to support COVID-19 pandemic response. *Nature Human Behaviour, 4*, 460–471.

Wade, D. M., Howell, D. C., Weinman, J. A., Hardy, R. J., Mythen, M. G., Brewin, C. R., . . . Raine, R. A. (2012). Investigating risk factors for psychological morbidity three months after intensive care: A prospective cohort study. *Critical Care, 16*(5), R192.

Wang, D., Hu, B., Hu, C., Zhu, F., Liu, X., Zhang, J., . . . Peng, Z. (2020). Clinical characteristics of 138 hospitalized patients with 2019 novel coronavirus-infected pneumonia in Wuhan, China. *Journal of the American Medical Association, 323*(11), 1061–1069.

World Health Organization. (2011). *Implementation of the International Health Regulations (2005): Report of the Review Committee on the Functioning of the International Health Regulations (2005) in relation to pandemic (H1N1) 2009.* World Health Organization.

World Health Organization. (2020). Shortage of personal protective equipment endangering health workers worldwide. https://www.who.int/news/item/03-03-2020-shortage-of-personal-protective-equipment-endangering-health-workers-worldwide

9 Unique Considerations for Psychologists Working in Pediatric Critical Care

Crystal L. Cederna-Meko, Shannon L. Dennis, and Rebecca E. H. Ellens

WITHIN THE UNITED STATES, roughly 230,000 children are hospitalized annually in critical care settings (Treble-Barna et al., 2019). Youth enter critical care with a variety of acute and chronic problems. Presenting issues span bodily systems and organs (e.g., respiratory, cardiovascular, endocrine, renal, neurologic, hematologic), infections and illness (e.g., pneumonia, sepsis, influenza), traumatic injuries (e.g., brain and spinal cord injuries, fractures, burns), and poisonings (e.g., substance ingestions). Studies suggest mortality rates in pediatric critical care (PCC) are declining to as low as 3% to 5%, owing, in part, to advances in cardiopulmonary resuscitation (Berg et al., 2016), mechanical ventilation, medications (Ong et al., 2016), and surgical interventions (Namachivayam et al., 2010).

While more youth survive critical illness, rates of new functional morbidity at hospital discharge and up to 2 years later are as high as 36% and 13%, respectively (Ong et al., 2016). In a study of youth with neurologic diagnoses in critical care, Williams, Eriksson, and colleagues (2019) found that 35% developed new disability(ies) involving sensory, motor, feeding, mental status, respiratory, and communication changes. Youth also experience adverse psychiatric sequelae following PCC admissions (e.g., Colville, 2015; Davydow et al., 2010; Kyösti et al., 2019). Thus, the risk is great of acquiring problems during a PCC stay that reduce quality of life and impair functioning beyond hospital discharge.

Crystal L. Cederna-Meko, Shannon L. Dennis, and Rebecca E. H. Ellens, *Unique Considerations for Psychologists Working in Pediatric Critical Care* In: *Critical Care Psychology and Rehabilitation.* Edited by: Kirk J. Stucky and Jennifer E. Jutte, Oxford University Press. © Oxford University Press 2022. DOI: 10.1093/oso/9780190077013.003.0009

In 2010, the Society of Critical Care Medicine coined the term "postintensive care syndrome" (PICS) to describe the onset or worsening of cognitive, social/emotional, and physical problems in adult patients after discharge from critical care (Needham et al., 2012). PICS has since been expanded to include family members (Davidson et al., 2012) and pediatric patients (e.g., Williams, Hartman, et al., 2019). Efforts are under way to enhance PICS assessment and management resources (e.g., Esses et al., 2019). Specifically, the following are advised: assessing for functional changes early and often, including at all transitions in care (Elliott et al., 2014), and routinely employing a multidisciplinary team in order to prevent and treat associated deficits (LaBuzetta et al., 2019; Williams, Hartman, et al., 2019).

Along with a growing appreciation for the functional morbidities that can follow critical care stays, psychologists have long been embedded within PCC settings; publications describing psychologists' consultation and liaison roles within PCC date back 40 years (e.g., Schenkenberg et al., 1981). Providing assessment and intervention, health promotion, interprofessional team support, and familial support through biopsychosocial and developmental frameworks, psychologists are valuable members of PCC teams. From this position, psychologists can initiate early contact, monitor and intervene throughout hospitalization, and support optimal transfers of care to outpatient-based specialty services.

In what follows, the key knowledge, skills, and attributes necessary for psychologists to function effectively within PCC settings will be reviewed. Thereafter, the needs of pediatric patients and families from PCC admission through discharge will be examined as well as the accompanying roles for psychologists. Throughout the chapter, opportunities for individualized adaptations will be highlighted. Of note, neonatal critical care settings are increasingly an area of practice for psychologists (Hynan et al., 2015) but are beyond the scope of this chapter; interested readers are encouraged to see Barbosa (2013).

Essential knowledge, skills, and attributes for psychologists

PCC settings involve high medical acuity, require more resources than non–critical care settings, and consequently can be emotionally charged and stressful environments (Tunick et al., 2013). Readiness to practice as a psychologist in PCC requires advanced knowledge, skills, and attributes derived from graduate-level coursework in addition to supervised practice in relevant clinical settings. In what follows, key areas for ensuring expertise prior to practicing as a psychologist within PCC are reviewed.

CHILD DEVELOPMENT AND PSYCHOPATHOLOGY

Children's thinking, reasoning, and behavior are a function of their developmental level. Consequently, pediatric patients' understanding of the illness, appreciation for the rationale behind necessary interventions, and ability to gain new skills in response will be limited by their development. A solid foundation in child development and the ability to differentiate typical from atypical development across the domains of cognition and self-help, expressive and receptive language, fine and gross motor, and social/emotional development are essential. Psychologists within PCC need to comfortably apply developmental theories to promote coping and develop effective interventions targeting identified abnormalities. Primary developmental theories span cognition, behavior, psychosocial, self-regulation, and attachment models. Children exist in and, in large part, are directed by their social environments. Therefore, psychologists must also be astute in the use of multi-informant, multimethod approaches to gathering data while conceptualizing through ecological and biopsychosocial lenses.

The capacity to apply knowledge of human learning to a variety of circumstances is also a requisite skill. Social learning theory, classical and operant conditioning theories, and the transtheoretical model of behavior change are employed for various reasons, including to (1) promote patient and family adaptation to circumstances following PCC admission, (2) increase desirable and decrease undesirable behaviors, and (3) support treatment and discharge goals. Psychologists in PCC are often asked to assist in reducing problematic or health-compromising behaviors and also to increase health-promoting and outcome-enhancing behaviors. As part of this work, psychologists need to efficiently identify the modifiable antecedents and consequences surrounding target behaviors as well as enlist the motivations of the patient or family. The aforementioned goals are also supported by skillfully identifying and creating opportunities for adaptive modeling while reducing patients' exposure to unintentional maladaptive modeling by family members and staff.

Expertise in child and adolescent psychopathology is also essential to PCC practice. With such knowledge comes appreciation for the variance in symptom presentation based on a child's age (e.g., depressed mood may manifest as irritability or somatic complaints; anxiety may present as freezing, agitation, disorganized thinking, and regression). Recognition of what might be a typical reaction within a PCC versus an outpatient setting, given the acuity of symptoms, loss of routine and sense of autonomy, and illness-associated consequences, is also important. Expertise in differentiating normal from abnormal phenomena allows the astute psychologist to either provide guidance to families that maintains health, or provide evidence-based interventions to treat clinically significant difficulties.

INTERPERSONAL AND COMMUNICATION SKILLS

A psychologist's interpersonal and communication skills support the patient, family, physicians, and others involved in the care of youth. Psychologists best support assessment and treatment goals when they can efficiently and effectively clarify consultation requests from a variety of referral sources (e.g., physician's assistants, resident physicians, intensivists, surgeons, neurologists) and then provide the rationale for their involvement to patients and families using family-centered language. Thereafter, psychologists need flexibility in their approach, paired with sufficient structure and organization, to ensure they gather necessary information during patient encounters. The psychologist must be able to quickly develop and maintain strong alliances (Colville, 2001) with the patient, family, and all members of the treatment team.

As previously noted, patients, family members, and others within the treatment team are susceptible to experiencing strong affective states. Consequently, keen emotion recognition skills ensure the early detection of strong emotional responses in oneself and others. Once identified, skill in self-emotion regulation, along with comfort in therapeutically managing the emotions of others in live time, is critical. Maintaining resilience and wellness over time is also imperative and likely best supported by the same strategies under exploration with physicians and nurses. Specifically, routine self-compassion (Mills & Chapman, 2016), developing and maintaining social connectedness (Zigelstein, 2018), and ensuring a sense of meaning in workplace activities (Gogo et al., 2019) are encouraged.

Psychologists often serve as a liaison for the patient/family and other individuals within the treatment team. Within the liaison role, psychologists enhance awareness of patient and family experiences, needs, and strategies to optimize psychosocial functioning and outcomes. Psychologists may also advise on communication strategies for a given patient or family as well as on strategies for delivering information to families in a retainable and useful manner (e.g., providing brief, recurring, developmentally tailored information; Colville, 2015). Effectively fulfilling liaison roles rests upon familiarity with commonly used medical terminology, the ability to apply health literacy principles to patient and family communication, and skill in tailoring communication to a wide variety of recipients, time constraints, and circumstances.

COMFORT AND CONTRIBUTIONS WITHIN
THE INTERPROFESSIONAL TEAM

Psychologists' comfort with and participation in the interprofessional PCC team yields many benefits (Buckloh & Schilling, 2017). Team integration increases first-person communication and supports efficient care coordination (Colville, 2001). Active team participation also supports awareness of, and respect for, the contributions of each team member, fosters the development and maintenance of shared treatment plans, and ensures that psychosocial considerations are routinely included within care plans. Opportunities for team participation will vary but can include interdisciplinary rounds, educational venues (e.g., trauma conference, morbidity and mortality conferences), staff training sessions (e.g., de-escalation training), departmental and clinical operations meetings, and family conferences (Tunick et al., 2013).

Interprofessional teams are further enhanced by clear delineation of roles for disciplines that are distinct but have the potential to overlap (Hynan et al., 2015). This applies most readily to psychologists as their work delves into domains where multiple providers may have expertise. Examples include end-of-life support; identification of sibling or parental-related psychosocial needs; and the assessment and management of risk for self-harm, neurodevelopmental concerns, or failure to thrive. Table 9.1 provides a summary of common disciplines that may overlap with psychology functions within PCC settings. Other disciplines apply on a case-by-case basis (e.g., occupational therapy when feeding-related issues emerge; pediatric neurology when new, uncharacteristic motoric movement episodes present in a child with a history of epilepsy). Of note, the scope of practice by specialty is likely to vary as a product of the institution, patient need, provider comfort and availability, and the totality of resources available. Thus, initiating team-based dialogue surrounding provider roles and associated workflows should occur early and then be revisited periodically thereafter.

Patients and family members are also central members of the treatment team (Committee on Hospital Care and Institute for Patient- and Family-Centered Care, 2012; Meert et al., 2013). Psychologists' awareness of the expertise that patients and families bring to the team (e.g., knowledge of the patient before hospitalization, social resources available to the patient and family outside of the hospital) supports their advocacy for routine patient/family involvement in care planning. Psychologists also must appreciate the diversity inherent in familial structure and dynamics, socioeconomic status, spiritual and religious affiliations, sources of support, and health beliefs and behaviors (Shudy et al., 2006). Respect for variations in the type and level of information preferred by various members of a family (e.g., patient vs. caregiver; older vs. younger) also supports optimal communication. In sum, by adhering to evidence-based yet culturally informed care practices, psychologists can support teams in taking account of patient/family preferences, navigating conflicts between health care and familial values, and assisting teams in identifying shared treatment priorities.

TABLE 9.1.

Common disciplines available in PCC settings (in alphabetical order)

Specialty service	Common roles
Art therapy	• Provision of sensory experiences that promote psychological and physiologic improvement
Case management	• Coordination with insurance providers to establish and maintain the medical necessity of hospital care
	• Facilitation of interprofessional and family meetings
	• Anticipation and arrangement of patient needs at hospital discharge (e.g., medical equipment, medication, appointments, transportation to/from appointments, therapy referrals)
Child and adolescent psychiatry	• Psychiatric evaluation
	• Psychiatric management recommendations
Child life	• Access to developmentally appropriate activities aligned with medical needs or restrictions
	• Comfort-promoting measures during procedures
	• Diversionary activities before, during, and after procedures
	• Promotion of sibling adjustment
	• Preprocedural education
Music therapy	• Provision of sensory experiences that promote psychological and physiologic improvement
Psychology team: pediatric psychology, neuropsychology, rehabilitation psychology	• Evaluation specific to the psychology specialty represented
	• Management recommendations specific to the psychology specialty represented
Social work	• Familial support
	• Mental health and social/environmental referrals
	• Social/environmental evaluation, resource acquisition, and referral coordination
Spiritual care	• Prayer
	• Spiritual and end-of-life support
Teachers/educators	• Specialized instruction aligned with pre-admission academics, developmental level, and medical needs or restrictions
	• Evaluation and recommendations for eventual return to academic environment

TELEHEALTH SERVICE DELIVERY

In some circumstances, in-person service delivery is contraindicated or unavailable (e.g., rural health settings where specialty providers are not geographically proximal, contact or patient isolation precautions in the absence of readily available personal protective equipment for providers, patients in an immunocompromised state amidst rapid transmission of novel communicable diseases). In such instances, the costs to organizations, patients, providers, and the public at large warrant identification of alternative care methods. One method that is increasingly encouraged and reimbursed (Owings-Fonner, 2020) is telehealth—the provision of patient care using video and/or audio (i.e., telephone) connection.

In addition to understanding relevant policies, laws, and regulations governing telehealth, psychologists must remain cognizant of the unique ethical considerations that telehealth with minors introduces (Kroll, 2020). At a minimum, the psychologist should abide by the American Psychological Association (APA, 2017)'s ethical principles concerning informed consent, privacy and confidentiality, and competence. Standards related to therapy and assessment also warrant review, as telehealth can lessen the applicability, benefit, and appropriateness of clinical services designed for in-person delivery (e.g., APA, 2020; Chenneville & Schwartz-Mette, 2020; Hewitt et al., 2020).

When selecting between telehealth and in-person care methods, consideration of patient- and family-specific factors is important. Accommodations will be needed for patients with sensory impairments, those with developmental delays or disabilities, individuals for whom English is an additional language, and those with limited prior exposure to related technologies or virtual means of communicating. Similarly, psychologists will benefit from planning in advance how best to adapt telehealth to preschool-aged youth, patients with compromised health status and altered mental status, and patients/families in need of individual interviews. Strategies to maximize telehealth success may include use of the services of an interpreter, use of closed captioning, additional attention to minimizing extraneous stimuli in the patient's room, ensuring the availability of a separate and private room for individual interviews, orienting the patient to the device and common controls, ensuring the presence of a staff member throughout the encounter, and placing the device out of a patient's reach yet close enough to maintain a visual and auditory connection.

Finally, psychologists' knowledge and comfort with telehealth in PCC contributes to the success of telehealth service delivery (Kroll, 2020). In vivo guidance to address access and connection issues alongside staff and families reduces frustrations, staff/family burden, and disruptions to clinical care. Periodically revisiting telehealth workflows with relevant parties promotes telehealth service effectiveness, while coordinating telehealth care with support staff and other providers improves service efficiency. Telehealth viability can also be expanded by advocating for additional resources, equipment, and technologies to improve telehealth benefit for PCC patients. Resources likely to help PCC patients include the following:

- Flexible equipment stands that accommodate varying heights, proximities to the patient, and orientations beyond portrait and landscape.
- Equipment to accommodate youth with varying levels of cognitive, motor, and speech/language ability.
- Access to one-time-use headphones with built-in microphones.
- Reliance upon a virtual video platform with built-in or installable engagement-enhancing features (e.g., screen sharing, drawing boards, virtual games).

Psychologists' activities on the PCC unit

PCC settings can vary from highly specialized (e.g., pediatric neurointensive or cardiac care unit) to broad and generalized (e.g., pediatric or neonatal intensive care unit; Buckloh & Schilling, 2017). Based on the PCC setting, the indications for referral, ages served, presenting problems addressed, and timing of psychologists' involvement may vary considerably. Regardless, all PCC psychologists serve in consultation and liaison roles (Carter et al., 2017) that can be initiated at any time during a PCC stay. Common psychologist activities and roles from PCC admission through discharge are discussed next.

CRITICAL CARE ADMISSION

Roles with families

When youth are admitted to a PCC setting, communication with the patient may be limited by mechanical ventilation, altered mental status, and other consequences of the presenting problem(s). At this time, psychologists' clinical roles may primarily involve work with family members (Lassen et al., 2014). Early interactions between the psychologist and family enable families to gain familiarity with the role of the psychology service and to receive education about what can be expected in the early days of admission. Psychologists can provide feedback to families about observed or anticipated changes in a patient's behavior, mood, and mental status. For example, children and adolescents may exhibit uncharacteristic mood states and behavior secondary to delirium (Colville, 2015), medication or illness-induced effects, moderate to high pain levels, and alterations in sleep and routine. While surveying the patient, psychologists can learn of changes observed by relatives and inform families of alterations in the patient's ability to communicate. For instance, as alertness returns, infants and young children may not be soothed as easily by their parents, and children with more developed verbal communication skills may not be able to respond to questions or directions in their typical manner. By educating family members about what may occur (Baker & Gledhill, 2017) and providing them with strategies for responding optimally, familial coping is improved and distress is reduced (Esses et al., 2019).

As the patient's level of alertness improves, family members can also learn strategies to optimize coping and address emerging psychosocial needs. Specifically, patients and siblings may need support to understand the presenting problem(s) and treatments that are under way, to support communication, to ensure that questions of importance to them are answered in developmentally appropriate yet matter-of-fact ways, and to cope with adjustments in daily routines and separations between family members (Meert et al., 2013). Delivery of caregiver support interventions that reduce parental and familial stress benefit the family and patient recovery process (Mills et al., 2018; Syngal & Giuliano, 2018). Of particular benefit are interventions that ensure caregivers maintain their own adequate nutrition, hydration, sleep quantity and quality, medication regimens, sources of support to fulfill outside-of-hospital responsibilities, and social support (see Baker & Gledhill, 2017, for a complete review). Finally, similar to the concept and use of ICU diaries (Mikkelsen, 2018), families can be encouraged to record questions as they arise to ensure they are retrievable and answered when the related specialists are available.

Psychologists should also elicit patient-related information from the family. Parents and others with personal knowledge of the patient can often provide information about the patient's medical history, presence/absence of sensory impairments, prenatal and perinatal history, current developmental level, psychiatric and behavioral health history (patient and family), psychosocial functioning, typical daily activities, prior response to stressors or distress, and historical sources of comfort. In young children, the following additional information is helpful: ages of developmental milestone attainment thus far, times of feeding/sleeping, and temperament. For school-aged youth, additional attention to academic functioning and in-school support (e.g., response to intervention, speech therapy, an individualized education plan, social work services) should be obtained. For adolescent patients, it is helpful to gather information regarding long-term goals and career aspirations, current activities outside of school (e.g., club participation, volunteer work, athletics, employment, social activities), and meaningful interpersonal relationships.

If a history of psychiatric diagnoses, mental health services, or use of psychotropic medications is endorsed, continuation of interventions within the context of the child's acute presentation and current hospitalization may be indicated. Similarly, if information provided suggests the presence of high future risk for harm to oneself or others before admission, then ongoing monitoring and related safety precautions (e.g., safety observation, restriction of access to unneeded potential means of harm) should be instituted.

Roles with patients

In children and adolescents who may be more responsive at PCC admission, brief assessments can be initiated. Areas to be assessed vary depending on the presenting problem and scope of the psychologist's PCC practice. Common foci include mental status, delirium, pain, mood and anxiety, behavior, coping and adaptation, adequacy of oral intake, sleep, treatment goal or intervention adherence, knowledge of illness, and risk for self-harm. Forms of assessment range from multi-informant questioning (e.g., "How has Janae been feeling in the past 2 hours?" "How are you feeling, Janae?") to standardized screener administration.

Several assessment instruments have been standardized for the biopsychosocial context and developmental level of patients admitted to PCC settings. For example, the Children's Orientation and Amnesia Test (COAT; Ewing-Cobbs et al., 1990) and Westmead Post Traumatic Amnesia Scale (Shores et al., 1986) aid in brief serial assessments of orientation (e.g., Briggs et al., 2016). The Faces, Legs, Arms, Crying and Consolability Scale (FLACC Scale; Merkel et al., 1997) can aid in pain assessment following surgical intervention. In addition, scales such as the Vanderbilt Assessment for Delirium in Infants and Children (VADIC; Gangopadhyay et al., 2017) are being validated to support a standardized approach to pediatric delirium assessment. Such measures aid in monitoring change over time and provide valuable information to the treatment team. Brief assessments that are appropriate within the PCC setting can be completed in little time and used repeatedly to monitor change over the course of a PCC stay.

If validated instruments are not available or contextual circumstances require deviation from standardized administration procedures, psychologists must appreciate the reduced representativeness of data obtained, consider the meaningfulness of resulting data to treatment planning, and modify interpretations of the data as indicated. Youth in PCC often exhibit significant fatigue that precludes their participation in lengthier assessments. Furthermore, fluctuations in cognitive functions can minimize the applicability of results found over time (Dodd et al., 2018). Thus, comprehensive assessment measures such as those used in an outpatient-based neuropsychological evaluation are generally contraindicated in the PCC setting.

After obtaining information through brief assessment, results should be shared with the treatment team and incorporated into treatment plans as indicated. For example, psychologists may recommend routine staff-initiated pain assessments when patients are observed to refrain from spontaneously reporting pain unless it is severe; they may also educate family members about signs of moderate to severe physical discomfort to ensure a timely response. For patients presenting with gradually resolving altered mental status involving behavioral agitation, psychologists may recommend de-escalating strategies, continuity in providers as possible, parental engagement in orienting activities, and a psychiatry consultation concerning possible pharmacologic management of agitation or contributing factors. Thus, psychologists can play an integral role in providing recovery-promoting education and recommendations during and after the PCC admission.

COURSE OF CRITICAL CARE STAY

As the patient's condition evolves and increased patient involvement becomes possible, psychologists' roles expand to include direct intervention. A cycle emerges of evaluation, followed by intervention, then re-evaluation. The cycle is informed by observational data, updated medical information, and reports from involved specialists, the patient, and relevant family members. After each consultation, tailored feedback is provided that includes what to expect and strategies to promote optimal outcomes. Documentation occurs within a medical record to ensure all team members can access the evaluation data obtained, interventions executed, patient response to intervention, and resulting interprofessional recommendations.

Psychologists' interventions in PCC are broad and tailored to the treatment targets of the team, including the patient and family. As a patient's health status evolves, so too do the areas of assessment and intervention. Psychoeducation is relied upon heavily to promote adaptation, anticipation of potential challenges, and strategies to overcome them (Wysocki et al., 2017). Interventions including motivational enhancement (Jeter et al., 2019), mindfulness (Lois et al., 2019), and a variety of cognitive and behavioral techniques may be used—for example, positive self-scripts, cognitive reframing, shaping, response-contingent reward systems, progressive muscle relaxation, and activity scheduling (Catarozoli et al., 2019; Law et al., 2017; Schurman et al., 2017). Liaison work with PCC staff to support developmentally informed care practices is also common (Tunick et al., 2013). For example, psychologists may promote the offering of choices to toddler-aged youth, when possible, to enhance their sense of autonomy, encourage the use of visual schedules to increase awareness of upcoming activities for early elementary-aged children, and suggest that staff complete checks of patient comprehension after sharing information with an adolescent.

As youth move beyond the acute phase of a PCC admission, psychologists with requisite expertise can apply their knowledge of the patient and the presenting condition(s) to inform patients and families of resulting neurocognitive impairments and changes in prior abilities. Potential alterations to the rate or acquisition of developmental progress and risk for psychosocial difficulties can also be reviewed in a manner that promotes reasonable expectations and outlines potential mitigating strategies. Psychologists can also monitor and offer strategies to promote adaptation to medically necessary alterations in daily activities and pre-admission routines (Hartung et al., 2015; Mills et al., 2018; Syngal & Giuliano, 2018). Available evidence suggests that earlier familial identification of the aforementioned risks and associated changes may reduce the probability of developing new psychosocial comorbidities (Dodd et al., 2018).

Psychologists with experience in hospital-based, pediatric psychology specialty services can also begin to identify what pre-admission developmental and psychiatric difficulties may affect a child's understanding of the illness, coping and cooperation during present hospitalization, and long-term adaptation and adherence. For example, an adolescent with a history of attention-deficit/hyperactivity disorder (ADHD) who is admitted to PCC to address the consequences of new-onset type 1 diabetes is at risk for poorer health outcomes related to nonadherence (Vinker-Shuster et al., 2019). As patients are better able to engage, psychologists can also begin evaluating and intervening to address psychiatric symptoms that emerge during a PCC admission such as sleep disturbance, acute stress disorder, anxiety, and depressive symptoms.

In settings where youth may not be able to follow up with specialty psychology services after PCC discharge, intensified evaluations or interventions provided during the course of PCC stay are of benefit. For example, the adolescent with ADHD described in the prior paragraph would benefit from more intensive efforts to identify feasible environmental accommodations and to collaboratively construct tailored behavior plans to increase the likelihood of cross-setting adherence. For youth believed to benefit from neuropsychological evaluation after discharge, but for whom specialty services may not be readily available, a brief neuropsychological evaluation could be conducted prior to PCC discharge. Such an evaluation could involve use of screening measures or selected subtests from larger assessment batteries, with test selection based upon specific areas of concern indicated by the presenting illness or injury and patient characteristics. As previously noted, caution is advised in using assessment measures outside of the circumstances in which they were validated. However, in the absence of outpatient-based follow-up, resulting data could be invaluable to promoting optimal functioning and ongoing recovery after PCC discharge.

CRITICAL CARE DISCHARGE

Although some youth are discharged home from a PCC unit, many are transferred to a rehabilitation program or less intensive medical unit within the same hospital. To ease the transition, families can be encouraged to learn about the new setting and to tour the facility or unit prior to transfer. Encouragement to remain active participants in the daily care of their child is also important and provides opportunities to learn the skills needed to more fully assume care once the patient is discharged home. Emphasizing the ongoing availability of a treatment team also provides reassurance to parents as they prepare for entry into a less intensive level of care. When psychologists in PCC also serve the general pediatric or rehabilitation unit(s), they can be a welcomed source of continuity for the patient and family. When psychologists do not cover the locations where youth are transferred following PCC unit discharge, ensuring sufficient familial education and enlisting social support aids their preparation and subsequent adjustment.

When youth are preparing for a PCC discharge to their place of residence, psychologists have several roles. Providing education on the developmental level of the child and corresponding strategies for promoting ongoing developmental progress (when not medically contraindicated) is essential. In early infancy, for example, high levels of responsivity, social reciprocity, and putting children to bed tired yet awake are generally advised. For toddlers, psychologists should encourage setting and upholding consistent limits while allowing choices (e.g., "Should we poke this finger or that finger?"; "Which shirt do you want to wear: this red shirt, or this blue shirt?"; "Do you want orange juice or apple juice after your medicine?"). With school-aged youth, it is of benefit to review behavior management strategies to increase desirable and decrease undesirable behaviors. For adolescents, collaboratively generating scripts for how best to discuss their conditions or medical needs with peers can ease related tensions and improve confidence about social reintegration. Finally, all youth benefit from re-establishing routines that incorporate sleep, feeding, medical-related regimens, and any other important daily life tasks of the family.

Parents and youth may experience a variety of emotional responses as PCC discharge approaches. Also, youth can experience difficulties adhering to ongoing interventions, coping with the impact of events, and adapting to life after the injury or illness. When patients exhibit or are at risk of developing psychiatric sequelae, psychologists or the relevant team member (e.g., social work) should provide referrals that take into account the patient's age, health status, and psychiatric needs. As part of the referral process, patients who are school-aged or older and their parents can be educated about the symptoms that warrant psychiatric or psychological care after PCC discharge. To prevent behavioral changes after PCC discharge associated with counterproductive parenting practices, it can be helpful to remind parents to maintain behavioral expectations and warmth, while avoiding adoption of an overly permissive parenting style (Baker & Gledhill, 2017).

Individual differences in the emotional experience of patients and family members are also common. Some youth experience adverse changes in behavior or mood during their PCC stay that resolve immediately upon returning to an approximation of their pre-admission routine and the home environment. In those same youth, parents may experience distress later in the hospital stay that remains long after hospital discharge (Colville, 2017). Families should be made aware that differing thoughts and feelings across individuals are to be expected. Psychologists must also monitor parental and sibling functioning, to the extent that this is within their role (vs. the roles of social work or child life), as children are dependent on their caregivers for care and emotional support (Baker & Gledhill, 2017).

For school-aged youth, psychologists can provide the school with information obtained from assessments, along with relevant recommendations for instructional needs and school-related accommodations (Wade & Walz, 2010). When youth can return immediately to the school setting, psychologists can assist the interprofessional team in developing school reentry plans that take into account the effects of the injury or illness on psychiatric and neurocognitive functioning. Components of a school reentry plan may include specifications around a gradual return to school, abbreviated attendance schedules, adjustments to academic work, and activity modifications.

Common school-based accommodations for youth with chronic medical conditions include excused absences for illness and related medical care, plans for making up work following medically related absences, supervision of medical regimens, access to nonpharmacologic means of symptom management (e.g., water bottles, bathroom passes, hot pads and cushions for pain management), and plans for management of symptom exacerbations (e.g., asthma attack, hyperglycemia, pain crisis, incontinence). Some schools may informally provide accommodations based upon hospital documentation (e.g., detailed discharge instructions, letter directed to the school). Other schools may require that accommodations are formally established through an individualized education program or 504 plan. When psychologists fulfill school-related roles as part of the interprofessional care team, they should support parents in knowing their child's educational rights and processes for gaining access to reasonable accommodations within the least restrictive school environment. This can be done by providing handouts, enlisting the assistance of social work, providing contact information for local school advocates, and offering verbal education.

In addition to coordinating academic supports, psychologists in PCC may recommend other outpatient-based specialty evaluations based upon their own assessment data. Referrals may include, but are not limited to, consultations with developmental-behavioral medicine; genetics; adolescent medicine; rehabilitation programs; audiology; and autism evaluation centers. Psychologists play a key role in ensuring that families appreciate the role of evaluation and treatment in maximizing functioning following illness or injury (Wade & Walz, 2010). At the same time, psychologists must appreciate a family's priorities and the entirety of illness-related follow-ups at PCC discharge, then collaborate with the treatment team to support the family in generating a feasible discharge plan.

Conclusion

Youth enter PCC settings for a variety of reasons. Owing to advances in technology and treatment, more children survive their hospitalizations than ever before. However, with increased survival comes increased risk of functional morbidities. Psychologists within PCC must possess knowledge, skills, and attributes unique to working with children and adolescents, in addition to those needed to function effectively within critical care settings. Those with PCC expertise can contribute to the treatment team from PCC admission through discharge. Roles for psychologists are broad, spanning assessment and monitoring, intervention and management, liaison, and clinician. Moreover, psychologists' activities are idiosyncratic—determined often by the setting and situation, and continuously evolving to match patient needs, family needs, and treatment team goals. Through their many roles, psychologists engage in health promotion, prevention, and treatment using culturally informed, evidence-based practices that are tailored to the PCC setting and unique constellation of presenting biopsychosocial factors. As a result of psychologists' contributions, interprofessional teams are strengthened, as are the outcomes for pediatric patients and their families.

References

American Academy of Pediatrics. (2014). Policy statement: Child life services. *Pediatrics, 133*(5), e1471–e1478. doi:10.1542/peds.2014-0556

American Psychological Association. (2017). Ethical principles of psychologists and code of conduct (2002, amended effective June 1, 2010, and January 1, 2017). http://www.apa.org/ethics/code/index.html

American Psychological Association. (2020, April 16). Telehealth testing with children: Important factors to consider. http://www.apaservices.org/practice/legal/technology/telehealth-testing-children-covid-19

Baker, S. C., & Gledhill, J. A., (2017). Systematic review of interventions to reduce psychiatric morbidity in parents and children after PICU admissions. *Pediatric Critical Care Medicine, 18*(4), 343–348. doi:10.1097/ICU.0000000000001096

Barbosa, V. M. (2013). Teamwork in the neonatal intensive care unit. *Physical Occupational Therapy Pediatrics, 33*(1), 5–26. doi:10.3109/01942638.2012.729556

Berg, R. A., Nadkarni, V. M., Clark, A. E., Moler, F., Meert, K., Harrison, R. E., . . . Eunice Kennedy Shriver National Institute of Child Health and Human Development Collaborative Pediatric Critical Care Research Network. (2016). Incidence and outcomes of cardiopulmonary resuscitation in PICUs. *Critical Care Medicine, 44*(4), 798–808. doi:10.1097/CCM.0000000000001484

Briggs, R., Birse, J., Tate, R., Brookes, N., Epps, A., & Lah, S. (2016). Natural sequence of recovery from child post-traumatic amnesia: A retrospective cohort study. *Child Neuropsychology, 22*(6), 666–678. doi:10.1080/09297049.2015.1038988

Buckloh, L., & Schilling, L. (2017). Professional development, roles and practice patterns. In M. C. Roberts & R. G. Steele (Eds.), *Handbook of pediatric psychology* (pp. 26–37). Guilford Press.

Carter, B. D., Kronenberger, W. G., Scott, E. L., Kullgren, K. A., Piazza-Waggoner, C., & Brady, C.E. (2017). Inpatient pediatric consultation-liaison. In M. C. Roberts & R. G. Steele (Eds.), *Handbook of pediatric psychology* (pp. 105–118). Guilford Press.

Catarozoli, C., Brodzinsky, L., Salley, C. G., Miller, S. P., Lois, B. H., & Carpenter, J. L. (2019). Necessary adaptations to CBT with pediatric patients. In R. Friedberg & J. Paternostro (Eds.), *Handbook of cognitive behavioral therapy for pediatric medical conditions* (pp. 103–118). Springer.

Chenneville, T., & Schwartz-Mette, R. (2020). Ethical considerations for psychologists in the time of COVID-19. *American Psychologist, 75*(5), 644–654. https://doi.org/10.1037/amp0000661

Colville, G. (2001). The role of a psychologist on the paediatric critical care unit. *Child Psychology & Psychiatry Review, 6*(2), 102–109.

Colville, G. A. (2015). Psychological aspects of care of the critically ill child. *Journal of Pediatric Critical Care, 4*(4), 182–187. doi:10.1055/s-0035-1563542

Colville, G. A. (2017). Supporting pediatric patients and their families during and after critical care treatment. In O. J. Bienvenu, C. Jones, & R. O. Hopkins (Eds.), *Psychological and cognitive impact of critical illness*. Oxford University Press.

Committee on Hospital Care and Institute for Patient- and Family-Centered Care. (2012). Patient- and family-centered care and the pediatrician's role. *Pediatrics, 129*(2), 394–404. doi:10.1542/peds.2011-3084

Davidson, J., Jones, C., & Bienvenu, O. (2012). Family response to critical illness: Postintensive care syndrome-family. *Critical Care Medicine, 40*(2), 618–624. doi:10.1097/CCM.0b013e318236ebf9

Davydow, D. S., Richardson, L. P., Zatzick, D. F., & Katon, W. J. (2010). Psychiatric morbidity in pediatric critical illness survivors: A comprehensive review of the literature. *Archives of Pediatrics & Adolescent Medicine, 164*(4), 377–385. doi:10.1001/archpediatrics. 2010.10

Dodd, J., Hall, T., Guilliams, K., Guerriero, R., Wagner, A., Malone, S., . . . Piantino, J. (2018). Optimizing neurocritical care follow-up through the integration of neuropsychology. *Pediatric Neurology, 89*, 58–62. doi:10.1016/j.pediatrneurol.2018.09.007

Elliott, D., Davidson, J., Harvey, M., Bemis-Dougherty, A., Hopkins, R., Iwashyna, T., . . . Needham, D. (2014). Exploring the scope of post-intensive care syndrome therapy and care: Engagement of non-critical care providers and survivors in a second stakeholders meeting. *Critical Care Medicine, 42*(12), 1518–2526. doi:10.1097/CCM.0000000000000525

Esses, S., Small, S., Rodemann, A., & Hartman, M. (2019). Post-intensive care syndrome: Educational interventions for parents of hospitalized children. *American Journal of Critical Care, 28*(1), 19–27. doi:10.4037/ajcc2019151

Ewing-Cobbs, L., Levin, H. S., Fletcher, J. M., Miner, M. E., & Eisenberg, H. M. (1990). The Children's Orientation and Amnesia Test: Relationship to severity of acute head injury and to recovery of memory. *Neurosurgery, 27*(5), 683–691.

Gangopadhyay, M., Smith, H., Pao, M., Silver, G., Deepmala, D., De Souza, C., . . . Fuchs, C. (2017). Development of the Vanderbilt Assessment for Delirium in Infants and Children to standardize pediatric delirium assessment by psychiatrists. *Psychosomatics, 58*(4), 355–363. doi:10.1016/j.psym.2017.03.006

Gogo, A., Osta, A., McClafferty, H., & Rana, D. T. (2019). Cultivating a way of being and doing: Individual strategies for physician well-being and resilience. *Current Problems in Pediatric and Adolescent Health Care, 49*(12), 100663. doi:10.1016/j.cppeds.2019.100663

Hartung, E. A., Laney, N., Kim, J. Y., Ruebner, R. L., Detre, J. A., Liu, H. S., . . . Furth, S. L., (2015). Design and methods of the NiCK study: Neurocognitive assessment and magnetic resonance imaging analysis of children and young adults with chronic kidney disease. *BMC Nephrology, 16*, Article 66. doi:10.1186/s12882-015-0061-1

Hewitt, K. C., Rodgin, S., Loring, D. W., Pritchard, A. E., & Jacobson, L. A. (2020). Transitioning to telehealth neuropsychology service: Considerations across adult and pediatric care settings. *Clinical Neuropsychologist, 34*(7–8), 1335–1351.

Hynan, M., Steinberg, Z., Baker, L., Cicco, R., Geller, P., Lassen, S., . . . Stuebe, L. (2015). Recommendations for mental health professionals in the NICU. *Journal of Perinatology, 35,* S14–S18. doi:10.1038/jp.2015.144

Jeter, K., Gillaspy, S., & Leffingwell, T. R. (2019) Motivational interviewing. In R. Friedberg & J. Paternostro (Eds.), *Handbook of cognitive behavioral therapy for pediatric medical conditions* (pp. 69–86). Springer.

Kroll, K. (2020). *Pediatric psychology in clinical practice: Empirically supported interventions.* Cambridge University Press.

Kyösti, E., Ala-Kokko, T., Ohtonen, P., Peltoniemi, O., Ebeling, H., Spalding, M., . . . Liisanantti, J. H. (2019). Strengths and Difficulties Questionnaire assessment of long-term psychological outcome in children after intensive care admission. *Pediatric Critical Care Medicine, 20*(11), e496–e502. doi:10.1097/PCC.0000000000002078

LaBuzetta, J., Rosand, J., & Vranceanu, A. (2019). Review: Post-intensive care syndrome: Unique challenges in the neurointensive care unit. *Neurocritical Care, 31*(3), 534–545. doi:10.1007/s12028-019-00826-0

Lassen, S., Wu, Y. P., & Roberts, M. C. (2014). Common presenting concerns and settings for pediatric psychology practice. In M. C. Roberts, B. S. Aylward, & Y. P. Wu (Eds.), *Clinical practice of pediatric psychology* (pp. 17–31). Guilford Press.

Law, E. F., Noel, M., Nagel, M. S., & Dahlquist, L. M. (2017). Chronic and recurrent pain. In M. C. Roberts & R. G. Steele (Eds.), *Handbook of pediatric psychology* (pp. 26–37). Guilford Press.

Lois, B. H., Corcoran, V. P., & Miller, A. L. (2019). DBT adaptations with pediatric patients. In R. Friedberg & J. Paternostro (Eds.), *Handbook of cognitive behavioral therapy for pediatric medical conditions* (pp. 137–150). Springer.

Meert, K. L., Clark, J., & Eggly, S. (2013). Family-centered care in the pediatric intensive care unit. *Pediatric Clinics, 60*(3), 761–772.

Merkel, S., Voepel-Lewis, T., Shayevitz, J., & Malviya, S. (1997). The FLACC: A behavioral scale for scoring postoperative pain in young children. *Pediatric Nursing, 23*(3), 293–297.

Mikkelsen, G. (2018). The meaning of personal diaries to children and families in the pediatric critical care unit: A qualitative study. *Critical & Critical Care Nursing, 45*, 25–30. doi:10.1016/j.iccn.2017.10.001

Mills, J., & Chapman, M. (2016). Compassion and self-compassion in medicine: Self-care for the caregiver. *Australasian Medical Journal, 9*(5), 87–91. doi:10.4066/AMJ.2016.2583

Mills, R., McCusker, C.G., Tennyson, C. & Hanna, D. (2018). Neuropsychological outcomes in CHD beyond childhood: A meta-analysis. *Cardiology in the Young, 28*, 421–431. doi:10.1017/S104795111700230X

Namachivayam, P., Shann, F., Shekerdemian, L., Taylor, A., van Sloten, I., Delzoppo, C., . . . Butt, W. (2010). Three decades of pediatric intensive care: Who was admitted, what happened in intensive care, and what happened afterward. *Pediatric Critical Care Medicine, 11*(5), 549–555.

Needham, D. M., Davidson, J., Cohen, H., Hopkins, R. O., Weinert, C., Wunsch, H., . . . Brady, S. L. (2012). Improving long-term outcomes after discharge from intensive care unit: Report from a stakeholders' conference. *Critical Care Medicine, 40*(2), 502–509.

Ong, C., Lee, J., Leow, M., & Puthucheary, Z. (2016). Functional outcomes and physical impairments in pediatric critical care survivors: A scoping review. *Pediatric Critical Care Medicine, 17*(5), 247–259. doi:10.1097/PCC.0000000000000706

Owings-Fonner, N. (2020, June). Telepsychology expands to meet demand. *Monitor on Psychology, 51*(4). http://www.apa.org/monitor/2020/06/covid-telepsychology

Schenkenberg, T., Peterson, L., Wood, D., & DaBell, R. (1981). Psychological consultation/liaison in a medical and neurological setting: Physicians' appraisal. *Professional Psychology, 12*(3), 309–317. doi:10.1037/0735-7028.12.3.309

Schurman, J. V., Maddux, M. H., Blossom, J. B., & Friesen, C. A. (2017). Abdominal pain-related gastrointestinal disorders: Irritable bowel syndrome and inflammatory bowel disease. In M. C. Roberts & R. G. Steele (Eds.), *Handbook of pediatric psychology* (pp. 375–390). Guilford Press.

Shores, E. A., Marosszeky, J. E., Sandanam, J., & Batchelor, J. (1986). Preliminary validation of a clinical scale for measuring the duration of post-traumatic amnesia. *Medical Journal of Australia, 144*, 569–572.

Shudy, M., de Almeida, M., Ly, S., Landon, C., Groft, S., Jenkins, T., . . . Nicholson, C. E. (2006). Impact of pediatric critical illness and injury on families: A systematic literature review. *Pediatrics, 111*(Suppl 3), S203–S218. doi:10.1542/peds.2006-0951B

Syngal, P. & Giuliano Jr., J. S. (2018). Health-related quality of life after pediatric severe sepsis. *Healthcare, 6*(3), 113. doi:10.3390/healthcare6030113

Treble-Barna, A., Beers, S. R., Houtrow, A. J., Ortiz-Aguayo, R., Valenta, C., Stanger, M., . . . Fink, E. L. (2019). PICU-based rehabilitation and outcomes assessment: A survey of pediatric critical care physicians. *Pediatric Critical Care Medicine, 20*(6), e274–e282. doi:10.1097/ICU.0000000000001940

Tunick, R. A., Gavin, J. A., DeMaso, D. R., & Meyer, E. C. (2013). Pediatric psychology critical care consultation: An emerging specialty. *Clinical Practice in Pediatric Psychology, 1*(1), 42–54. doi:10.1037/ccpp0000006

Vinker-Shuster, M., Golan-Cohen, A., Merhasin, I., & Merzon, E. (2019). Attention-deficit hyperactivity disorder in pediatric patients with type 1 diabetes mellitus: Clinical outcomes and diabetes control. *Journal of Developmental and Behavioral Pediatrics, 40*(5), 330–334. doi:10.1097/DBP.0000000000000670

Wade, S. L., & Walz, N. C. (2010). Family, school, and community: Their role in rehabilitation of children. In R. G. Frank, M. Rosenthal, & B. Caplan (Eds.), *Handbook of rehabilitation psychology* (2nd ed., pp. 345–354). American Psychological Association.

Williams, C., Eriksson, C., Kirby, A., Piantino, J., Hall, T., Luther, M., & McEvoy, C. (2019). Hospital mortality and functional outcomes in pediatric neurocritical care. *Hospital Pediatrics, 9*(12), 958–966. doi:10.1542/hpeds.2019-0173

Williams, C., Hartman, M., Guilliams, K., Rejean, M., Guerriero, D., Piantino, J., Bosworth, M., . . . Hall, T. (2019). Postintensive care syndrome in pediatric critical care survivors: Therapeutic options to improve outcomes after acquired brain injury. *Current Treatment Options in Neurology, 21*(10), 49. doi:10.1007/s11940-019-0586-x

Wysocki, T., Buckloh, L. M., & Greco, P. (2017). The psychological context of diabetes mellitus in youths. In M. C. Roberts & R. G. Steele (Eds.), *Handbook of pediatric psychology* (pp. 287–302). Guilford Press.

Ziegelstein, R. (2018). Creating structured opportunities for social engagement to promote well-being and avoid burnout in medical students and residents. *Academic Medicine, 93*(4), 537–539. doi:10.1097/ACM.0000000000002117

10 Caring for Older Adults During and After Critical Illness
Maria C. Duggan, Julie Van, and E. Wesley Ely

Introduction

Older adults (>65 years) are the fastest-growing age cohort in the United States, projected to make up 16% of the population by 2050 (Ortman et al., 2014). Persons aged 85 and older make up about 1.5% of the U.S. population, a figure predicted to rise to 5% of the population by 2050 (Ortman et al., 2014). The number of older adults admitted to intensive care units (ICUs) has been increasing due to increased life expectancy and advances in medical care. Older adults account for over half of all ICU days and ICU admissions in the United States (Kahn et al., 2015). This population is complex and requires a unique approach to optimize not only survival but also functional status and quality of life (QoL) after critical illness. The integration of geriatric principles into the care of older adults has been associated with reduced mortality, fewer hospital complications, and shorter length of stay (Barnes et al., 2012; Ellis et al., 2017). All health care providers should ideally be familiar with these principles, since there is a massive shortage of professionals to care for the aging population.

The objectives of this chapter are (1) to provide an overview of the effects of aging on multiple domains of an older person with critical illness and (2) to describe evidence-based approaches to caring for older adults with critical illness.

Maria C. Duggan, Julie Van, and E. Wesley Ely, *Caring for Older Adults During and After Critical Illness* In: *Critical Care Psychology and Rehabilitation.* Edited by: Kirk J. Stucky and Jennifer E. Jutte, Oxford University Press. © Oxford University Press 2022.
DOI: 10.1093/oso/9780190077013.003.0010

Aging's impact on the person with critical illness

Aging is a universal process, a set of predictable, gradual, and inevitable changes in biologic function that occur with the passage of time. Because aging increases the complexity of individuals, it can be helpful to consider the multiple domains of an older person's health state to guide the most effective care during and after critical illness (Figure 10.1). The World Health Organization (1995)'s QoL assessment framework shaped our development of this multidimensional conceptualization of an older adult's health state. By considering all these domains, providers can more easily assess an older patient's goals and values to align treatment plans with the patient's most important goals and avoid overly burdensome treatments.

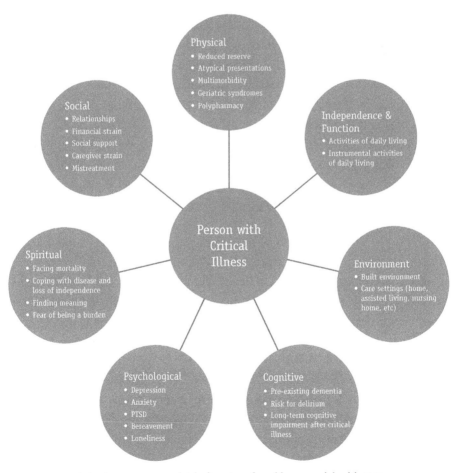

FIGURE 10.1. Aging issues among multiple domains of an older person's health state.

Understanding these domains in the context of a person's goals and values can help providers with prognostication, medical decision-making, and identifying unmet psychosocial needs that may impair recovery after critical illness.

Next we will discuss the various domains of older adults. While we discuss each domain separately, each often directly affects and interacts with others and should not be considered in isolation.

PHYSICAL

Although age alone is not a consistent independent predictor of mortality, older adults are, for many reasons, physically vulnerable to complications during critical illness.

First, normal physiologic changes of aging result in homeostenosis, a narrowing of the body's ability to maintain homeostatic equilibrium in the face of stress (Becker & Cohen, 1984). This reduced reserve is clinically relevant to older patients in the ICU. For example, older adults have reduced cognitive reserve, making them more prone to developing delirium with fewer precipitating factors (Inouye et al., 2014); with aging comes a decline in glomerular filtration rate, making older adults more susceptible to acute kidney injury (Himmelfarb, 2009).

Second, older adults also present uniquely in part due to reduced immune and inflammatory responses (Weyand & Goronzy, 2016). Because conditions in the elderly may not present like descriptions of diseases in textbooks, erroneous diagnoses may be made, leading to inappropriate treatments, delayed correct diagnoses, and changes to appropriate treatments.

Third, aging is associated with multimorbidity, which can further complicate the primary problem precipitating a person's ICU admission. These can be diseases of aging (e.g., aortic stenosis, congestive heart failure, Alzheimer's disease) and geriatric syndromes (frailty, dementia, malnutrition, pressure injury, falls, delirium, urinary incontinence, hearing and vision impairments) (Inouye et al., 2007).

Geriatric syndromes result from an interaction of predisposing and precipitating factors. They are usually multifactorial, often due to a combination of physiologic changes of aging, multiple diseases, and external factors like medications. Geriatric syndromes often go unrecognized in older adults, yet they are associated with morbidity and mortality. One syndrome that is the subject of increasing research is frailty, manifested by shrinking, weakness, slowness, low physical activity, and exhaustion (Fried et al., 2001). Since frailty is independently associated with mortality and disability among people with critical illness, recognizing it can aid in prognostication and risk stratification (Muscedere et al., 2017).

Lastly, inadequate medication management can cause harm with older adults. Medication errors and adverse drug events are common among adults of all ages, but these can be particularly harmful in older adults. With age comes polypharmacy, which makes it even more important to complete a thorough medication reconciliation upon admission to the hospital and at discharge.

Polypharmacy has countless definitions, the most common being the use of four or more chronic medications, more than 10 medications, or more medications than are necessary (Masnoon et al., 2017). Regardless of definition, polypharmacy is common among critically ill older adults and is associated with increased adverse events, higher rates of drug interactions, and increased costs (Garpestad & Devlin, 2017). Older adults also respond to drugs differently than younger persons due to changes in drug absorption, distribution, metabolism, and elimination that occur with aging (McLean & Le Couteur, 2004). In addition, older adults have more disease–drug interactions, in which a medication worsens the symptoms of a disease. This is commonly seen with anticholinergic medications like diphenhydramine, which often worsen such common geriatric problems as constipation, urinary retention, orthostatic hypotension, and cognitive impairment. Beyond classic anticholinergics like diphenhydramine, multiple classes of medications can have anticholinergic effects, and higher cumulative anticholinergic burden is associated with greater risk of morbidity and mortality, longer length of stay, discharge to nursing home, functional decline, and cognitive decline (Salahudeen et al., 2015).

To address the problem of polypharmacy, many experts and researchers have developed tools for assessing the appropriateness of medications, including the American Geriatrics Society Beers criteria for potentially inappropriate medications (American Geriatrics Society Beers Criteria Update Expert Panel, 2019), Screening Tool of Older Person's Potentially Inappropriate Prescriptions (STOPP) (Gallagher et al., 2008), and Rationalization of Home Medication by an Adjusted STOPP List in Older Patients (RASP) (Van der Linden et al., 2014).

The Beers criteria are the most widely used by medical professionals, educators, researchers, and administrators. The aims of the Beers criteria are to improve medication selection, reduce adverse drug events, and educate clinicians and patients alike about medications best suited for older adults. The Beers criteria also serve as a tool for practicing clinicians to evaluate the quality of care and patterns of drug use in this group of patients. These criteria include medications that are potentially contraindicated for most older adults, those that should be avoided in older adults with certain diseases and conditions, drugs to use with caution, drug–drug interactions, and drug dose adjustments based on kidney function.

INDEPENDENCE AND FUNCTION

Functional status, also known as the "sixth vital sign" for older adults, is the ability to function in everyday life and depends on both a person's physical ability and surrounding environment. Functional status can be characterized by basic activities of daily living (ADLs; dressing, eating, ambulating, toileting, bathing) and instrumental activities of daily living (IADLs; shopping, finances, medication management, housekeeping, cooking, driving) (Katz, 1983; Lawton & Brody, 1969).

Understanding a person's baseline functional status is important for a number of reasons. First, it can be a helpful prognostic indicator. Trajectory of functional status before ICU admission strongly influences functional trajectory and risk of death in the subsequent year (Ferrante et al., 2015).Furthermore, older adults with poor baseline functional status are at greater risk of increased health care utilization, including readmission and nursing home placement.

Second, functional status should have a direct influence on treatment plans. Understanding baseline function can help providers set realistic functional goals on a daily basis in an effort to maximize functional recovery and discuss whether return to baseline status is possible.

Third, the possibility of functional recovery matters greatly to many older adults. Functional status often carries significant weight on their QoL ratings (Iyasere et al., 2016; van Leeuwen et al., 2019). It is also important to consider that each patient has a unique perception of what degree of function is acceptable to them, and there is evidence that older adults maintain QoL despite functional limitations, in part due to adapting their expectations and values (van Leeuwen et al., 2019). In fact, older adults tend to report better QoL than younger patients despite having more functional impairments (Pisani, 2009). Health care providers should never assume that functionally dependent individuals have poor QoL. In fact, health care providers are prone to judging individuals' QoL to be lower than patients themselves; this can lead to bias and unintentional discriminatory practices. Health care providers can help patients and families navigate treatment decisions by counseling them about possible functional outcomes (the "best case, worst case, and most likely case scenario" can be a useful tool) and factoring in patients' values and preferences.

ENVIRONMENT

An older adult's environment plays a large role in their independence and well-being. Older adults receive care in various care settings (home, independent living, assisted living, long-term care, post-acute care) with different levels of support services provided. Older adults commonly acquire new disabilities during critical illness and may require adaptive equipment if judged fit to return home or post-acute care at a skilled nursing facility or inpatient rehabilitation unit if too debilitated currently but there remain prospects for additional recovery. These care transitions are a risky period where medication errors, poor education, or suboptimal understanding by patients can occur (Ziaeian et al., 2012).

COGNITION

In older adults, cognitive impairment is common but underrecognized (Livingston et al., 2017). Cognitive decline is associated with institutionalization, hospitalization, and significant societal expenses (Chodosh et al., 2004). Older adults with dementia are vulnerable to adverse events due to nonadherence with medication, motor vehicle collisions, and usual complications of dementia like aspiration pneumonia and pressure injuries that often result in critical illness (Livingston et al., 2017). It is important to recognize cognitive impairment in order to identify those at highest risk for complications (e.g., delirium, falls) and to ensure that staff understand a patient's goals of care. Cognitive assessment can be challenging for critically ill older adults who may have limited communication; in such cases, history provided by surrogates is often most helpful. A tool like the Ascertain Dementia 8 (AD8) is an easy and efficient measure that has high sensitivity for detecting dementia by relying on surrogate report (Galvin et al., 2005; Jackson et al., 2016).

Cognitive impairment is also commonly acquired during critical illness and can persist for years (Hopkins & Jackson, 2006). Delirium is an independent risk factor for developing cognitive impairment (Pandharipande et al., 2014). While we will discuss delirium in more detail later in this chapter, it is important to note that patients who experience delirium should undergo cognitive assessment prior to discharge. No one tool is recommended to assess cognition after critical illness; however, the Mini-Cog offers a quick measure with high sensitivity for detecting cognitive impairment in older adults (Tsoi et al., 2015). If cognitive impairment is present, families and caregivers should be counseled about assisting with ADLs, especially managing medications, cooking, and driving, as these can be dangerous activities for people with cognitive impairment. For more information on cognitive impairment, see Chapter 6.

PSYCHOLOGICAL

Psychological issues common in older adults include depression and anxiety as well as issues unique to aging like bereavement and loneliness. Mental health problems are associated with morbidity and mortality and are important to recognize, as they are usually treatable. Depression often goes unrecognized in older adults, in part because it does not present with the classic symptoms of sadness; rather, somatic complaints are more common (Drayer et al., 2005). Understanding an older adult's psychological state is important, because many medical illnesses and medications can cause psychiatric side effects, some of which may be treatable. For example, depressive symptoms may result from hypothyroidism or frailty as well as beta blockers. Critical care also imposes new psychological insults and challenges for older adults. For more on this, please see Chapter 5.

SPIRITUAL

Spirituality and religion are common ways of coping with disease and can influence medical decisions for seriously ill older adults. Common spiritual issues that older adults may encounter include facing mortality, coping with morbidity, finding meaning in one's life, loss of independence, and fear of becoming a burden to others. Health care professionals are committed to healing, and often the greatest treatable need is spiritual. It is important to inquire about spiritual/religious history with all patients so that care aligns with their values and goals.

There is growing evidence demonstrating a connection between spiritual involvement and other aspects of mental and physical health in later life (Koenig, 2012). Assessing and addressing the spiritual needs of older adult patients, especially in those with disabling psychiatric or mental impairments, is well within the scope of health professionals who integrate principles outside of just the patient illness and critical care setting alone. Individual spirituality is common in later life and many times is used as a way to cope with health issues that arise (Peteet et al., 2019). This may affect patient and family decisions about interventions and therapies, so health professionals must be empathetic and familiar with these beliefs.

SOCIAL

An older adult's social situation has direct impact on health and well-being. Older adults are more likely to be impoverished and unable to afford needed health care (Lynn, 2019). Older adults are also more prone to abuse and mistreatment, especially among those with cognitive impairment (Acierno et al., 2010). Identifying primary relationships, caregivers, financial strain, community- or government-based social support, and any unmet social needs will be important to preventing readmission and ensuring the patient can follow up and adhere to various treatment recommendations. Issues such as caregiver strain or burnout are common in those who care for physically or mentally disabled older adults. Social isolation is also common and is associated with poor health outcomes like falls, hospital readmission, and mortality (Nicholson, 2012). Early identification of such social issues would allow for referrals to community agencies and home health services to try to prevent poor outcomes. Engagement of social workers and case managers is crucial to ensuring optimization of older adults' health and well-being.

Approaches to critically ill older adults

ABCDEF: AN EVIDENCE-BASED BUNDLE OF ICU LIBERATION

Older adults are predisposed to newly acquired deficits and diseases when they experience critical illness. They are admitted with pneumonia or appendicitis, and the vast majority leave with new problems that greatly affect functioning and QoL (Brummel et al., 2015). These new or worsening impairments in a patient's physical, cognitive, or mental health after critical illness are known as postintensive care syndrome (PICS) (Needham et al., 2012). To address this problem, a comprehensive program was developed known as the ABCDEF model of ICU liberation (Ely, 2017):

> **A**ssess, prevent, and manage pain
> **B**oth spontaneous awakening trial (SAT) and spontaneous breathing trial (SBT)
> **C**hoice of sedation and analgesia
> **D**elirium assessment, prevention, and management
> **E**arly mobility and Exercise
> **F**amily engagement.

Although the ABCDEF bundle is not specific to older adults, it improves quality and safety and is beneficial to reduce PICS in older adults.

For a complete review of the ABCDEF bundle's philosophy and science, please see a thorough review in Ely (2017). In brief, adequate performance of the bundle is associated with lower likelihood of hospital death within 7 days, next-day mechanical ventilation, coma, delirium, physical restraint use, immobility, ICU readmission, and discharge to a facility. Higher adherence to the bundle is associated with greater improvements in each of these outcomes. For maximal effectiveness, this multicomponent approach requires coordination of an interprofessional team including family members and the patient. Next we will highlight the major features of the ABCDEF bundle in the context of caring for older adults.

ASSESS, PREVENT, AND MANAGE PAIN

Pain should be routinely monitored in all patients. Inadequate pain management contributes to impaired mobility and delirium and increases the risk for nosocomial infections, prolonged mechanical ventilation, chronic pain, posttraumatic stress disorder (PTSD), and impaired QoL after hospitalization (Erstad et al., 2009). In older adults, pain may be underrecognized due to the false belief that pain is a normal part of aging (Thielke et al., 2012).

Identifying pain in older adults with cognitive impairment can be particularly challenging. Over 35 pain assessment tools for patients with dementia exist; they incorporate a variety of self-report, observation, caregiver rating, and patient-interactive information. Each tool's utility depends on severity of dementia. In patients with early dementia, self-report can be reliable, making the Present Pain Intensity (PPI) scale a good tool to evaluate pain (Corbett et al., 2012). For patients with advanced dementia who may be noncommunicative, pain scales are based on observing pain-related behaviors. Scales intended for caregiver use include the Pain Assessment for the Dementing Elderly (Villanueva et al., 2003) and Pain Assessment in Noncommunicative Elderly Persons (Cohen-Mansfield, 2006). A variety of rating tools require intensive observation by the health care team. The observational tool with the highest reliability, validity, and feasibility is the Mobilization-Observation-Behaviour-Intensity-Dementia Pain Scale, which detects pain-related behavior after a series of prescribed physical movements (Husebo et al., 2010).

Guidelines from the American Geriatrics Society on pharmacologic management of persistent pain in older adults can guide clinicians about which medications to use for older adults (2009). General approaches involve starting drugs at the lowest dose possible and gradually titrating up as necessary, avoiding highly anticholinergic medications, and avoiding excessive nonsteroidal anti-inflammatory drug (NSAID) use due to increased risk of renal failure and gastric ulcers (American Geriatrics Society Panel on Pharmacological Management of Persistent Pain in Older, 2009). For more information on pain in patients with critical illness, please see Chapter 7.

BOTH SAT AND SBT

Respiratory disease is common among older adults, and its incidence increases 10-fold from ages 55 to 85 years (Behrendt, 2000). Patients with respiratory failure who are older than 70 years were shown to have twice the duration of mechanical ventilation and reintubation rates compared to younger patients (Ely et al., 2002). The prolongation of mechanical ventilation in older adults is often due to extrapulmonary processes (e.g., infection other than pneumonia), delirium, or neuromuscular diseases, rather than worse respiratory function, as time to pass SBT in older patients is similar to that of younger patients (Ely et al., 1999, 2002).

Daily SATs consist of stopping narcotics (as long as pain is managed) and sedatives every day. Data from a randomized, controlled trial involving adult patients receiving mechanical ventilation and infusions of sedative drugs suggest that daily SAT uses less analgosedation while still improving ICU outcomes, including less time on mechanical ventilation and shorter time to follow commands, a surrogate for delirium duration (Kress et al., 2000). While SATs are used to promote wakefulness and reduce exposure to sedation, SBTs aim to decrease the effects of exposure to mechanical ventilation. Combining SATs with SBTs results in more days with unassisted breathing, earlier discharge from the hospital, and lower 1-year mortality (Girard et al., 2008).

CHOICE OF ANALGESIA AND SEDATION

Analgesia and sedation are particularly dangerous in older adults, as they are at a high risk of delirium and complications from polypharmacy and medication interactions (Cahir et al., 2010). Goal-directed administration of psychoactive medications is important to avoid oversedation and adverse effects and to promote earlier extubation. The Richmond Agitation-Sedation Scale (RASS) (Sessler et al., 2002) and the Riker Sedation-Agitation Scale (SAS) (Riker et al., 1999), both validated and reliable methods to measure patients' level of sedation in the ICU, can be used to determine and monitor levels of sedation. Analgosedation is used for the relief of both pain and anxiety and may be enough to reach target level of consciousness.

When choosing sedation for an older person, providers should be aware of certain physiologic changes with aging that affect drug pharmacokinetics and pharmacodynamics. Mangoni and Jackson review this topic thoroughly (2004). Briefly, body composition changes in older individuals, with an increase in fat-to-lean body mass ratio, resulting in an increase in the effective half-life of lipophilic medications (e.g., propofol or diazepam). Reduced glomerular filtration rate (GFR) requires reduced dosages and/or frequencies of renally eliminated medications to avoid excessive drug levels. Also, older adults have an increased sensitivity to psychoactive drugs, which should be used with caution.

Benzodiazepines should be avoided in older adults because they increase the risk for delirium, falls, and urinary retention (Fraser et al., 2013). Upon evaluating mechanically ventilated patients and the probabilities of their daily transition to delirium, every unit dose of lorazepam was correlated with a higher risk for daily transition to delirium (Pandharipande et al., 2006). In contrast, other sedatives besides benzodiazepines (like propofol or dexmedetomidine) were associated with less time on ventilation, shorter length of stay, and reduced health care costs when compared to benzodiazepine strategies (Pandharipande et al., 2007).

DELIRIUM ASSESSMENT

Delirium is an acute disturbance of consciousness with inattention accompanied by a change in cognition or perceptual disturbance that fluctuates over time. Delirium is associated with poor clinical outcomes: prolonged mechanical ventilation, longer ICU stay, discharge to a nursing home, and higher mortality up to 2 years after discharge (Ely et al., 2004). Even for survivors who physically recover from critical illness, delirium can have longstanding neuropsychiatric effects. Delirium itself may last for months and for some patients may unmask or lead to the development of dementia with substantial declines in memory and executive functioning. Psychiatric illness can also arise, including depression and signs of PTSD combined with flashbacks and hallucinations.

Older adults are particularly prone to experiencing delirium, which affects up to 80% of critically ill older adults; each year of age above 65 increases the odds of delirium by 2% (Pandharipande et al., 2006). Without formal delirium screening, up to 75% of cases of delirium are missed (Spronk et al., 2009). All patients in the ICU should be regularly screened for delirium via the Confusion Assessment Method ICU (CAM-ICU) (Ely et al., 2001) or the Intensive Care Delirium Screening Checklist (ICDSC) (Bergeron et al., 2001). Since delirium often persists beyond the ICU stay, hospital wards and post-acute care facilities should have delirium protocols in place for recognizing and managing delirium. Validated screening tools and more information on optimizing delirium care in settings outside of the ICU can be found on the Age-Friendly Health Systems initiative's website (Institute for Healthcare Improvement, 2020).

Nonpharmacologic management is the best strategy for preventing and treating delirium. A robust body of evidence shows that nonpharmacologic protocols (e.g., Hospital Elder Life Program, Nurses Improving Care for Healthsystem Elders, and ABCDEF bundle) are effective at reducing delirium (Hshieh et al., 2015). All of these programs have excellent summaries that are beyond the scope of this chapter, but suffice it to say that the idea common among them is that we must spend more time with the patient and less time writing for medications to artificially "fix" the delirium, and subsequently the delirium will resolve more quickly and more completely. In addition, a robust evidence base shows that antipsychotic medications (e.g., haloperidol, ziprasidone) do not shorten time in delirium or reduce mortality, length of stay, or other clinical outcomes (Girard et al., 2018). Thus, we can no longer conclude that we must rely on medication to treat delirium. Instead, we should be

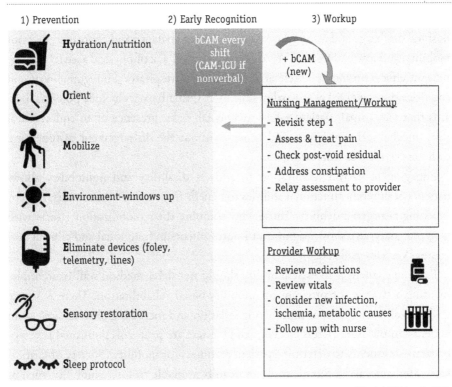

1) Prevention   2) Early Recognition   3) Workup

Hydration/nutrition

Orient

Mobilize

Environment-windows up

Eliminate devices (foley, telemetry, lines)

Sensory restoration

Sleep protocol

bCAM every shift (CAM-ICU if nonverbal)

+ bCAM (new)

Nursing Management/Workup
- Revisit step 1
- Assess & treat pain
- Check post-void residual
- Address constipation
- Relay assessment to provider

Provider Workup
- Review medications
- Review vitals
- Consider new infection, ischemia, metabolic causes
- Follow up with nurse

© Vanderbilt University 2019

FIGURE 10.2. Sample delirium protocol for a hospital ward or skilled nursing facility.

orienting non-sedated patients, getting them out of bed to walk and exercise earlier, and avoiding rather than prescribing psychoactive medications. A sample delirium protocol with a focus on nonpharmacologic prevention and treatment is provided in Figure 10.2.

EARLY MOBILITY AND EXERCISE

Older adults are particularly vulnerable to the hazards of immobility that often accompany critical illness. With age, muscle strength and function are reduced, also known as sarcopenia. Sarcopenia is a strong predictor of disability and mortality in older adults (Fielding et al., 2011). Because older adults have less physiologic reserve, it is imperative for them to maintain muscle strength and function.

ICU patients of all ages risk losing up to 25% of peripheral muscle within 4 days when mechanically ventilated and 18% in body weight by the time of discharge (Marra et al., 2017). ICU-acquired weakness may be caused by several pathophysiologic mechanisms, not all of which are mutually exclusive; they include the diseases leading to critical illness, drugs administered during treatment, and outcomes of prolonged immobility (Kress & Hall, 2014). These deficits commonly persist beyond hospital discharge and result in weakness, impaired balance and coordination, poor mobility, and low endurance (Verceles et al., 2012). Lack of physical activity has significant effects on musculoskeletal, cardiovascular, respiratory, integumentary, and cognitive systems (Dirkes & Kozlowski, 2019). Other barriers include potential hazards that may impair patient safety such as fall risks, presence of an endotracheal tube, mechanical ventilation, and concerns about the dislodgement of tubes and catheters (Dirkes & Kozlowski, 2019).

Engaging in early rehabilitation to address disability and immobility allows patients of different functional abilities to benefit from exercise maneuvers, thereby lessening iatrogenic debility. Those who combine their mobilization efforts with targeted goals have shown significant improvements in functional and clinical outcomes (Verceles et al., 2018).

Existing challenges to early mobility should not deter medical staff from implementing a strategy or program for mobility-based rehabilitation. There is strong evidence of the benefits of minimizing sedation and increasing physical activity in patients on the ICU (Kress & Hall, 2014). There are protocols published for step-by-step assessments to determine patient readiness for mobility (Society of Critical Care Medicine, n.d.). Simple tools are readily available to foster mobility, such as using the high Fowler upright position in bed to improve ventilation (Richard et al., 2006).

FAMILY ENGAGEMENT/EMPOWERMENT

Success in patient recovery after discharge largely depends on the care they receive from their families. Critical illness affects not only an individual but an entire support system of friends and family members who are actively engaged in these roles. Provider communication with a patient's support system is especially crucial at this time, as families frequently set unrealistic expectations for their loved one's rehabilitation. Another purpose of these interactions is for providers to educate families on the potential barriers and psychological difficulties they may experience themselves, addressing both the physical and psychological needs of caregivers who are at risk of burnout from caring for critically ill patients (please see Chapter 12 for more discussion regarding common family issues).

Conclusion

As the aging population continues to grow, it will become more important for all health care providers to understand the complexities of caring for older adults during and after critical illness. Care models, like HELP for wards and the ABCDEF bundle for the ICU, delivered with an understanding of older adults' multifaceted complexities, are critical to delivering effective interdisciplinary care.

References

Acierno, R., Hernandez, M. A., Amstadter, A. B., Resnick, H. S., Steve, K., Muzzy, W., & Kilpatrick, D. G. (2010). Prevalence and correlates of emotional, physical, sexual, and financial abuse and potential neglect in the United States: The National Elder Mistreatment Study. *American Journal of Public Health, 100*(2), 292–297. doi:10.2105/AJPH.2009.163089

American Geriatrics Society Beers Criteria Update Expert Panel. (2019). American Geriatrics Society 2019 Updated AGS Beers Criteria® for potentially inappropriate medication use in older adults. *Journal of the American Geriatrics Society, 67*(4), 674–694. doi:10.1111/jgs.15767

American Geriatrics Society Panel on Pharmacological Management of Persistent Pain in Older Persons. (2009). Pharmacological management of persistent pain in older persons. *Journal of the American Geriatrics Society, 57*(8), 1331–1346. doi:10.1111/j.1532-5415.2009.02376.x

Barnes, D. E., Palmer, R. M., Kresevic, D. M., Fortinsky, R. H., Kowal, J., Chren, M. M., & Landefeld, C. S. (2012). Acute care for elders units produced shorter hospital stays at lower cost while maintaining patients' functional status. *Health Affairs, 31*(6), 1227–1236. doi:10.1377/hlthaff.2012.0142

Becker, P. M., & Cohen, H. J. (1984). The functional approach to the care of the elderly: A conceptual framework. *Journal of the American Geriatrics Society, 32*(12), 923–929. doi:10.1111/j.1532-5415.1984.tb00894.x

Behrendt, C. E. (2000). Acute respiratory failure in the United States: Incidence and 31-day survival. *Chest, 118*(4), 1100–1105.

Bergeron, N., Dubois, M. J., Dumont, M., Dial, S., & Skrobik, Y. (2001). Intensive Care Delirium Screening Checklist: Evaluation of a new screening tool. *Intensive Care Medicine, 27*(5), 859–864.

Brummel, N. E., Balas, M. C., Morandi, A., Ferrante, L. E., Gill, T. M., & Ely, E. W. (2015). Understanding and reducing disability in older adults following critical illness. *Critical Care Medicine, 43*(6), 1265–1275. doi:10.1097/ccm.0000000000000924

Cahir, C., Fahey, T., Teeling, M., Teljeur, C., Feely, J., & Bennett, K. (2010). Potentially inappropriate prescribing and cost outcomes for older people: A national population study. *British Journal of Clinical Pharmacology, 69*(5), 543–552. doi:10.1111/j.1365-2125.2010.03628.x

Chodosh, J., Seeman, T. E., Keeler, E., Sewall, A., Hirsch, S. H., Guralnik, J. M., & Reuben, D. B. (2004). Cognitive decline in high-functioning older persons is associated with an increased risk of hospitalization. *Journal of the American Geriatrics Society, 52*(9), 1456–1462. doi:10.1111/j.1532-5415.2004.52407.x

Cohen-Mansfield, J. (2006). Pain Assessment in Noncommunicative Elderly persons: PAINE. *Clinical Journal of Pain, 22*(6), 569–575. doi:10.1097/01.ajp.0000210899.83096.0b

Corbett, A., Husebo, B., Malcangio, M., Staniland, A., Cohen-Mansfield, J., Aarsland, D., & Ballard, C. (2012). Assessment and treatment of pain in people with dementia. *Nature Reviews: Neurology, 8*(5), 264–274. doi:10.1038/nrneurol.2012.53

Dirkes, S. M., & Kozlowski, C. (2019). Early mobility in the intensive care unit: Evidence, barriers, and future directions. *Critical Care Nurse, 39*(3), 33–42. doi:10.4037/ccn2019654

Drayer, R. A., Mulsant, B. H., Lenze, E. J., Rollman, B. L., Dew, M. A., Kelleher, K., . . . Reynolds, C. F., 3rd. (2005). Somatic symptoms of depression in elderly patients with medical comorbidities. *International Journal of Geriatric Psychiatry, 20*(10), 973–982. doi:10.1002/gps.1389

Ellis, G., Gardner, M., Tsiachristas, A., Langhorne, P., Burke, O., Harwood, R. H., . . . Shepperd, S. (2017). Comprehensive geriatric assessment for older adults admitted to hospital. *Cochrane Database of Systematic Reviews, 9*, CD006211. doi:10.1002/14651858.CD006211.pub3

Ely, E. W. (2017). The ABCDEF bundle: Science and philosophy of how ICU liberation serves patients and families. *Critical Care Medicine, 45*(2), 321–330. doi:10.1097/CCM.0000000000002175

Ely, E. W., Evans, G. W., & Haponik, E. F. (1999). Mechanical ventilation in a cohort of elderly patients admitted to an intensive care unit. *Annals of Internal Medicine, 131*(2), 96–104.

Ely, E. W., Shintani, A., Truman, B., Speroff, T., Gordon, S. M., Harrell, F. E., Jr., . . . Dittus, R. S. (2004). Delirium as a predictor of mortality in mechanically ventilated patients in the intensive care unit. *Journal of the American Medical Association, 291*(14), 1753–1762. doi:10.1001/jama.291.14.1753

Ely, E. W., Truman, B., May, L., Gordon, S., Francis, J., Margolin, R., . . . Inouye, S. K. (2001). Validation of the CAM-ICU for delirium assessment in mechanically ventilated patients. *Journal of the American Geriatrics Society, 49*(4), S2.

Ely, E. W., Wheeler, A. P., Thompson, B. T., Ancukiewicz, M., Steinberg, K. P., & Bernard, G. R. (2002). Recovery rate and prognosis in older persons who develop acute lung injury and the acute respiratory distress syndrome. *Annals of Internal Medicine, 136*(1), 25–36.

Erstad, B. L., Puntillo, K., Gilbert, H. C., Grap, M. J., Li, D., Medina, J., . . . Sessler, C. N. (2009). Pain management principles in the critically ill. *Chest, 135*(4), 1075–1086. doi:10.1378/chest.08-2264

Ferrante, L. E., Pisani, M. A., Murphy, T. E., Gahbauer, E. A., Leo-Summers, L. S., & Gill, T. M. (2015). Functional trajectories among older persons before and after critical illness. *JAMA Internal Medicine, 175*(4), 523–529. doi:10.1001/jamainternmed.2014.7889

Fielding, R. A., Vellas, B., Evans, W. J., Bhasin, S., Morley, J. E., Newman, A. B., . . . Zamboni, M. (2011). Sarcopenia: An undiagnosed condition in older adults. Current consensus definition: Prevalence, etiology, and consequences. International Working Group on Sarcopenia. *Journal of the American Medical Directors Association, 12*(4), 249–256. doi:10.1016/j.jamda.2011.01.003

Fraser, G. L., Devlin, J. W., Worby, C. P., Alhazzani, W., Barr, J., Dasta, J. F., . . . Spencer, F. A. (2013). Benzodiazepine versus nonbenzodiazepine-based sedation for mechanically ventilated, critically ill adults: A systematic review and meta-analysis of randomized trials. *Critical Care Medicine, 41*(9 Suppl 1), S30–S38. doi:10.1097/CCM.0b013e3182a16898

Fried, L. P., Tangen, C. M., Walston, J., Newman, A. B., Hirsch, C., Gottdiener, J., . . . Cardiovascular Health Study Collaborative Research Group. (2001). Frailty in older adults: Evidence for a phenotype. *Journals of Gerontology. Series A: Biological Sciences and Medical Sciences, 56*(3), M146–M156.

Gallagher, P., Ryan, C., Byrne, S., Kennedy, J., & O'Mahony, D. (2008). STOPP (Screening Tool of Older Person's Prescriptions) and START (Screening Tool to Alert Doctors to

Right Treatment). Consensus validation. *International Journal of Clinical Pharmacology and Therapeutics, 46*(2), 72–83.

Galvin, J. E., Roe, C. M., Powlishta, K. K., Coats, M. A., Muich, S. J., Grant, E., . . . Morris, J. C. (2005). The AD8: A brief informant interview to detect dementia. *Neurology, 65*(4), 559–564. doi:10.1212/01.wnl.0000172958.95282.2a

Garpestad, E., & Devlin, J. W. (2017). Polypharmacy and delirium in critically ill older adults: Recognition and prevention. *Clinics in Geriatric Medicine, 33*(2), 189–203. doi:10.1016/j.cger.2017.01.002

Girard, T. D., Exline, M. C., Carson, S. S., Hough, C. L., Rock, P., Gong, M. N., . . . MindUSA Investigators. (2018). Haloperidol and ziprasidone for treatment of delirium in critical illness. *New England Journal of Medicine, 379*(26), 2506–2516. doi:10.1056/NEJMoa1808217

Girard, T. D., Kress, J. P., Fuchs, B. D., Thomason, J. W., Schweickert, W. D., Pun, B. T., . . . Ely, E. W. (2008). Efficacy and safety of a paired sedation and ventilator weaning protocol for mechanically ventilated patients in intensive care (Awakening and Breathing Controlled trial): A randomised controlled trial. *Lancet, 371*(9607), 126–134. doi:10.1016/S0140-6736(08)60105-1

Himmelfarb, J. (2009). Acute kidney injury in the elderly: Problems and prospects. *Seminars in Nephrology, 29*(6), 658–664. doi:10.1016/j.semnephrol.2009.07.008

Hopkins, R. O., & Jackson, J. C. (2006). Long-term neurocognitive function after critical illness. *Chest, 130*(3), 869–878. doi:10.1378/chest.130.3.869

Hshieh, T. T., Yue, J., Oh, E., Puelle, M., Dowal, S., Travison, T., & Inouye, S. K. (2015). Effectiveness of multicomponent nonpharmacological delirium interventions: A meta-analysis. *JAMA Internal Medicine, 175*(4), 512–520. doi:10.1001/jamainternmed.2014.7779

Husebo, B. S., Strand, L. I., Moe-Nilssen, R., Husebo, S. B., & Ljunggren, A. E. (2010). Pain in older persons with severe dementia. Psychometric properties of the Mobilization-Observation-Behaviour-Intensity-Dementia (MOBID-2) Pain Scale in a clinical setting. *Scandinavian Journal of Caring Sciences, 24*(2), 380–391. doi:10.1111/j.1471-6712.2009.00710.x

Inouye, S. K., Studenski, S., Tinetti, M. E., & Kuchel, G. A. (2007). Geriatric syndromes: Clinical, research, and policy implications of a core geriatric concept. *Journal of the American Geriatrics Society, 55*(5), 780–791. doi:10.1111/j.1532-5415.2007.01156.x

Inouye, S. K., Westendorp, R. G., & Saczynski, J. S. (2014). Delirium in elderly people. *Lancet, 383*(9920), 911–922. doi:10.1016/S0140-6736(13)60688-1

Institute for Healthcare Improvement. (2020, July). Age-Friendly Health Systems guide to using the 4Ms in the care of older adults. http://www.ihi.org/Engage/Initiatives/Age-Friendly-Health-Systems/Documents/IHIAgeFriendlyHealthSystems_GuidetoUsing4MsCare.pdf

Iyasere, O. U., Brown, E. A., Johansson, L., Huson, L., Smee, J., Maxwell, A. P., . . . Davenport, A. (2016). Quality of life and physical function in older patients on dialysis: A comparison of assisted peritoneal dialysis with hemodialysis. *Clinical Journal of the American Society of Nephrology, 11*(3), 423–430. doi:10.2215/CJN.01050115

Jackson, T. A., MacLullich, A. M., Gladman, J. R., Lord, J. M., & Sheehan, B. (2016). Diagnostic test accuracy of informant-based tools to diagnose dementia in older hospital patients with delirium: A prospective cohort study. *Age and Ageing, 45*(4), 505–511. doi:10.1093/ageing/afw065

Kahn, J. M., Le, T., Angus, D. C., Cox, C. E., Hough, C. L., White, D. B., . . . ProVent Study Group Investigators. (2015). The epidemiology of chronic critical illness in the United States. *Critical Care Medicine, 43*(2), 282–287. doi:10.1097/CCM.0000000000000710

Katz, S. (1983). Assessing self-maintenance: Activities of daily living, mobility, and instrumental activities of daily living. *Journal of the American Geriatrics Society, 31*(12), 721–727.

Koenig, H. G., King, D. E. and Carson, V. B. (2012). *Handbook of religion and health* (2nd ed.). Oxford University Press.

Kress, J. P., & Hall, J. B. (2014). ICU-acquired weakness and recovery from critical illness. *New England Journal of Medicine, 371*(3), 287–288. doi:10.1056/NEJMc1406274

Kress, J. P., Pohlman, A. S., O'Connor, M. F., & Hall, J. B. (2000). Daily interruption of sedative infusions in critically ill patients undergoing mechanical ventilation. *New England Journal of Medicine, 342*(20), 1471–1477. doi:10.1056/NEJM200005183422002

Lawton, M. P., & Brody, E. M. (1969). Assessment of older people: self-maintaining and instrumental activities of daily living. *Gerontologist, 9*(3), 179–186.

Livingston, G., Sommerlad, A., Orgeta, V., Costafreda, S. G., Huntley, J., Ames, D., . . . Mukadam, N. (2017). Dementia prevention, intervention, and care. *Lancet, 390*(10113), 2673–2734. doi:10.1016/S0140-6736(17)31363-6

Lynn, J. (2019). The "fierce urgency of now": Geriatrics professionals speaking up for older adult care in the United States. *Journal of the American Geriatrics Society, 67*(10), 2001–2003. doi:10.1111/jgs.16116

Mangoni, A. A., & Jackson, S. H. (2004). Age-related changes in pharmacokinetics and pharmacodynamics: Basic principles and practical applications. *British Journal of Clinical Pharmacology, 57*(1), 6–14. doi:10.1046/j.1365-2125.2003.02007.x

Marra, A., Ely, E. W., Pandharipande, P. P., & Patel, M. B. (2017). The ABCDEF bundle in critical care. *Critical Care Clinics, 33*(2), 225–243. doi:10.1016/j.ccc.2016.12.005

Masnoon, N., Shakib, S., Kalisch-Ellett, L., & Caughey, G. E. (2017). What is polypharmacy? A systematic review of definitions. *BMC Geriatrics, 17*(1), 230. doi:10.1186/s12877-017-0621-2

McLean, A. J., & Le Couteur, D. G. (2004). Aging biology and geriatric clinical pharmacology. *Pharmacological Reviews, 56*(2), 163–184. doi:10.1124/pr.56.2.4

Muscedere, J., Waters, B., Varambally, A., Bagshaw, S. M., Boyd, J. G., Maslove, D., . . . Rockwood, K. (2017). The impact of frailty on intensive care unit outcomes: A systematic review and meta-analysis. *Intensive Care Medicine, 43*(8), 1105–1122. doi:10.1007/s00134-017-4867-0

Needham, D. M., Davidson, J., Cohen, H., Hopkins, R. O., Weinert, C., Wunsch, H., . . . Harvey, M. A. (2012). Improving long-term outcomes after discharge from intensive care unit: Report from a stakeholders' conference. *Critical Care Medicine, 40*(2), 502–509. doi:10.1097/CCM.0b013e318232da75

Nicholson, N. R. (2012). A review of social isolation: An important but underassessed condition in older adults. *Journal of Primary Prevention, 33*(2–3), 137–152. doi:10.1007/s10935-012-0271-2

Ortman, J. M., Velkoff, V. A., & Hogan, H. (2014, May). An aging nation: The older population in the United States. U.S. Census Bureau, Current Population Reports, pp. 25–114. http://usd-apps.usd.edu/coglab/schieber/psyc423/pdf/AgingNation.pdf

Pandharipande, P., Shintani, A., Peterson, J., Pun, B. T., Wilkinson, G. R., Dittus, R. S., . . . Ely, E. W. (2006). Lorazepam is an independent risk factor for transitioning to delirium in intensive care unit patients. *Anesthesiology, 104*(1), 21–26.

Pandharipande, P. P., Girard, T. D., & Ely, E. W. (2014). Long-term cognitive impairment after critical illness. *New England Journal of Medicine, 370*(2), 185–186. doi:10.1056/NEJMc1313886

Pandharipande, P. P., Pun, B. T., Herr, D. L., Maze, M., Girard, T. D., Miller, R. R., . . . Ely, E. W. (2007). Effect of sedation with dexmedetomidine vs lorazepam on acute brain dysfunction in mechanically ventilated patients: The MENDS randomized controlled trial. *Journal of the American Medical Association, 298*(22), 2644–2653. doi:10.1001/jama.298.22.2644

Peteet, J. R., Zaben, F. A., & Koenig, H. G. (2019). Integrating spirituality into the care of older adults. *International Psychogeriatrics, 31*(1), 31–38. doi:10.1017/S1041610218000716

Pisani, M. A. (2009). Considerations in caring for the critically ill older patient. *Journal of Intensive Care Medicine, 24*(2), 83–95. doi:10.1177/0885066608329942

Richard, J. C., Maggiore, S. M., Mancebo, J., Lemaire, F., Jonson, B., & Brochard, L. (2006). Effects of vertical positioning on gas exchange and lung volumes in acute respiratory distress syndrome. *Intensive Care Medicine, 32*(10), 1623–1626. doi:10.1007/s00134-006-0299-y

Riker, R. R., Picard, J. T., & Fraser, G. L. (1999). Prospective evaluation of the Sedation-Agitation Scale for adult critically ill patients. *Critical Care Medicine, 27*(7), 1325–1329.

Salahudeen, M. S., Hilmer, S. N., & Nishtala, P. S. (2015). Comparison of anticholinergic risk scales and associations with adverse health outcomes in older people. *Journal of the American Geriatrics Society, 63*(1), 85–90. doi:10.1111/jgs.13206

Society of Critical Care Medicine. Early mobility and exercise. https://www.sccm.org/getattachment/7265d851-d6b5-4df8-9554-513c4f280239/Implementing-the-E-component-of-the-ABCDEF-bundle

Sessler, C. N., Gosnell, M. S., Grap, M. J., Brophy, G. M., O'Neal, P. V., Keane, K. A., . . . Elswick, R. K. (2002). The Richmond Agitation-Sedation Scale: Validity and reliability in adult intensive care unit patients. *American Journal of Respiratory and Critical Care Medicine, 166*(10), 1338–1344. doi:10.1164/rccm.2107138

Spronk, P. E., Riekerk, B., Hofhuis, J., & Rommes, J. H. (2009). Occurrence of delirium is severely underestimated in the ICU during daily care. *Intensive Care Medicine, 35*(7), 1276–1280. doi:10.1007/s00134-009-1466-8

Thielke, S., Sale, J., & Reid, M. C. (2012). Aging: Are these 4 pain myths complicating care? *Journal of Family Practice, 61*(11), 666–670.

Tsoi, K. K., Chan, J. Y., Hirai, H. W., Wong, S. Y., & Kwok, T. C. (2015). Cognitive tests to detect dementia: A systematic review and meta-analysis. *JAMA Internal Medicine, 175*(9), 1450–1458. doi:10.1001/jamainternmed.2015.2152

Van der Linden, L., Decoutere, L., Flamaing, J., Spriet, I., Willems, L., Milisen, K., . . . Tournoy, J. (2014). Development and validation of the RASP list (Rationalization of Home Medication by an Adjusted STOPP list in Older Patients): A novel tool in the management of geriatric polypharmacy. *European Geriatric Medicine, 5*(3), 175–180. doi:10.1016/j.eurger.2013.12.005

van Leeuwen, K. M., van Loon, M. S., van Nes, F. A., Bosmans, J. E., de Vet, H. C. W., Ket, J. C. F., . . . Ostelo, R. (2019). What does quality of life mean to older adults? A thematic synthesis. *PLoS One, 14*(3), e0213263. doi:10.1371/journal.pone.0213263

Verceles, A. C., Diaz-Abad, M., Geiger-Brown, J., & Scharf, S. M. (2012). Testing the prognostic value of the rapid shallow breathing index in predicting successful weaning in patients requiring prolonged mechanical ventilation. *Heart & Lung, 41*(6), 546–552. doi:10.1016/j.hrtlng.2012.06.003

Verceles, A. C., Wells, C. L., Sorkin, J. D., Terrin, M. L., Beans, J., Jenkins, T., & Goldberg, A. P. (2018). A multimodal rehabilitation program for patients with ICU acquired weakness improves ventilator weaning and discharge home. *Journal of Critical Care, 47*, 204–210. doi:10.1016/j.jcrc.2018.07.006

Villanueva, M. R., Smith, T. L., Erickson, J. S., Lee, A. C., & Singer, C. M. (2003). Pain Assessment for the Dementing Elderly (PADE): Reliability and validity of a new measure. *Journal of the American Medical Directors Association, 4*(1), 1–8. doi:10.1097/01.JAM.0000043419.51772.A3

Weyand, C. M., & Goronzy, J. J. (2016). Aging of the immune system: Mechanisms and therapeutic targets. *Annals of the American Thoracic Society, 13*(Suppl 5), S422–S428. doi:10.1513/AnnalsATS.201602-095AW

World Health Organization. (1995). World Health Organization Quality of Life assessment (WHOQOL): Position paper. *Social Science and Medicine, 41*(10), 1403–1409. doi:10.1016/0277-9536(95)00112-k

Ziaeian, B., Araujo, K. L., Van Ness, P. H., & Horwitz, L. I. (2012). Medication reconciliation accuracy and patient understanding of intended medication changes on hospital discharge. *Journal of General Internal Medicine, 27*(11), 1513–1520. doi:10.1007/s11606-012-2168-4

11 Psychopharmacology in the Critical Care Setting

Sandeep Nayak, Jonathan Brigham, Ted Avi Gerstenblith, and
Elizabeth Prince

Introduction

Psychotropic medications can be a powerful treatment of critically ill patients. However, a careful approach to psychopharmacology is necessary in the critical care setting. Special considerations include interactions with other medications and treatments, high levels of physiologic stress that alter metabolism, and the challenges of obtaining diagnostic clarity due to limitations in assessment and confounding factors during critical illness.

In an effort to be practical and useful, we have chosen to organize this chapter by common consult questions posed by intensive care teams to the psychiatry consultation service: (1) management of agitation and sedation, (2) poor participation in care, (3) anxiety, (4) continuation of outpatient medication regimens, and (5) alternatives to oral medication.

Agitation and sedation

Agitation, or excessive psychomotor activity with psychological distress, can clearly be harmful in the critical care setting. It can interfere with the provision of lifesaving

Sandeep Nayak, Jonathan Brigham, Ted Avi Gerstenblith, and Elizabeth Prince, *Psychopharmacology in the Critical Care Setting* In: *Critical Care Psychology and Rehabilitation*. Edited by: Kirk J. Stucky and Jennifer E. Jutte, Oxford University Press. © Oxford University Press 2022. DOI: 10.1093/oso/9780190077013.003.0011 care, increase metabolic demand, be physically dangerous to both the patient and staff, and be a harbinger of life-threatening conditions. Agitation has been reported in 46% to 52% of patients in a medical-surgical intensive care unit (ICU) (Fraser et al., 2000; Jaber et al., 2005). Pharmacologic means of suppressing agitation may be required if patient behavior interferes with lifesaving medical care or endangers the patient or others such as family and hospital staff.

The first step in management of agitation is to identify which patient behaviors are disruptive and/or problematic. The term "agitation" is a vague descriptor that is used to refer to a variety of psychomotor manifestations ranging from mild to severe in degree. We therefore prefer to identify specific descriptions of patient behaviors (e.g., yelling, attempting to disconnect ventilator, swinging at staff members) and their associated factors (e.g., precipitated vs. spontaneous, rapid vs. gradual escalation, frequency) when documenting and delineating agitation. Descriptions assist in understanding potential underlying contributors to agitation. Furthermore, when ordering the use of "as needed" (PRN) medication, it is important to identify what behaviors warrant medication administration as opposed to nonpharmacologic interventions.

Targeted treatment of the underlying etiology is the most effective management strategy. Pain, delirium, and anxiety are common drivers of agitation (Siegel, 2003). For instance, the hyperactive subtype of delirium, various withdrawal syndromes (such as alcohol, benzodiazepine, or opioid withdrawal), and acute pain can all independently manifest with agitation. Primary psychiatric disorders such as decompensated affective or psychotic disorders can also drive agitation but should be considered only after excluding other life-threatening causes of agitation. While treatment directed at the underlying cause of agitation is preferable to simply sedating a patient, this is not always possible in an acute care setting. See Table 11.1 for a review of common classes of medications used for agitation and sedation.

Because this chapter is focused on pharmacology, we will not discuss behavioral and nonpharmacologic interventions or the use of safety observers and physical restraints when patients are posing a threat to themselves or others. It should be noted, however, that in some circumstances, these nonpharmacologic approaches may be more effective, associated with lower risk of morbidity, or a useful adjunct to the use of medications.

HYPERACTIVE DELIRIUM

Delirium is a multifactorial cerebral process that stems from a variety of illnesses, medications, and withdrawal/intoxication syndromes. Delirium is common in the

TABLE 11.1.

Common medications used for agitation

Class	Example	Risks	Benefits/applications
Alpha agonists	Dexmedetomidine	Dose-dependent hypotension, bradycardia	Opioid, alcohol, and benzodiazepine withdrawal
Anesthetics	Propofol	Respiratory depression	Alcohol and benzodiazepine withdrawal
Anticholinergic agents	Diphenhydramine	Potential to worsen delirium	Cholinergic toxicity or EPS-related agitation
Antiepileptics	Valproate	Liver toxicity	Agitation related to seizure activity
Antipsychotics	Haloperidol	NMS, extrapyramidal symptoms (EPS), dystonic reactions	Multiple formulations and routes of administration
Benzodiazepines	Lorazepam	Potential to worsen delirium or develop dependence, respiratory depression particularly when in combination with opioids	Alcohol and benzodiazepine withdrawal
Opioids	Fentanyl	Can cause serotonin syndrome	Pain management Air hunger

For more detailed discussion please see Levenson, J. L. (2019). *The American Psychiatric Association Publishing textbook of psychosomatic medicine and consultation-liaison psychiatry* (3rd ed.). American Psychiatric Association Publishing.

critical care setting, with some studies suggesting that up to 32.3% of patients will develop delirium in the ICU (Salluh et al., 2010), with the rate increasing to 83% for those patients who are mechanically ventilated (Ely et al., 2001). Though not a formal part of the classification system, it is useful to divide delirium into different subtypes: (1) hyperactive (excited or agitated) delirium, which includes agitation; (2) hypoactive delirium, which does not include agitation; and (3) a mixed hypo- and hyper-active delirium with fluctuations in agitation. Delirium is associated with a higher risk for mortality (Inouye et al., 1998), and there are even case reports of agitated delirium leading to sudden death (Vilke et al., 2012).

In the event of agitation that interferes with care or poses safety risks, medications may be administered to reduce disruptions to care. Medications may not only minimize disruptions to medical care but may also reduce a patient's subjective sense of suffering. However, it is important to note that medications are not treatment for the syndrome of delirium itself, but they will assist with its associated feature of agitation. There is no known medication that invariably eliminates delirium or reduces the duration of delirium (see the section on hypoactive delirium later in the chapter).

WITHDRAWAL

Alcohol

Alcohol and/or benzodiazepine withdrawal can be a special contributor to delirium that should always be considered. Chronic alcohol or benzodiazepine use results in receptor adaptation that, upon cessation, can cause withdrawal symptoms ranging from troublesome to fatal. Alcohol withdrawal can also cause agitation in the ICU setting (Awissi et al., 2013). However, it is unclear what portion of agitation in the ICU is attributable to withdrawal.

Identification of withdrawal occurs through careful history gathering (if possible) and attention to the well-known signs and symptoms of alcohol withdrawal. The withdrawal syndrome spans the gamut from mild and self-limited to severe and potentially fatal. Alcohol withdrawal begins 6 to 24 hours after cessation and may include a variety of signs and symptoms, such as autonomic hyperactivity, tremor, anxiety, gastrointestinal distress, hallucinations, and seizures. Ten percent to 31% of patients in the ICU setting may have an alcohol use disorder (Baldwin et al., 1993; Gacouin et al., 2008), and 18% of patients in the ICU setting develop alcohol withdrawal (de Wit et al., 2010). Despite this estimated frequency, there are no best-practice guidelines for identification, prevention, and treatment of alcohol withdrawal in the ICU setting. Either scheduled doses or symptom-triggered doses of benzodiazepines may be appropriate. A symptom-triggered approach may require a lesser amount of the drug (Daeppen et al., 2002; Saitz et al., 1994; Spies et al., 2003). The Clinical Institute Withdrawal Assessment (CIWA-Ar) is a commonly used scale for a symptom-triggered approach (Sullivan et al., 1989), though it may be confounded by other conditions with overlapping symptoms such as paroxysmal sweats in opioid withdrawal or sepsis.

Alcohol withdrawal may manifest later than expected in the critical care setting, given the routine use of benzodiazepines and propofol that may mask, or delay, withdrawal onset. Benzodiazepines are the mainstay of treatment of the agitation related to alcohol withdrawal. However, care must be taken so that treatment of alcohol withdrawal will not lead to benzodiazepine toxicity, which can itself be deliriogenic (Johnson et al., 2013). For this reason, benzodiazepine-sparing medications such as dexmedetomidine and/or valproate may be useful in the management of alcohol withdrawal. (Crispo et al., 2014; Darrouj et al., 2008; Maldonado, 2017).

Nicotine

Individuals who regularly use tobacco products or other nicotine-containing substances may be at higher risk for agitation in the ICU setting (Lucidarme et al., 2010). However, it is not precisely clear whether this is due to nicotine withdrawal or cravings for nicotine. Kowalski and colleagues (2016) reviewed the literature on nicotine replacement therapy in the management of agitation and delirium in smokers on the ICU and concluded that there is a lack of quality evidence as to whether nicotine replacement is helpful in attenuating agitation in heavy smokers in the critical care setting.

INTOXICATION SYNDROMES

Intoxication syndromes, which may lead to a state of delirium, are another possible cause for agitation. Clues to drug intoxication–related agitation include rapid mental status changes without other clear explanation, similarity to a specific intoxication syndrome, and temporal association with visitors at the bedside. Urine toxicology and a careful room search can help identify objective evidence of substance use. It is important to note that intoxication with opioids and benzodiazepines generally does not cause agitation, but withdrawal from these substances can do so. See Table 11.2 for some examples of drugs and their potential intoxication effects and duration of action.

SEROTONIN SYNDROME

Serotonin syndrome is characterized by a triad of mental status changes, neuromuscular abnormalities, and dysautonomia. Serotonin toxicity is typically caused by a combination of multiple serotonergic medications or overdose (Boyer & Shannon, 2005). Autonomic abnormalities include tachycardia, hypertension, and markedly elevated body temperature. Neuromuscular abnormalities include hyperreflexia, sustained clonus, and increased tone. Other clinical features include mydriasis, diaphoresis, shivering, and hyperactive bowel sounds. Psychomotor agitation is also a frequent aspect of serotonin syndrome.

TABLE 11.2.

Intoxication effects and duration of action for select drugs of abuse

	Effects	Duration
Amphetamines (meth, Ecstasy)	Psychomotor agitation, sympathetic hyperactivity, mydriasis, possibly psychosis	Depends on formulation
Synthetic cannabinoids (K2, Spice)	Psychosis, slurred speech, ataxia, nystagmus, tachycardia, physical agitation, seizures	Hours to days
Phencyclidine (PCP)	Acute psychosis, bizarre behavior, physical agitation, sedation, nystagmus, disorientation	1–3 hours, though depends on route of administration
Alcohol	Disinhibition, slurred speech, ataxia, mood lability	Typically clears at a rate of 0.015 g/100 mL/hour
Cocaine	Physical agitation, euphoria, seizures, tachycardia, hypertension	30–120 minutes
Methylenedioxypyrovalerone (MDPV, bath salts)	Physical agitation, agitated delirium, tachycardia, mydriasis, diaphoresis, seizures	Up to 48 hours; highly variable given several different drugs commonly used

Serotonin syndrome typically occurs within hours after the addition of the offending agent. Therefore, a careful medication history may assist in identification of the cause. One should note the addition of not only serotonergic medications but also medications that are cytochrome P450 inhibitors, as these may increase the levels of other serotonergic drugs. Commonly used drugs in the intensive care setting (e.g., fentanyl, tramadol) are serotonergic and have been associated with serotonin syndrome. Linezolid has weak monoamine oxidase inhibitor (MAOI) activity and may contribute to serotonin syndrome in the presence of other serotonergic drugs as well.

Recognition of the serotonin syndrome is the most important step in treatment. It may be missed due to lack of awareness of the condition and heterogeneity of presentation. In a patient with agitation, a history of serotonergic drug use, and other suggestive features as just listed, a diagnosis of serotonin syndrome should be considered and appropriate care initiated. Treatment begins with cessation of serotonergic agents as well as supportive care and possibly addition of a serotonin antagonist such as cyproheptadine.

NEUROLEPTIC MALIGNANT SYNDROME

Neuroleptic malignant syndrome (NMS) is an atypical drug reaction to dopamine antagonists (antipsychotics, some anti-nausea agents). It may cause agitation and is characterized by muscle rigidity (sometimes extreme), elevated body temperatures, delirium, and dysautonomia. Unlike serotonin syndrome, gastrointestinal effects are not common. Prompt identification and treatment are essential, as NMS has a mortality rate as high as 10% (Tse et al., 2015). Risk factors for NMS include high doses of neuroleptics, use of multiple neuroleptics, initiation of neuroleptics, intramuscular administration, and agitation. As such, there have been cases of NMS following neuroleptic treatment for agitation (Seitz & Gill, 2009). Due to potential lethality and overlapping characteristics with critical illness, the astute clinician should keep NMS in the differential calculation in patients who are delirious and have had any recent exposure to neuroleptic medications.

PAIN

Untreated pain and opioid withdrawal may result in agitation (Clegg & Young, 2011; Das et al., 2017; Feast et al., 2018). Careful history, review of medication administration, and examination of the patient will determine how pain and pain medications may contribute to agitation in a patient. Antipsychotics may also be used to assist in addressing pain by decreasing pain salience (Fishbain, 2000). Ketamine, a medication with increasing application for a multitude of conditions, can decrease the need for opioids, which can thereby decrease chances of opioid side effects and toxicity (Subramaniam et al., 2004). However, as an NMDA receptor antagonist, psychotic symptoms are a potential side effect of ketamine and may limit its use (Patanwala et al., 2017).

AGITATION INTERFERING WITH VENTILATOR WEANING AND EXTUBATION

Agitation may impede the process of weaning from mechanical ventilation, but use of sedating medications to manage agitation can also prevent extubation. A certain level of alertness and cooperation is needed for successful extubation and resumption of normal respiration. It is critical to identify and address as much as possible the underlying cause of agitation, which may include delirium, pain, withdrawal, and ventilatory adequacy.

Dupuis and colleagues (2019) performed a systematic review of interventions to facilitate extubation in patients having difficulty weaning due to agitation, delirium, or anxiety. In this study, dexmedetomidine was the only drug found to facilitate ventilator weaning and therefore should be considered in these cases. Dexmedetomidine is an alpha-2 agonist that produces conscious sedation and decreases sympathetic nerve activity (Keating, 2015). Sympatholytic effect may also explain its beneficial role in alcohol and benzodiazepine withdrawal. Whether or not dexmedetomidine is indeed an effective intervention for benzodiazepine and alcohol withdrawal, it can reduce the benzodiazepine requirement in these patients (Bielka et al., 2015; Rayner et al., 2012). Dexmedetomidine's sedative-sparing effect may also result in the use of fewer deliriogenic medications and lead to a lower chance of withdrawal from other sedatives. Either of these may partially explain why dexmedetomidine has been observed to shorten duration of intubation. Moreover, dexmedetomidine does not suppress respiratory drive, unlike other common sedatives, including benzodiazepines and opioids (Dupuis et al., 2019). This may lead to less ventilator asynchrony, which may also facilitate extubation. Thus, dexmedetomidine's pharmacologic properties may render it less harmful than common alternatives.

OTHER

Active delirium precludes the diagnosis of a primary psychiatric illness. Delirium, "the great imitator," can masquerade as a multitude of psychiatric diagnoses. Hallmarks of primary psychiatric illness, including delusions, hallucinations, mood lability, and cognitive changes, can all be seen in delirium. In cases where the patient is agitated but not delirious, assess for psychiatric illness. Mania and psychosis are the most likely psychiatric diagnoses to lead to agitation. However, arriving at diagnostic clarity requires time, collateral informants, and serial assessments. Antipsychotics are first-line medications for the management of agitation in this context. However, caution must be taken with these drugs, particularly for specific patient groups. For example, antipsychotics might impair motor recovery in brain injury and may carry greater risks of extrapyramidal side effects (Feeney, Gonzalez, & Law, 1982; Wolf & Wertenschlag, 1989).

Poor participation

While agitation can interfere with provision of necessary care in the critical care setting, so can poor patient participation. An example would be a patient declining or refusing interventions or displaying poor effort with physical and/or occupational therapy. The differential for poor participation in rehabilitation includes hypoactive delirium, demoralization, depression, and/or anxiety. Miscommunication or misunderstandings between the patient and treatment team can also impede patient participation. Again, the underlying etiology guides treatment, but it must be recognized that assessment can be impaired and limited in the critical illness setting.

HYPOACTIVE DELIRIUM

Medications, including sedatives, analgesics, and anticholinergics, can contribute to delirium. However, as referenced earlier in the section on hyperactive delirium, there is no evidence that any medication will prevent or reduce duration of delirium in critical illness (Girard et al., 2018; Neufeld et al., 2016).

We first encourage environmental (otherwise classified as nonpharmacologic) interventions, including regulation of sleep–wake cycles, followed by minimization of exposure to deliriogenic medications before initiating additional medications. Medications like trazodone, melatonin, or ramelteon may be of use for promoting sleep. There is some evidence that disruption of melatonin (an endogenous circadian hormone) may be involved in the pathogenesis of delirium (Yoshitaka et al., 2013). There is mixed evidence that melatonin supplementation may protect against the development of delirium (Lewis et al., 2018; Ng et al., 2020).

DEMORALIZATION AND DEPRESSION

Poor participation in care can be driven by low mood, fatigue, hopelessness, apathy, or even suicidality. Accurate diagnosis and differentiation of demoralization and/ or depression can be confounded by critical illness. Furthermore, medications may induce symptoms of depression—for example, both steroids and steroid withdrawal.

While antidepressant medications are effective treatments for depression, they do not have a role in the management of demoralization or delirium. The use of antidepressant medications in the critical care setting is also challenging, as the majority of antidepressants take weeks to become effective (Hashmi et al., 2017). In addition, antidepressant medications are not without risk, including the precipitation of hyponatremia, antiplatelet effects, cardiac effects (including prolonged QT), serotonin syndrome, and interaction with other medications.

In some cases of depressive disorder, administration of psychostimulants (e.g., methylphenidate, modafinil) can produce more rapid improvement in depressive symptoms than more conventional antidepressants like selective serotonin reuptake inhibitors (SSRIs), though these improvements may only sustain for a short time. Under close monitoring and in low doses, a stimulant may improve engagement with rehabilitation, although there are limited studies (Hashemian & Farhadi, 2020). Risks include tachycardia, changes in sleep and appetite, or worsening of delirium.

Anxiety

Anxiety is common in the critical care setting and may result from dyspnea, pain, withdrawal, fear and uncertainty surrounding a procedure, separation from loved ones, disorientation, and delusions. Avoidance is a manifestation of anxiety that can impair participation in care. There is no one-size-fits-all pharmacologic approach to anxiety. As with any clinically significant neuropsychiatric phenomenon in the critical care setting, it is essential that an attempt be made to identify the cause so that effective treatment can be initiated.

Benzodiazepines are commonly used to treat anxiety, though they risk respiratory suppression, delirium, and dependency. Benzodiazepines are also associated with the subsequent development of psychiatric morbidity in the form of postintensive care syndrome (Prince et al., 2018). Non-benzodiazepine medications that may help with management of anxiety include buspirone, hydroxyzine, and low-dose antipsychotics (Eisendrath & Shim, 2006). While SSRIs are effective treatment for anxiety disorders, efficacy may not be observed for weeks to months; therefore, they do not have a role in acute anxiolysis.

AIR HUNGER

Air hunger, or the sensation of not being able to breathe sufficiently, can be a horrific experience that causes a great deal of distress. It is triggered by excess, unventilated carbon dioxide. Air hunger is so unpleasant that it has been used as torture in the form of waterboarding (Başoğlu, 2017). In the critical care setting, treatment of the underlying cause is the primary directive for addressing air hunger. Treatments may include antibiotics for pneumonia or beta-2 agonists for asthma. Opioids very effectively suppress air hunger but also suppress respiratory drive; thus, they are often inadvisable in patients experiencing air hunger with a treatable respiratory process (Banzett et al., 2011). There are cases, however, in which treating air hunger with opioids is appropriate. The most obvious use is in the palliative care setting, where comfort trumps treating the underlying respiratory process.

It is important to recognize that mechanically ventilated individuals are at times ventilated with a low inspiratory volume and pressure as a lung protective strategy. This can lead to buildup of carbon dioxide, which can be a contributor to the sensation of air hunger. Air hunger can be difficult to assess in an intubated patient and is likely an underrecognized cause of suffering in the critical care setting for which opioids may be underused (Schmidt et al., 2014; Worsham et al., 2020). It is also important to note that benzodiazepines are not effective in reducing air hunger (Simon et al., 2016). Air hunger can be assessed in conversant patients by asking whether they are feeling shortness of breath, rating their shortness of breath from 0 to 10, or using a visual analog scale (Powers & Bennett, 1999). Air hunger is subjective, and it has no well-validated physiologic surrogates.

DELUSIONS/HALLUCINATIONS

Delirium in the critical care setting can result in distressing delusions and hallucinations. Treatment involves first diagnosing and managing the underlying etiology, which is often multifactorial. Treating anxiety secondary to delirium with deliriogenic anxiolytics (e.g., benzodiazepines) risks worsening the problem. For clinically significant anxiety in the setting of delirium, a low-dose antipsychotic may be appropriate to reduce patient distress and potential interference with necessary care. However, this should be thought of as a stopgap measure rather than a solution. As such, antipsychotics in the setting of delirium should be given with a harm-reduction mentality and used with the lowest dose possible and for the shortest duration necessary.

PROCEDURE-RELATED DISTRESS

Common procedures on the ICU such as wound and tracheostomy care can be painful and anxiety-provoking. A cycle of anticipatory anxiety can build up related to these interventions over time. Judicious use of as-needed medications can assist with providing needed care, but it is important to keep in mind that benzodiazepines and opioids in particular can contribute to dependence and addition. Of course, nonpharmacologic measures, including clear communication with the patient and reassurance, are essential.

Continuation of prior medications

For patients who had a previously effective psychiatric medication regimen, physicians will have to weigh the risks and benefits of continuing these agents in the critical care setting. This involves consideration of medication interactions, changes in metabolism (renal/hepatic impairment), cardiac impairment (QTc prolongation, arrhythmia), platelet/bleeding effects, routes of administration (see section on alternative routes of administration later in the chapter), and severity of prior symptoms.

In the case of discontinuation or reinitiation of psychiatric medications, it is ideal for a critical care physician to collaborate with psychiatrists. Given the unpredictable course during and following critical illness, we do not typically recommend continuation of long-acting injectable medications for critical care patients.

In some patients a reduction in dose or gradual taper rather than abrupt discontinuation is preferable. Certain medications (e.g., lamotrigine, clozapine), should be restarted gradually with careful monitoring. In any case, the decision to hold or resume psychiatric medications should be carefully reasoned through with consideration of risks of withdrawal, risks of decompensated psychiatric disorder, and risks of home psychiatric medications negatively affecting the patient's new critical condition.

Alternative routes of administration

Lack of enteral access can limit administration of psychiatric medications. Table 11.3 offers an overview, but not a complete list, of psychiatric medications with non-oral

TABLE 11.3.

Psychiatric medications with non-oral preparations

Medication name	Route	Notes
Aripiprazole	IM	Not the long-acting formulation
Asenapine	SL	Oral mucosal absorption
Chlorpromazine	IV	May cause hypotension
Diazepam	PR	Typically used for seizures
Diazepam	IV	Long half-life benzodiazepine
Diphenhydramine	IM	May be co-administered with antipsychotics to counteract extrapyramidal symptoms (EPS)
Fluphenazine	IM	
Haloperidol	IV	May require cardiac monitoring
Haloperidol	IM	
Lorazepam	IM	Short half-life benzodiazepine
Lorazepam	IV	
Loxapine	Inhaled powder	Risk of bronchospasm
Olanzapine	IM	Cannot co-administer with benzodiazepines
Olanzapine	IV	Cannot co-administer with benzodiazepines; not widely available
Selegiline	Transdermal	Caution with drug/food interactions
Valproate	IV	Risk of liver toxicity
Ziprasidone	IM	Monitor for QTc prolongation
Ziprasidone	IV	Monitor for QTc prolongation; not widely available

IM = intramuscular; IV = intravenous, SL = sublingual, PR = per rectum routes of administration (Kaminsky et al., 2015). As formularies and policies differ across hospital settings, we advise collaboration with pharmacists to determine availability.

Conclusion

Psychotropic medications in critically ill patients are safest and most effective when rationally directed. Agitation, poor participation in care, and anxiety can be manifestations of a variety of underlying conditions. Optimal management of psychopharmacologic treatment in the critical care setting is best achieved through collaboration with consultation liaison psychiatrists, pharmacists, rehabilitation therapists, and psychologists, as well as critical care nurses and physicians.

References

Awissi, D. K., Lebrun, G., Coursin, D. B., Riker, R. R., & Skrobik, Y. (2013). Alcohol withdrawal and delirium tremens in the critically ill: a systematic review and commentary. *Intensive Care Medicine, 39*(1), 16–30. doi:10.1007/s00134-012-2758-y

Baldwin, W. A., Rosenfeld, B. A., Breslow, M. J., Buchman, T. G., Deutschman, C. S., & Moore, R. D. (1993). Substance abuse-related admissions to adult intensive care. *Chest, 103*(1), 21–25. doi:10.1378/chest.103.1.21

Banzett, R. B., Adams, L., O'Donnell, C. R., Gilman, S. A., Lansing, R. W., & Schwartzstein, R. M. (2011). Using laboratory models to test treatment: Morphine reduces dyspnea and hypercapnic ventilatory response. *American Journal of Respiratory and Critical Care Medicine, 184*(8), 920–927. doi:10.1164/rccm.201101-0005OC

Başoğlu, M. (2017). Effective management of breathlessness: A review of potential human rights issues. European Respiratory Journal, *49*, 1602099.

Bielka, K., Kuchyn, I., & Glumcher, F. (2015). Addition of dexmedetomidine to benzodiazepines for patients with alcohol withdrawal syndrome in the intensive care unit: A randomized controlled study. *Annals of Intensive Care, 5*, 33. doi:10.1186/s13613-015-0075-7

Boyer, E. W., & Shannon, M. (2005). The serotonin syndrome—Reply. *New England Journal of Medicine, 352*(23), 2455–2456.

Clegg, A., & Young, J. B. (2011). Which medications to avoid in people at risk of delirium: A systematic review. *Age and Ageing, 40*(1), 23–29. doi:10.1093/ageing/afq140

Crispo, A. L., Daley, M. J., Pepin, J. L., Harford, P. H., & Brown, C. V. (2014). Comparison of clinical outcomes in nonintubated patients with severe alcohol withdrawal syndrome treated with continuous-infusion sedatives: Dexmedetomidine versus benzodiazepines. *Pharmacotherapy, 34*(9), 910–917. doi:10.1002/phar.1448

Daeppen, J. B., Gache, P., Landry, U., Sekera, E., Schweizer, V., Gloor, S., & Yersin, B. (2002). Symptom-triggered vs fixed-schedule doses of benzodiazepine for alcohol withdrawal: a randomized treatment trial. *Archives of Internal Medicine, 162*(10), 1117–1121. doi:10.1001/archinte.162.10.1117.

Darrouj, J., Puri, N., Prince, E., Lomonaco, A., Spevetz, A., & Gerber, D. R. (2008). Dexmedetomidine infusion as adjunctive therapy to benzodiazepines for acute alcohol withdrawal. *Annals of Pharmacotherapy, 42*(11), 1703–1705. doi:10.1345/aph.1K678

Das, S., Sah, D., Nandi, S., & Das, P. (2017). Opioid withdrawal presenting as delirium and role of buprenorphine: A case series. *Indian Journal of Psychological Medicine, 39*(5), 665–667. doi:10.4103/0253-7176.217027

de Wit, M., Jones, D. G., Sessler, C. N., Zilberberg, M. D., & Weaver, M. F. (2010). Alcohol-use disorders in the critically ill patient. *Chest, 138*(4), 994–1003. doi:10.1378/chest.09-1425

Dupuis, S., Brindamour, D., Karzon, S., Frenette, A. J., Charbonney, E., Perreault, M. M., . . . Williamson, D. R. (2019). A systematic review of interventions to facilitate extubation in patients difficult-to-wean due to delirium, agitation, or anxiety and a meta-analysis of the effect of dexmedetomidine. *Canadian Journal of Anesthesia, 66*(3), 318–327. doi:10.1007/s12630-018-01289-1

Eisendrath, S. J., & Shim, J. J. (2006). Management of psychiatric problems in critically ill patients. *American Journal of Medicine, 119*(1), 22–29. doi:10.1016/j.amjmed.2005.05.033

Ely, E. W., Inouye, S. K., Bernard, G. R., Gordon, S., Francis, J., May, L., . . . Dittus, R. (2001). Delirium in mechanically ventilated patients: Validity and reliability of the Confusion Assessment Method for the intensive care unit (CAM-ICU). *Journal of the American Medical Association, 286*(21), 2703–2710. doi:10.1001/jama.286.21.2703

Feast, A. R., White, N., Lord, K., Kupeli, N., Vickerstaff, V., & Sampson, E. L. (2018). Pain and delirium in people with dementia in the acute general hospital setting. *Age and Ageing, 47*(6), 841–846. doi:10.1093/ageing/afy112

Feeney, D. M., Gonzalez, A., & Law, W. A. (1982). Amphetamine, haloperidol, and experience interact to affect rate of recovery after motor cortex injury. *Science, 217*(4562), 855–857. doi:10.1126/science.7100929.

Fishbain, D. (2000). Evidence-based data on pain relief with antidepressants. *Annals of Medicine, 32*(5), 305–316. doi:10.3109/07853890008995932

Fraser, G. L., Prato, S., Riker, R. R., Berthiaume, D., & Wilkins, M. L. (2000). Frequency, severity, and treatment of agitation in young versus elderly patients in the ICU. *Pharmacotherapy, 20*(1), 75–82. doi:10.1592/phco.20.1.75.34663

Gacouin, A., Legay, F., Camus, C., Volatron, A. C., Barbarot, N., Donnio, P. Y., . . . Le Tulzo, Y. (2008). At-risk drinkers are at higher risk to acquire a bacterial infection during an intensive care unit stay than abstinent or moderate drinkers. *Critical Care Medicine, 36*(6), 1735–1741. doi:10.1097/CCM.0b013e318174dd75

Girard, T. D., Exline, M. C., Carson, S. S., Hough, C. L., Rock, P., Gong, M. N., . . . MindUSA Investigators. (2018). Haloperidol and ziprasidone for treatment of delirium in critical illness. *New England Journal of Medicine, 379*(26), 2506–2516. doi:10.1056/NEJMoa1808217

Hashemian, S. M., & Farhadi, T. (2020). A review on modafinil: The characteristics, function, and use in critical care. *Journal of Drug Assessment, 9*(1), 82–86. doi:10.1080/21556660.2020.1745209

Hashmi, A. M., Han, J. Y., & Demla, V. (2017). Intensive care and its discontents: Psychiatric illness in the critically ill. *Psychiatric Clinics of North America, 40*(3), 487–500. doi:10.1016/j.psc.2017.05.011

Inouye, S. K., Rushing, J. T., Foreman, M. D., Palmer, R. M., & Pompei, P. (1998). Does delirium contribute to poor hospital outcomes? A three-site epidemiologic study. *Journal of General Internal Medicine, 13*(4), 234–242. doi:10.1046/j.1525-1497.1998.00073.x

Jaber, S., Chanques, G., Altairac, C., Sebbane, M., Vergne, C., Perrigault, P. F., & Eledjam, J. J. (2005). A prospective study of agitation in a medical-surgical ICU: Incidence, risk factors, and outcomes. *Chest, 128*(4), 2749–2757. doi:10.1378/chest.128.4.2749

Johnson, M. T., Yamanaka, T. T., Fraidenburg, D. R., & Kane, S. P. (2013). Benzodiazepine misadventure in acute alcohol withdrawal: The transition from delirium tremens to ICU delirium. *Journal of Anesthesia, 27*(1), 135–136. doi:10.1007/s00540-012-1458-7

Kaminsky, B. M., Bostwick, J. R., & Guthrie, S. K. (2015). Alternate routes of administration of antidepressant and antipsychotic medications. *Annals of Pharmacotherapy, 49*(7), 808–817. doi:10.1177/1060028015583893

Keating, G. M. (2015). Dexmedetomidine: A review of its use for sedation in the intensive care setting. *Drugs, 75*(10), 1119–1130. doi:10.1007/s40265-015-0419-5

Kowalski, M., Udy, A. A., McRobbie, H. J., & Dooley, M. J. (2016). Nicotine replacement therapy for agitation and delirium management in the intensive care unit: A systematic review of the literature. *Journal of Intensive Care, 4*, 69. doi:10.1186/s40560-016-0184-x

Levenson, J. L. (2019). *The American Psychiatric Association Publishing textbook of psychosomatic medicine and consultation-liaison psychiatry* (3rd ed.). American Psychiatric Association Publishing.

Lewis, S. R., Pritchard, M. W., Schofield-Robinson, O. J., Alderson, P., & Smith, A. F. (2018). Melatonin for the promotion of sleep in adults in the intensive care unit. *Cochrane Database of Systematic Reviews, 5*, CD012455. doi:10.1002/14651858.CD012455.pub2

Lucidarme, O., Seguin, A., Daubin, C., Ramakers, M., Terzi, N., Beck, P., . . . du Cheyron, D. (2010). Nicotine withdrawal and agitation in ventilated critically ill patients. *Critical Care, 14*(2), R58. doi:10.1186/cc8954

Maldonado, J. R. (2017). Novel algorithms for the prophylaxis and management of alcohol withdrawal syndromes: Beyond benzodiazepines. *Critical Care Clinics, 33*(3), 559–599. doi:10.1016/j.ccc.2017.03.012

Neufeld, K. J., Yue, J., Robinson, T. N., Inouye, S. K., & Needham, D. M. (2016). Antipsychotic medication for prevention and treatment of delirium in hospitalized adults: A systematic review and meta-analysis. *Journal of the American Geriatric Society, 64*(4), 705–714. doi:10.1111/jgs.14076

Ng, K. T., Teoh, W. Y., & Khor, A. J. (2020). The effect of melatonin on delirium in hospitalised patients: A systematic review and meta-analyses with trial sequential analysis. *Journal of Clinical Anesthesia, 59*, 74–81. doi:10.1016/j.jclinane.2019.06.027

Patanwala, A. E., Martin, J. R., & Erstad, B. L. (2017). Ketamine for analgosedation in the intensive care unit: A systematic review. *Journal of Intensive Care Medicine, 32*(6), 387–395. doi:10.1177/0885066615620592

Powers, J., & Bennett, S. J. (1999). Measurement of dyspnea in patients treated with mechanical ventilation. *American Journal of Critical Care, 8*(4), 254–261.

Prince, E., Gerstenblith, T. A., Davydow, D., & Bienvenu, O. J. (2018). Psychiatric morbidity after critical illness. *Critical Care Clinics, 34*(4), 599–608. doi:10.1016/j.ccc.2018.06.006

Rayner, S. G., Weinert, C. R., Peng, H., Jepsen, S., Broccard, A. F., & Inst, S. (2012). Dexmedetomidine as adjunct treatment for severe alcohol withdrawal in the ICU. *Annals of Intensive Care, 2*, 12. doi:10.1186/2110-5820-2-12

Saitz, R., Mayo-Smith, M. F., Roberts, M. S., Redmond, H. A., Bernard, D. R., & Calkins, D. R. (1994). Individualized treatment for alcohol withdrawal. A randomized double-blind controlled trial. *JAMA, 272*(7), 519–523.

Salluh, J. I., Soares, M., Teles, J. M., Ceraso, D., Raimondi, N., Nava, V. S., . . . Delirium Epidemiology in Critical Care Study Group. (2010). Delirium Epidemiology in Critical Care (DECCA): An international study. *Critical Care*, *14*(6), R210. doi:10.1186/cc9333

Schmidt, M., Banzett, R. B., Raux, M., Morelot-Panzini, C., Dangers, L., Similowski, T., & Demoule, A. (2014). Unrecognized suffering in the ICU: Addressing dyspnea in mechanically ventilated patients. *Intensive Care Medicine*, *40*(1), 1–10. doi:10.1007/s00134-013-3117-3

Seitz, D. P., & Gill, S. S. (2009). Neuroleptic malignant syndrome complicating antipsychotic treatment of delirium or agitation in medical and surgical patients: Case reports and a review of the literature. *Psychosomatics*, *50*(1), 8–15. doi:10.1176/appi.psy.50.1.8

Siegel, M. D. (2003). Management of agitation in the intensive care unit. *Clinics in Chest Medicine*, *24*(4), 713–725. doi:10.1016/s0272-5231(03)00104-7

Simon, S. T., Higginson, I. J., Booth, S., Harding, R., Weingartner, V., & Bausewein, C. (2016). Benzodiazepines for the relief of breathlessness in advanced malignant and non-malignant diseases in adults. *Cochrane Database of Systematic Reviews*, *10*, CD007354. doi:10.1002/14651858. CD007354.pub3

Spies, C. D., Otter, H. E., Hüske, B., Sinha, P., Neumann, T., Rettig, J., Lenzenhuber, E., Kox, W. J., & Sellers, E. M. (2003). Alcohol withdrawal severity is decreased by symptom-orientated adjusted bolus therapy in the ICU. *Intensive Care Medicine*, *29*(12), 2230–2238. doi:10.1007/s00134-003-2033-3.

Subramaniam, K., Subramaniam, B., & Steinbrook, R. A. (2004). Ketamine as adjuvant analgesic to opioids: A quantitative and qualitative systematic review. *Anesthesia and Analgesia*, *99*(2), 482–495. doi:10.1213/01.Ane.0000118109.12855.07

Sullivan, J. T., Sykora, K., Schneiderman, J., Naranjo, C. A., & Sellers, E. M. (1989). Assessment of alcohol withdrawal: The revised clinical institute withdrawal assessment for alcohol scale (CIWA-Ar). *British Journal of Addiction*, *84*(11), 1353–1357. doi:10.1111/j.1360-0443.1989. tb00737.x.

Tse, L., Barr, A. M., Scarapicchia, V., & Vila-Rodriguez, F. (2015). Neuroleptic malignant syndrome: A review from a clinically oriented perspective. *Current Neuropharmacology*, *13*(3), 395–406. doi:10.2174/1570159X13999150424113345

Vilke, G. M., DeBard, M. L., Chan, T. C., Ho, J. D., Dawes, D. M., Hall, C., . . . Bozeman, W. P. (2012). Excited delirium syndrome (ExDS): Defining based on a review of the literature. *Journal of Emergency Medicine*, *43*(5), 897–905. doi:10.1016/j.jemermed.2011.02.017

Wolf, M. A., & Wertenschlag, N. (1989). Facteurs de risque et prévention des dyskinésies tardives [Risk factors and prevention of tardive dyskinesias]. *The Canadian Journal of Psychiatry*, *34*(3), 77–81. French. doi:10.1177/070674378903400303.

Worsham, C. M., Banzett, R. B., & Schwartzstein, R. M. (2020). Air hunger and psychological trauma in ventilated COVID-19 patients: An urgent problem. *Annals of the American Thoracic Society*, *17*(8), 926–927. doi:10.1513/AnnalsATS.202004-322VP

Yoshitaka, S., Egi, M., Morimatsu, H., Kanazawa, T., Toda, Y., & Morita, K. (2013). Perioperative plasma melatonin concentration in postoperative critically ill patients: Its association with delirium. *Journal of Critical Care*, *28*(3), 236–242. doi:10.1016/j.jcrc.2012.11.004

12 Family and Psychosocial Considerations in Critical Care

Macarena Gálvez Herrer, Judy E. Davidson, and Gabriel Heras La Calle

Humanization of intensive care units: working framework for studying families'
psychosocial needs Theoretical framework for the humanization of the health
care system

The term "humanize" means:

> to refer to humans in everything that is done to promote and protect health,
> cure diseases, guarantee an ambience that contributes to health and harmoni-
> ous lives at physical, emotional, social and spiritual levels. Speaking of human-
> ization claims the intrinsic dignity of all human beings and the rights stemming
> from this fact. And this makes it a need of vital importance and transcendence.
> (Bermejo, 2014, p. 79)

Since the 1990s, clinicians internationally have attempted to focus health care on
humanization (Delbanco et al., 2001; Harvey et al., 1993). Now, patients, families,
and professionals, along with health care managers and authorities, urge the redesign
of health care systems to focus on all of these stakeholders (Heras et al., 2020).[1] This
initiative is intended to overcome dehumanization in hospitals and health centers,

Macarena Gálvez Herrer, Judy E. Davidson, and Gabriel Heras La Calle, *Family and Psychosocial Considerations in Critical Care*
In: *Critical Care Psychology and Rehabilitation*. Edited by: Kirk J. Stucky and Jennifer E. Jutte, Oxford University Press. © Oxford
University Press 2022. DOI: 10.1093/oso/9780190077013.003.0012

with social interest at the core. Caring for all parties—including patients' families—is critical to building an excellent health service. To do so, we believe the particular problems of all parties must be heeded; responding to their needs and understanding that balance should be everyone's responsibility.

Therefore, and by way of summary, we believe that:

- Humanizing health care involves transforming hospitals and health care systems into friendlier and more pleasant people-centric places.
- Humanizing is paramount in the pursuit of service excellence as well as understanding and accepting that as professionals, we are fallible, we are vulnerable, and we have the right to express our emotions.
- Humanizing involves becoming more aware of ourselves: It is a significant personal commitment to improve our relationships and the environment starting with ourselves. We are humanized from the inside out.
- Humanizing means personalizing care, listening to what patients and family members need, not what we *think* they need, and converting it into a clinical process where humanized attitudes are essential. Health care systems will be humanized when they are at the service of all people and centered in dignity.
- Humanizing is not merely *gutmensch*, or do-gooding; it is the promotion of professional excellence with the necessary human, technological, behavioral, and economic resources (Heras et al., 2020).

HUMANIZATION OF INTENSIVE CARE UNITS

In February 2014, the international research project for the Humanization of Intensive Care Units (Project HU-CI) was founded (Heras et al., 2020). Through the creation of an interdisciplinary group consisting of patients; families; health care professionals (e.g., physicians, nurses, assistant nurses, psychologists); and professionals not in care (e.g., architects, computer technicians, designers, teachers), a collaborative research group was established based on the premises set out in the following sections, with the aim of redesigning health care service.

After listening to thousands of opinions collected via the blog for the Project HU-CI, which was co-created by all of the main stakeholders, eight lines of research for the project were defined (Heras et al., 2017) (Figure 12.1). The plan is to research and use networking to evaluate different areas and to implement the pertinent improvement actions. All these lines of research are interrelated,

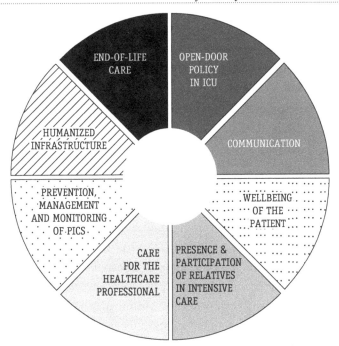

FIGURE 12.1. Lines of research for Project HU-CI.

so that working on one or the other affects the final outcome to improve patient and family care.

To date, this research group has published more than 100 articles in high-impact international journals (Davidson et al., 2020) about improvement projects for each line of research, with results that support the need for modifying practices toward a more people-centric management model. In November 2017, the first "Best Practices Guide for Humanizing Intensive Care Units" was published, later updated in May 2019 (Grupo de trabajo de certificación de Proyecto HU-CI, 2019).

In critical care settings, the emotional care of people has often been neglected, owing partly to a biomedical model that emphasizes saving lives and the extraordinary medical needs of critical care patients. As stated in a landmark World Health Organization (1948) document: "Health is a state of complete physical, mental and social wellbeing, and not merely the absence of disease or infirmity." To follow this directive, we need stronger efforts to humanize care and make managing patients' emotional responses to critical care a priority.

Going into greater depth in each of the lines of research, we have realized the need to work toward caring for both the patient and family as well as the care of intensive care unit (ICU) professionals, who are the true engines for humanization.

OPEN DOORS TO ICU AND FAMILIES' PARTICIPATION

No matter how empathetic we may be as health care providers, we will never replace the loving relationship between patients and their families. To capitalize on this relationship, it is advisable to make visiting hours flexible and involve family members in patient care (Davidson et al., 2017). The aim is to eliminate the concept of "visit" so that family roles can be restored—caring for the patient, being with the patient, and feeling like they are part of the recovery process. The family should be considered a partner in care delivery. In this model, policies on visiting hours, which are traditionally based more on restrictions than on flexibility and more about tradition than scientific evidence, are transformed into philosophies that welcome family presence and engagement. Holistically welcoming families, as well as their input and engagement at the bedside, allows practitioners to detect families' emotional and social needs, thus completing the care cycle and making care more comprehensive (Stress cause of nurse suicide, rules coroner, 2014).

During unique times such as a pandemic, visiting may be restricted due to necessary public health strategies for containing the infection. In these situations attention needs to be paid to tele-visits, phone calls, and other creative approaches to maintaining connection between patients and their family. Family needs should also be assessed regarding coping and spiritual and financial factors, and referrals should be made as indicated. Maintaining family integrity during the added crisis of a pandemic is essential. Isolation rooms can be constructed with windows for family viewing in the event that the risk of entering the room prohibits their physical presence (Papadimos et al., 2018). Furthermore, restriction of visits should be carried out on a purely scientific basis. For example, at the time of SARS-CoV-2 (COVID-19), specific training was needed for families about preventive measures such as hand hygiene and individual protection equipment. This was critical in facilitating specific interactions such as encouraging family members' presence when patients were dying.

COMMUNICATION

Improved communication is another key to humanization. Effective, interdisciplinary, and shared communication prevents mistakes and improves safety (Müller et al., 2018). To this end, we urge training clinicians in nontechnical skills such as active listening and empathic communication with a focus on cultivating compassion. Practical information is one of the main needs expressed by patients and families in the ICU (Alonso-Ovies et al., 2014). Clear communication with patients and families promotes a climate of trust and respect and facilitates mutually acceptable decision-making (Lewis et al., 2018). For patients who may not have decisional capacity, information is typically provided to family members. Difficulty in communicating can be a source of stress and frustration for patients, family members, and professionals (Trotta et al., 2020). Communication that is adapted to each patient's specific needs (through augmentative and alternative communication systems as needed) is essential for humanizing care and creating pathways that foster patients' and families' participation in critical processes (Garry et al., 2016).

PATIENT WELL-BEING

Many factors can contribute to suffering and discomfort for both patients and their family members (Alonso-Ovies & La Calle, 2016). Addressing all of these, in addition to management of pain, sedation, and acute delirium (Devlin et al., 2018), is essential for improving the level of comfort and the perceived experience of patients and families in the ICU. Psychological and emotional distress may be extremely high for patients and families in the ICU. Patients in the ICU often experience loneliness, isolation, fear, loss of identity, reduced privacy and dignity, a feeling of dependency on others, doubts due to poor communication, and incomprehension/confusion, among others (Cutler et al., 2013). Identifying, evaluating, and addressing these needs must be considered a core area of a quality health care service (Vincent et al., 2016).

CARING FOR THE CAREGIVER

It is difficult to administer good care if the caregivers themselves do not feel well treated and well cared for (Baggett et al., 2016; Dyrbye et al., 2017; Moss et al., 2016). The stress on ICU staff is intensified by continuous contact with suffering, death, fear, and uncertainty. In addition, long hours and shift work can take a toll on clinicians and their family life as well, further increasing cumulative stress. When this leads to burnout, downstream effects include decreased quality of care, reduced patient safety resulting from increased medical errors and missed care, and decreased ability to connect with patients and families. The consequences of clinician burden include low satisfaction of patients and their families but reach much further to decrease the ability to provide humanized care, resulting in an erosion of the health of the community (Moss et al., 2016).

PREVENTION, DETECTION, AND MONITORING OF POSTINTENSIVE CARE SYNDROME (PICS)

After leaving the ICU, 30% to 50% of patients continue to have physical problems (persistent pain, weakness acquired during hospitalization, malnutrition, bed sores, sleep alterations, need to use devices), neuropsychological problems (cognitive deficits, memory and/or attention loss, decreased mental processing speed), and emotional problems (anxiety, depression, or posttraumatic stress) (Needham et al., 2012). These medium- and long-term consequences affect the quality of life of patients and their families. Families can also be affected by feelings of worry and confusion that can lead them to neglect their own health (Johnson et al., 2019). The care team must be aware of these common issues in order to attend to the needs of the patient–family dyad.

HUMANIZED ARCHITECTURE AND INFRASTRUCTURE

Physical spaces should also accord with this change in management model and must be designed by and for the people who use them. There are recommendations focused on reducing stress and maximizing comfort by centering on architectural and structural improvements to ICUs. These changes consider suitable locations as well as adaptations to users and workflows in environmental conditions with adequate ambient light, comfortable temperature and humidity, controlled noise, and adapted furniture, if needed (Gómez-Tello & Ferrero, 2016; Hamilton, 2020). These modifications can have a positive influence on feelings and emotions by respecting privacy, dignity, and intimacy, with regard to not only patients and families but also professionals (Hamilton, 2020). It should also be noted that all hospital-grade furniture and surfaces, including areas for family and visitors, have to be made with materials and fabrics that can be easily cleaned and sanitized regularly. The importance of this intentional design is even more apparent during a pandemic.

END-OF-LIFE CARE

Staff in ICUs are often required to provide support during the dying process. Limiting life support, frequent in critically ill patients, must follow the guidelines and recommendations established by scientific communities (Estella et al., 2020). Shifting from goals of cure to palliative care should be done in an interdisciplinary fashion, with the aim of meeting the needs—physical, psychosocial, and spiritual— of both patients and family members (Cook & Rocker, 2014). There should be specific protocols and regular evaluation of the care provided to ensure that it is consonant with established goals. The complex decisions that are made about end-of-life care can lead to disagreements among health care professionals and between health care professionals and family members. Moral suffering of clinicians can occur (Mealer & Moss, 2016), particularly when care is perceived as nonbeneficial, poorly coordinated, or inappropriate (Kon et al., 2016). Left unresolved, these moral dilemmas may result in compassion fatigue (Sinclair et al., 2017) and contribute to professional burnout, with negative consequences for the patient, the family, professionals, and institutions (Costa & Moss, 2018). Ethics consults are indicated in cases where there may be conflict at end of life and to make sure the values of clinicians and the family are considered to minimize psychological trauma (Davidson et al., 2017).

Emotional challenges and risks for families in the ICU

The admission of a loved one into an ICU is an extremely stressful event for the family. It is a critical situation in which family caregivers often accompany patients with the aim of providing them with emotional support, upholding family integrity despite adversity, and providing logistic support. Having the patient admitted and receiving treatment can create a degree of family satisfaction as they will have ensured that the patient is where his or her condition dictates. However, in turn, there will often be emotional upset, with family members varying according to their level of psychological adjustment to the situation. According to Roy's adaptation model, the events during this period need to be managed to help families adapt. Maladaptation can result in poor family outcomes (Roy & Zhan, 2006).

FACILITATED SENSEMAKING

A specific strategy to support this adaptation is proposed in the facilitated sensemaking model (Figure 12.2). This midrange theory, derived from Roy's model, posits that we, as clinicians, can affect this period of adjustment to optimize the perceived experience and the family's ability to support the patient, participate in decision-making, and eventually maximize emotional adjustment after the ICU stay (Davidson & Zisook, 2017).

In facilitated sensemaking, we help the family members make sense of their role as caregivers while also making sense of what is happening with respect to the critical illness or injury. There are four key elements to facilitating family sensemaking: (1) role modeling caring behaviors; (2) welcoming family presence and engagement; (3) optimizing communication and information sharing; and (4) encouraging family-desired involvement in decision-making. It is theorized that when these actions are performed in a structured manner, families will experience less disturbance in those mental health, physical, and social consequences that have been known to occur following exposure to critical illness (Davidson & Zisook, 2017).

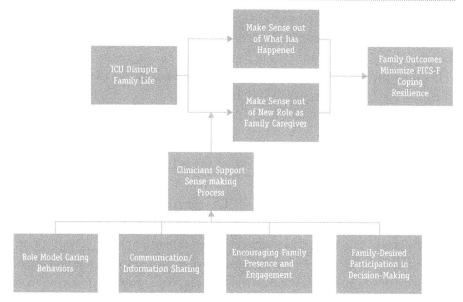

FIGURE 12.2. Facilitated sensemaking. Postintensive care syndrome—family (PICS-F) is a set of outcomes associated with family members' exposure to intensive care and can include mental health (e.g., posttraumatic stress, acute stress disorder, depression, anxiety), physical (e.g., sleep disorders, deterioration of previous health conditions), and social (e.g., financial and marital strain) consequences.

To illuminate the importance of family needs during admission, consider a study of the stress on family members of ICU patients. When asked to rate their stress level from 0 to 100 (where 100 is the highest level), families indicated an average of 63 (interquartile range 43–84), consistent with an overall stress level that is considered moderate to severe (Dziadzko et al., 2017). However, it has been demonstrated that with a structured approach to family care according to the facilitated sensemaking model (helping families make sense of the situation and their new role), making strategic efforts to communicate, connect, and engage, the anxiety of families can be minimized (Skoog et al., 2016).

FAMILY RESPONSE TO CRITICAL ILLNESS

There are key issues in ICU admission that should be assessed to minimize the development of emotional disorders and their chronicity. From the first days in the ICU, family members will cope with handling new life situations related to the pathology, their new role as caregiver, and the transformation of the family structure and roles. Coping with these new life situations can trigger various adverse reactions, including stress, fear, rage, and fatigue (Hopkins, 2018), all of which can increase due to factors like inability to communicate with patients due to their physical condition and the perception that their own medical or psychological needs are not adequately attended to by medical staff (Dziadzko et al., 2017). In turn, these emotional reactions in patients, family members, and caregivers will interact with problems related to sleep deficit, poor eating habits while in the hospital, and physical exhaustion (Haines et al., 2015; Netzer & Sullivan, 2014).

The entire physical and emotional process can wear down family members. Some authors speak of the caregiver burden (van Beusekom et al., 2015), which typically does not diminish after patients leave the ICU but can worsen and become chronic afterwards. Van Beusekom and colleagues (2015) suggest that family members who provide care often experience symptoms of anxiety, depression, and posttraumatic stress disorder (PTSD); 8% to 32% of caregivers are prescribed psychotropic medication (antidepressants, anxiolytics, and/or hypnotics). Emotional adjustment issues in family members can persist for months—even years—after patients leave the ICU and include symptoms like worry, sadness, concentration and sleep problems, and extreme nervousness (Alfheim et al., 2018). With regard to depressive symptoms, rates tend to be higher among caregivers when patients are first admitted to the ICU and caregivers must cope with the loss of health and the consequent living conditions, although symptoms tend to decrease over time (van Beusekom et al., 2015). However, there are circumstances that can slow and even prevent this decrease. For example, in a Canadian 1-year longitudinal study of family members of patients who had spent at least 7 days on mechanical ventilation, two differentiated groups were identified—those whose depressive symptoms decreased over time (84% of family members) and those for whom symptomatology persisted after 1 year (16%). Several factors were related to a greater number of symptoms among caregivers: younger age, lack of a social support system, and a lower sense of control over their own lives (Cameron et al., 2016). Moreover, issues related to patients are also key to caregivers' emotional states. For example, a Portuguese study revealed that persistent anxiety and depression in an ICU survivor were two factors that most influenced the caregiver burden, even above physical sequelae (Torres et al., 2017).

The emotional impact on family members who provide care, both during and after the ICU stay, has been termed postintensive care syndrome—family (PICS-F) (Needham et al., 2012). Its original definition included only symptoms related to mental health (anxiety, depression, PTSD, and complicated grief), yet psychosocial responses as well are now considered: physical problems (functional ability, sleep deprivation, fatigue), cognitive problems (reduced decision-making capacity), social tension problems (family, work, financial) factors that determine the person's quality of life (Davidson et al., 2017).

The way in which the family copes with critical illness is related to several factors, including each individual's relationship with the patient, whether or not the past family system was healthy, the way in which each family member copes with adversity, and the types of support offered between family members (Neves et al., 2018).

In a qualitative study about the experiences of the partners of ICU survivors (Nelderup & Samuelson, 2019), the people interviewed acknowledged the situation as "chaotic for the partner," with great support difficulties. In contrast, when partners perceive strong support, they view the experience as an opportunity to strengthen the relationship and their bond.

With regard to the patient's children, their age is a key factor in determining how they construct the experience. Depressive or anxious symptoms can occur as an understandable response to a stressful and unexpected situation such as ICU hospitalization and its aftermath. Studies of adolescents reveal this (Fergé et al., 2018), also finding that suitable identification and handling can prevent psychiatric sequelae from becoming chronic.

Interactions between family and medical professionals in critical illness

Given the impact of stress on the family, clinicians can be helpful in providing structured family care to optimize the family's adaptation to stress and mediate the stress reaction. Through facilitated sensemaking we can help families learn how to function in their new role as a caregiver while present in the ICU, and also prepare them for their future role as caregiver in the long term after the patient leaves this protected environment (Davidson & Zisook, 2017). Family members may need information repeated and provided in multiple formats, given that the ability to process information while under stress is limited. The more they are permitted to be omnipresent on the unit, the more they can absorb what is going on, which may lead to decreased fear of the unknown.

With family present, every action at the bedside can be transformed into meaning by talking through each motion and explaining in plain language the purpose of every treatment and piece of equipment and pertinent assessment findings. With time, the family members will become accustomed to the health care team's work and duties and understand our actions and the environment and in turn may exhibit fewer fear-based responses. Including family members in open dialogue is akin to teaching a junior colleague in a manner that is mutually beneficial. Families generally appreciate receiving information, even if they cannot fully integrate it at the time because of distraction due to stress. By speaking to them in caring tones, we believe they see that we care. The vision imprinted upon them of being surrounded by caring clinicians provides families with reassurance that everything is being done that can be done.

Even when there is uncertainty about the outcome, families appreciate when told that there is uncertainty. Silence, on the other hand, is often interpreted as secrecy. Further, in response to silence or limited information, families often generate their own reality of what is happening, which can be a dramatic distortion of the truth (Papadimos et al., 2018). Staff silence when rounding or providing direct care can also build a wall of separation, with the family watching and witnessing while being excluded. Worse yet is to round outside the patient room while the family is inside the room. This creates both a verbal and physical wall that family members can easily misinterpret as being unwelcome and not part of the team. Two-way communication, listening as well as speaking, creates a bond and a sense of "you matter." Establishing eye contact prior to any discussion and when entering and leaving signals that you have recognized their presence (Davidson, 2013; Strathdee et al., 2019; Young et al., 2017).

When family members are present in the room, they witness every staff action. This scrutiny can be unsettling for a provider because it can feel as though you are an actor on a stage. However, clinicians also have an opportunity here to model calm, strength, confidence, and caring. In a qualitative study of the factors that contribute to family members feeling cared for during hospitalization, provider characteristics including knowledge, confidence, and comportment (the way we carry ourselves) were identified as factors that translate into caring (Davidson, 2010). What we say is just as important as how we say it. It has been reported that families have fewer psychologically adverse outcomes months after discharge or death if physicians and staff were perceived as caring during the ICU stay (Siegel et al., 2008). Further, our actions constitute modeling of acceptable behaviors for the family. If you hold the hands of a comatose patient and talk to him as if he were listening, the family will, too. If you take a washcloth and wipe the patient's sweaty brow, so will the family once you are gone. If you invite them to help with positioning or reading to the patient, these simple acts of engagement will give them a purpose that may decrease their feelings of helplessness that arise when looking on uninvolved. In his seminal work, Weick (1995) informed us that we make sense of a crisis by what we do during that crisis, by looking back at our actions. By encouraging families to engage in meaningful tasks, the provider can help create important memories for them of what they did during the crisis. This engagement has the potential to help family members form a more constructive and positive adaptation to the situation (Davidson & Zisook, 2017).

A feasibility study of the provision of family support revealed that families appreciated the opportunity to help with communication, applying lip balm, providing range of motion, talking to the patient about daily events, engaging the awake patient cognitively in simple games, providing music, or praying (Davidson et al., 2009). Families also benefit from participating in a patient's early mobility program

(Rukstele & Gagnon, 2013) as well as monitoring of new-onset delirium (Krewulak et al., 2019).

There are many occasions for improving communication with family members: daily rounds, family meetings, when performing assessments, and while providing care. Though some worry that allowing family members to be present at rounds will detract from medical teaching and increase rounding time, studies have found that this is not true. Where rounds were lengthened by 1 to 3 minutes, time was actually saved later by avoiding unnecessary phone calls and other communication (Davidson, 2013). We have personally found that the more families are integrated into rounds, the fewer family meetings and ethics consultations are needed. Moreover, in humanizing the ICU, nothing is more important than cultivating the ability of trainees to speak in plain language so that families can understand what is happening. To do this while teaching requires skill and practice (Sullivan et al., 2016; Zaga et al., 2019). Families do appreciate the need for medical teaching, and witnessing the knowledge imparted during these times will build trust and respect, decreasing the likelihood of friction. The more the family is integrated into the system, the less alien they feel, and the less likelihood that conflict will occur (Strathdee et al., 2019).

For families who cannot be present, or for times when presence is restricted due to a pandemic, a structured approach to updating families is needed so that they are included in communication and can add information or ask questions. Scheduled teleconferences with family members will also help them receive the information they need and decrease the fear of the unknown.

Some worry that families will be oppositional, rude, and disruptive if allowed liberal presence in the ICU. In a humanized experience, it is important to evaluate negative behavior as a cry for help or expression of emotional angst. It is likely that more information and/or more reassurance are needed. Even-tempered people can lash out with anger when fearful or feeling threatened. When these behaviors arise, ask the family member in an open-ended manner whether they have enough information. Are their needs being met? What has frightened or threatened them? Have they had a negative experience in the past that has been triggered, opening up old wounds? Have they witnessed infighting among the team, causing them to lose faith? Have their voices been heard? Have we asked them about their concerns? An empathic approach will likely do more to solve the problem than confrontation or putting up walls that may escalate feelings of isolation. When all attempts at improving communication and de-escalation of the behaviors have failed, boundary setting will be necessary. However, question first whether more or better communication might help rather than responding immediately by adding rules or restrictions (Strathdee et al., 2019).

Family meetings are another form of communication. When there is any chance that the patient will die or there is conflict between providers or between providers and staff, a family meeting attended by the nurse, medical social worker, attending physician, and other disciplines involved in care can promote an atmosphere of open communication. We have found that fewer family meetings are needed when families receive daily information during rounds.

Psychological interventions with the family in the ICU

Throughout this chapter, we have set out essential issues that justify psychological interventions with the family in the ICU. Having shown why this is so, we now discuss when and how to implement helpful interventions.

KEY STAGES OF PSYCHOLOGICAL INTERVENTION

Pre-ICU

Due to the nature of acute issues and medical emergencies, the possibility of intervention in this phase is limited. However, this time is essential to prepare the family emotionally for the ICU admission process and collaboration with the interdisciplinary team for information and communication actions. When family members are notified of the need to admit their loved one to the ICU, applying an interdisciplinary protocol for the reception of family members is recommended. Also of value is a written guide describing the main characteristics of the ICU, the most common situations that could arise, and the resources they have available during the patient's stay (Velasco et al., 2017). Unfortunately, no evidence-based best practice for preparing a family for ICU admission exists; this remains an opportunity for improvement for most critical care settings.

In the ICU

Here, the main idea is to provide emotional support during the family members' adaptation process, facilitating the emotional and cognitive processing of everything they experience, empowerment via collaboration in care and feeling of some sense of control, acting on the emotional factors that make all these processes difficult, and maximizing healthy responses to them.

A key intervention is to begin preparation for discharge when patients are to be moved to general care rooms. Family members' emotional ambivalence at this time can be extremely high, although they may experience satisfaction and relief that the most immediate danger is over. There may also be the uncertainty and feeling of loss after transitioning from the highly controlled environment of the ICU. Fear of the unknown and the feeling of insecurity then create a state of alertness and anxiety that can cause the transfer to be experienced as something negative (Hughes et al., 2005). The emotional state at this time has been related to difficulty understanding and remembering verbal information (Paul et al., 2004). Therefore, this information should be disseminated by different means (verbal and written), but staff must also work to actively listen, have empathy, and detect the family members' emotional state to help them with emotional regulation and understanding of the message.

Post-ICU

The transition out of the ICU is a difficult one, and best practices for helping the family to adjust have not been identified. The decreased staffing and physiologic monitoring can create uneasiness, despite the fact that transfer generally means improvement in the patient's condition (de Grood et al., 2018; Mitchell et al., 2016). Post-ICU family intervention is essential to provide ongoing support and preparation for reincorporation into daily life (personal and professional roles, family dynamics, etc.), progressive acquisition of autonomy, coexistence and rehabilitation from possible sequelae after supporting a family member in the ICU, as well as early detection and intervention for PICS-F. Support groups are an excellent means of early detection of these needs and their intervention (Haines et al., 2018, 2019).

EVALUATING IN ORDER TO INTERVENE

Without evaluation, it would be impossible to determine a proper diagnosis, which is necessary for subsequent and effective family intervention. However, when family psychological needs are detected, any member of the team could refer for a psychological evaluation. An optimal ICU team would include psychology professionals. There are many tools that can be used to this end; we will focus on the interview with these objectives:

- Definition of the problem and coping strategies the family group can apply in their situation
- Evaluation of availability of various resources, explaining the care provided and how it will affect the primary caregiver
- Whether or not there is an emotional support network or support group

- Detection of emotional responses in the caregiver, including signs of anxiety and depression such as low mood, difficulty paying attention, sobbing, irritability, and agitation
- Existence of recent losses (deaths, significant life changes) and coping with the evolution of the current illness
- Existence of prior mental health issues
- System of values, beliefs, dynamics, and relationships within the family
- Difficulty sleeping, eating, or conducting daily activities
- Difficulty with focus and making decisions.

Another psychological methodology used with families involves genograms and ecograms (Belio & Vivar, 2012). Constructing a genogram is a method of understanding family dynamics through attachment theory. Acquiring the information for a genogram can provide an in-depth understanding of the family that can aid in understanding their response to exposure to critical illness, strengthen the bond between the family and the clinician, and guide suggestions for management of emotions during this stressful time (DeMaria et al., 2017). These strategies may be more welcomed or effective in certain countries or cultures. However, it may be difficult to employ such techniques if the critical care team does not have a psychologist or clinician who is comfortable in this role.

LINES OF ACTION

We believe that the support methods set out next are particularly relevant in critical care settings.

Psychological support

Depending on how emotions are mobilized in the care setting, attitudes of flexibility and resilience will be facilitated or not as well as adaptive and well-being processes. To be effective, a relationship must be created in which the person feels accepted and respected and not judged. This therapeutic bond will make it possible to seek objectives, including improved self-awareness, emotional identification and expression, enhancing sense of control over their decisions and behaviors, balancing emotional demands and resources, resolving situational crises, acquiring skills and competencies in the new relationship of caring for their loved ones (which will also benefit the patient), preventing the caregiver from becoming overburdened, facilitating self-care behaviors, and providing a setting for listening and respite.

"Schools" for families

Schools are also called support groups or family education sessions, depending on the international context. The psychoeducational model is widely implemented in the field of health care, though its use in ICUs is still uncommon and represents a challenge for present and future research. Schools for families provide intervention through education, advice, and instruction; they contribute to decreasing stress in family members and enhancing caregiving competencies and skills. In ICUs, the priority is to convey information (about treatments, technology, states of the critical disease, tips for taking part in care) for interacting with the critically ill patient and guidelines on how the unit operates. These interventions increase family caregivers' perceived control and provide coping strategies and emotional support. The organization of these educational interventions will depend on each hospital and the needs and resources available to provide them, although a few general recommendations for setting them up are as follows:

- Assign scheduling and facilitation to ICU nurses.
- Establish concrete and measurable objectives.
- Introduce the health care team and family members who are participating in the first session.
- Recommend a preliminary evaluation to detect needs (which can be revised in post-intervention evaluations).
- Create a satisfaction scale for this support method to permit suggestions for improvement (Haines et al., 2018).

ICU diaries

ICU diaries are beneficial for families as well as patients. Families' participation in writing them leads to establishing a narrative of the disease process from their viewpoint as caregivers and is also a vehicle for emotional expression. Some studies have identified a correlation between the use of ICU diaries and reduced effects of PTSD in the family (Garrouste-Orgeas et al., 2014; Jones et al., 2012). When family caregivers share their diary entries with their loved ones, besides letting them give voice to their experiences, it also strengthens the relationship between them. Even when patients do not want to share these experiences, the diary opens up an opportunity to speak of the illness process. However, in this case, family members will need support and guidance on how to accept and cope with this experience (Nielsen et al., 2019). When patients do not survive, the diary may help in the rational and emotional processing of the death and create a bond of union and commitment between caregivers and health care professionals (Johansson et al., 2018). Thus, the care team can do the following:

- Introduce the idea of keeping a diary.
- Provide support for family members while they are writing in the diary.
- Offer suggestions on what may be of interest to include (both caregivers and patients).
- Give advice on how to share what they have written with loved ones (not simply giving it to patients to read).
- Prepare them for patients' possible rejection or difficulty in integrating what is written in the diary.

The reader is referred to Chapter 5 for additional information about ICU diaries.

Post-ICU support groups

Initiatives like the Ítaca Group in Spain and Latin America (Grupo Ítaca, 2019) and Thrive by the Society of Critical Care Medicine (Thrive, 2020) in English-speaking countries are pioneers in providing group support for patients and family after ICU stays. Thrive has conducted a descriptive study of the different intervention models of peer support groups for PICS (McPeake et al., 2019). This work includes 17 teams in the United States, Great Britain, and Australia. Their conclusions produced five action models describing the general lines of action being carried out. Most are focused on former ICU patients, although some also include simultaneously working with the family (as in the community model, post-ICU follow-up queries, and groups conducted during stays in the ICU). The study found that the main barriers to implementing these support models were difficulty recruiting participants; the training of staff facilitators for the groups; sustainability and funding; risk management; and evaluation of their efficacy and success.

In other models, such as that of the Fuenlabrada University Hospital in Madrid, Spain (a member of the Ítaca Group), there are different groups for family members and for former patients, thus attending to each group's particular needs. For families, these needs include facilitating continuity for post-ICU care; handling post-ICU cognitive and emotional problems; early detection of symptomatology related to emotional problems and PICS-F; developing coping skills in family and personal life after the ICU experience; handling difficult situations related to the burden of care and/or emotional changes in their family member after the ICU stay; and caring for intrafamily bonds and communication (Grupo Ítaca, 2019).

In this model, the selection of caregivers to participate in the support groups is done at the post-ICU follow-up consultations by the intensive care physicians. Participants are referred to psychologists, who conduct interviews and evaluations (which are repeated when they leave the group). Finally, they join open support groups in which there are expert family members and psychologists acting as facilitators who also provide support and psychoeducation as necessary.

Support groups have proven efficacy in decreasing psychological morbidity, in working out the experiences, and in adjusting in a healthy fashion to the new situations of stress after ICU stays. However, research and intervention models are still needed with strict action guidelines so we can better comprehend their effects and continue improving how they help families at these vital times (Haines et al., 2018).

Conclusion

The experience of having a loved one in the ICU can be distressing. The focus of this chapter has been on humanizing the health care system in a manner that reduces the odds of adverse outcomes for family caregivers and promotes positive outcomes, when possible. We have reviewed several significant needs of family members, including the need for proximity, reassurance, information, and attention to their emotional health. As health care professionals working from an interdisciplinary focus, we are obligated to care for and strengthen positive emotions that are also present. Person-focused care is a humanized perspective that elevates the importance of the family experience and offers suitable lines of action in difficult and emotionally taxing situations.

Note

1. The lead (MGH) and last (GHLC) author of this chapter are members of the modern Humanizing the ICU movement created by GHLC in Spain.

References

Alfheim, H. B., Rosseland, L. A., Hofsø, K., Småstuen, M. C., & Rustøen, T. (2018). Multiple symptoms in family caregivers of intensive care unit patients. *Journal of Pain and Symptom Management*, 55(2), 387–394.

Alonso-Ovies, A., Álvarez, J., Velayos, C., García, M., & Luengo, M. (2014). Expectativas de los familiares de pacientes críticos respecto a la información médica. Estudio de investigación cualitativa. *Revista de Calidad Asistencial*, 29(6), 325–333.

Alonso-Ovies, Á., & La Calle, G. H. (2016). ICU: A branch of hell? *Intensive Care Medicine,* *42*(4), 591.

Baggett, M., Giambattista, L., Lobbestael, L., Pfeiffer, J., Madani, C., Modir, R., . . . Davidson, J. E. (2016). Exploring the human emotion of feeling cared for in the workplace. *Journal of Nursing Management, 24*(6), 816–824. doi:10.1111/jonm.12388

Belio, M. P., & Vivar, C. (2012). Necesidades de la familia en las unidades de cuidados intensivos. Revisión de la literatura. *Enfermería Intensiva, 23*(2), 51–67.

Bermejo, J. C. (2014). *Humanizar la asistencia sanitaria.* Desclée de Brouwer.

Cameron, J. I., Chu, L. M., Matte, A., Tomlinson, G., Chan, L., Thomas, C., . . . Levasseur, M. (2016). One-year outcomes in caregivers of critically ill patients. *New England Journal of Medicine, 374*(19), 1831–1841.

Cook, D., & Rocker, G. (2014). Dying with dignity in the intensive care unit. *New England Journal of Medicine, 370*(26), 2506–2514.

Costa, D. K., & Moss, M. (2018). The cost of caring: Emotion, burnout, and psychological distress in critical care clinicians. *Annals of the American Thoracic Society, 15*(7), 787–790.

Cutler, L. R., Hayter, M., & Ryan, T. (2013). A critical review and synthesis of qualitative research on patient experiences of critical illness. *Intensive and Critical Care Nursing, 29*(3), 147–157.

Davidson, J. E. (2010). Facilitated sensemaking: A strategy and new middle-range theory to support families of intensive care unit patients. *Critical Care Nurse, 30*(6), 28–39. doi:10.4037/ccn2010410

Davidson, J. E. (2013). Family presence on rounds in neonatal, pediatric, and adult intensive care units. *Annals of the American Thoracic Society, 10*(2), 152–156. doi:10.1513/AnnalsATS.201301-006PS

Davidson, J. E., Aslakson, R. A., Long, A. C., Puntillo, K. A., Kross, E. K., Hart, J., . . . Nunnally, M. E. (2017). Guidelines for family-centered care in the neonatal, pediatric, and adult ICU. *Critical Care Medicine, 45*(1), 103–128.

Davidson, J. E., Daly, B. J., Agan, D., Brady, N. R., & Higgins, P. A. (2009). Facilitated sensemaking: Testing of a mid-range theory of family support. *Communicating Nursing Research, 42,* 353.

Davidson, J. E., Hudson, C. A., Bueno, J. M. V., & Heras, G. (2020). Patient and family experience in the ICU. *Critical Care Nursing Clinics of North America, 32*(2), i.

Davidson, J., McDuffie, M., & Campbell, K. (2017). Family-centered care. In S. Goldsworthy, R. Kleinpell, & G. E. Speed (Eds.), *International best practices in critical care* (pp. 311–368). World Federation of Critical Care Nursing.

Davidson, J. E., & Zisook, S. (2017). Implementing family-centered care through facilitated sensemaking. *AACN Advanced Critical Care, 28*(2), 200–209.

de Grood, C., Leigh, J. P., Bagshaw, S. M., Dodek, P. M., Fowler, R. A., Forster, A. J., . . . Stelfox, H. T. (2018). Patient, family and provider experiences with transfers from intensive care unit to hospital ward: A multicentre qualitative study. *Canadian Medical Association Journal, 190*(22), E669–E676.

Delbanco, T., Berwick, D. M., Boufford, J. I., Edgman-Levitan, S., Ollenschlager, G., Plamping, D., & Rockefeller, R. G. (2001). Healthcare in a land called PeoplePower: Nothing about me without me. *Health Expectations, 4*(3), 144–150.

DeMaria, R., Weeks, G. R., & Twist, M. L. (2017). Focused genograms: Intergenerational assessment of individuals, couples, and families. Taylor & Francis.

Devlin, J. W., Skrobik, Y., Gélinas, C., Needham, D. M., Slooter, A. J., Pandharipande, P. P., . . . Rochwerg, B. (2018). Clinical practice guidelines for the prevention and management of pain, agitation/sedation, delirium, immobility, and sleep disruption in adult patients in the ICU. *Critical Care Medicine, 46*(9), e825–e873.

Dyrbye, L. N., Shanafelt, T. D., Sinsky, C. A., Cipriano, P., Bhatt, J., Ommaya, A., West, C. P., & Meyers, D. (2017). Burnout among health care professionals: A call to explore and address this underrecognized threat to safe, high-quality care. *NAM Perspectives.* Discussion Paper, National Academy of Medicine, Washington, DC. https://doi.org/10.31478/201707b

Dziadzko, V., Dziadzko, M. A., Johnson, M. M., Gajic, O., & Karnatovskaia, L. V. (2017). Acute psychological trauma in the critically ill: Patient and family perspectives. *General Hospital Psychiatry, 47*, 68–74.

Estella, Á., Saralegui, I., Sanchiz, O. R., Hernández-Tejedor, A., Camps, V. L., Martín, M., . . . Monzón, J. (2020). Update and recommendations in decision making referred to limitation of advanced life support treatment. *Medicina Intensiva (English Edition), 44*(2), 101–112.

Fergé, J.-L., Le Terrier, C., Banydeen, R., Kentish-Barnes, N., Derancourt, C., Jehel, L., . . . Mehdaoui, H. (2018). Prevalence of anxiety and depression symptomatology in adolescents faced with the hospitalization of a loved one in the ICU. *Critical Care Medicine, 46*(4), e330–e333.

Garrouste-Orgeas, M., Perier, A., Mouricou, P., Gregoire, C., Bruel, C., Brochon, S., . . . Misset, B. (2014). Writing in and reading ICU diaries: Qualitative study of families' experience in the ICU. *PLoS One, 9*(10), e110146. doi:10.1371/journal.pone.0110146

Garry, J., Casey, K., Cole, T. K., Regensburg, A., McElroy, C., Schneider, E., . . . Chi, A. (2016). A pilot study of eye-tracking devices in intensive care. *Surgery, 159*(3), 938–944.

Gómez-Tello, V., & Ferrero, M. (2016). Humanised infrastructure in the ICU: A challenge within our reach. *Enfermeria Intensiva, 27*(4), 135–137.

Grupo de trabajo de certificación de Proyecto HU-CI. (2019). *Manual de buenas prácticas de humanización en Unidades de Cuidados Intensivos.* https://humanizandoloscuidadosintensivos.com/es/buenas-practicas/

Grupo Ítaca. (2019). https://proyectohuci.com/es/nace-el-grupo-itaca/

Haines, K. J., Beesley, S. J., Hopkins, R. O., McPeake, J., Quasim, T., Ritchie, K., & Iwashyna, T. J. (2018). Peer support in critical care: A systematic review. *Critical Care Medicine, 46*(9), 1522–1531. doi:10.1097/ccm.0000000000003293

Haines, K. J., Denehy, L., Skinner, E. H., Warrillow, S., & Berney, S. (2015). Psychosocial outcomes in informal caregivers of the critically ill: A systematic review. *Critical Care Medicine, 43*(5), 1112–1120. doi:10.1097/ccm.0000000000000865

Haines, K. J., Sevin, C. M., Hibbert, E., Boehm, L. M., Aparanji, K., Bakhru, R. N., . . . Drumright, K. (2019). Key mechanisms by which post-ICU activities can improve in-ICU care: Results of the international THRIVE collaboratives. *Intensive Care Medicine, 45*(7), 939–947.

Hamilton, D. K. (2020). Design for critical care. In A. Sethumadhavan & F. Sasangohar (Eds.), *Design for health* (pp. 129–145). Elsevier.

Harvey, M. A., Ninos, N. P., Adler, D. C., Goodnough-Hanneman, S. K., Kaye, W. E., & Nikas, D. L. (1993). Results of the consensus conference on fostering more humane critical care: Creating a healing environment. *AACN Advanced Critical Care, 4*(3), 484–507.

Heras La Calle, G. (2018). My Favorite Slide: The ICU and the Human Care Bundle. NEJM Catalyst. April 5.

Heras La Calle, G., Oviés, Á. A., & Tello, V. G. (2017). A plan for improving the humanization of intensive care units. *Intensive Care Medicine, 43*(4), 547–549. doi: 10.1007/s00134-017-4705-4.

Heras, G., Zimmerman, J., & Hidalgo, J. (2020). Humanizing critical care. In J. Hidalgo, J. Pérez-Fernández, & G. Rodríguez-Vega (Eds.), *Critical care administration: A comprehensive clinical guide* (pp. 189–197). Springer.

Hopkins, R. O. (2018). Emotional processing/psychological morbidity in the ICU. In G. Netzer (Ed.), *Families in the intensive care unit: A guide to understanding, engaging, and supporting at the bedside* (pp. 31–47). Springer.

Hughes, F., Bryan, K., & Robbins, I. (2005). Relatives' experiences of critical care. *Nursing in Critical Care, 10*(1), 23–30.

Johansson, M., Wåhlin, I., Magnusson, L., Runeson, I., & Hanson, E. (2018). Family members' experiences with intensive care unit diaries when the patient does not survive. *Scandinavian Journal of Caring Sciences, 32*(1), 233–240.

Johnson, C. C., Suchyta, M. R., Darowski, E. S., Collar, E. M., Kiehl, A. L., Van, J., . . . Hopkins, R. O. (2019). Psychological sequelae in family caregivers of critically ill intensive care unit patients. A systematic review. *Annals of the American Thoracic Society, 16*(7), 894–909.

Jones, C., Backman, C., & Griffiths, R. D. (2012). Intensive care diaries and relatives' symptoms of posttraumatic stress disorder after critical illness: A pilot study. *American Journal of Critical Care, 21*(3), 172–176. doi:10.4037/ajcc2012569

Kon, A. A., Shepard, E. K., Sederstrom, N. O., Swoboda, S. M., Marshall, M. F., Birriel, B., & Rincon, F. (2016). Defining futile and potentially inappropriate interventions: A policy statement from the Society of Critical Care Medicine Ethics Committee. *Critical Care Medicine, 44*(9), 1769–1774. doi:10.1097/ccm.0000000000001965

Krewulak, K. D., Sept, B. G., Stelfox, H. T., Ely, E., Davidson, J. E., Ismail, Z., & Fiest, K. M. (2019). Feasibility and acceptability of family administration of delirium detection tools in the intensive care unit: A patient-oriented pilot study. *Canadian Medical Association Journal Open, 7*(2), E294.

La Calle, G. H. (2018). My favorite slide: The ICU and the human care bundle. *New England Journal of Medicine Catalyst, 4*(2). https://catalyst.nejm.org/doi/full/10.1056/CAT.18.0215

La Calle, G. H., Oviés, Á. A., & Tello, V. G. (2017). A plan for improving the humanisation of intensive care units. *Intensive Care Medicine, 43*(4), 547–549.

Lewis, S. R., Pritchard, M. W., Schofield-Robinson, O. J., Evans, D. J., Alderson, P., & Smith, A. F. (2018). Information or education interventions for adult intensive care unit (ICU) patients and their carers. *Cochrane Database of Systematic Reviews, 10*(*10*), CD012471.

McPeake, J., Hirshberg, E. L., Christie, L. M., Drumright, K., Haines, K., Hough, C. L., . . . Bakhru, R. (2019). Models of peer support to remediate post-intensive care syndrome: A report developed by the Society of Critical Care Medicine Thrive International Peer Support Collaborative. *Critical Care Medicine, 47*(1), e21–e27.

Mealer, M., & Moss, M. (2016). Moral distress in ICU nurses. *Intensive Care Medicine, 42*(10), 1615–1617.

Mitchell, M. L., Coyer, F., Kean, S., Stone, R., Murfield, J., & Dwan, T. (2016). Patient, family-centred care interventions within the adult ICU setting: An integrative review. *Australian Critical Care, 29*(4), 179–193.

Moss, M., Good, V. S., Gozal, D., Kleinpell, R., & Sessler, C. N. (2016). An official critical care societies collaborative statement: Burnout syndrome in critical care health care professionals: A call for action. *American Journal of Critical Care, 25*(4), 368–376.

Müller, M., Jürgens, J., Redaèlli, M., Klingberg, K., Hautz, W. E., & Stock, S. (2018). Impact of the communication and patient hand-off tool SBAR on patient safety: A systematic review. *BMJ Open, 8*(8), e022202. doi:10.1136/bmjopen-2018-022202

Needham, D. M., Davidson, J., Cohen, H., Hopkins, R. O., Weinert, C., Wunsch, H., . . . Harvey, M. A. (2012). Improving long-term outcomes after discharge from intensive care unit: Report from a stakeholders' conference. *Critical Care Medicine, 40*, 502–509. doi:10.1097/CCM.0b013e318232da75

Nelderup, M., & Samuelson, K. (2019). Experiences of partners of intensive care survivors and their need for support after intensive care. *Nursing in Critical Care, 25*(4), 245–252.

Netzer, G., & Sullivan, D. R. (2014). Recognizing, naming, and measuring a family intensive care unit syndrome. *Annals of the American Thoracic Society, 11*(3), 435–441. doi:10.1513/AnnalsATS.201309-308OT

Neves, L., Gondim, A. A., Soares, S. C. M. R., Coelho, D. P., & Pinheiro, J. A. M. (2018). O impacto do processo de hospitalização para o acompanhante familiar do paciente crítico crônico internado em Unidade de Terapia Semi-Intensiva. *Escola Anna Nery, 22*(2).

Nielsen, A. H., Egerod, I., Hansen, T. B., & Angel, S. (2019). Intensive care unit diaries: Developing a shared story strengthens relationships between critically ill patients and their relatives: A hermeneutic-phenomenological study. *International Journal of Nursing Studies, 92*, 90–96.

Papadimos, T. J., Marcolini, E. G., Hadian, M., Hardart, G. E., Ward, N., Levy, M. M., . . . Davidson, J. E. (2018). Ethics of outbreaks position statement. Part 2: Family-centered care. *Critical Care Medicine, 46*(11), 1856–1860.

Paul, F., Hendry, C., & Cabrelli, L. (2004). Meeting patient and relatives' information needs upon transfer from an intensive care unit: The development and evaluation of an information booklet. *Journal of Clinical Nursing, 13*(3), 396–405.

Roy, C., & Zhan, L. (2006). Sister Callista Roy's adaptation model and its applications. In M. E. Parker (Ed.), *Nursing theories & nursing practice* (pp. 268–280). F. A. Davis.

Rukstele, C. D., & Gagnon, M. M. (2013). Making strides in preventing ICU-acquired weakness: Involving family in early progressive mobility. *Critical Care Nursing Quarterly, 36*(1), 141–147.

Siegel, M. D., Hayes, E., Vanderwerker, L. C., Loseth, D. B., & Prigerson, H. G. (2008). Psychiatric illness in the next of kin of patients who die in the intensive care unit. *Critical Care Medicine, 36*(6), 1722–1728.

Sinclair, S., Raffin-Bouchal, S., Venturato, L., Mijovic-Kondejewski, J., & Smith-MacDonald, L. (2017). Compassion fatigue: A meta-narrative review of the healthcare literature. *International Journal of Nursing Studies, 69*, 9–24.

Skoog, M., Milner, K. A., Gatti-Petito, J., & Dintyala, K. (2016). The impact of family engagement on anxiety levels in a cardiothoracic intensive care unit. *Critical Care Nurse, 36*(2), 84–89. doi:10.4037/ccn2016246

Strathdee, S. A., Hellyar M., Montesa C., & Davidson, J. E. (2019). The power of family engagement in rounds: An exemplar with global outcomes. *Critical Care Nurse, 39*(5), 14–20.

Stress cause of nurse suicide, rules coroner. (2014). *Nursing Times, 110*(48), 5.

Sullivan, A. M., Rock, L. K., Gadmer, N. M., Norwich, D. E., & Schwartzstein, R. M. (2016). The impact of resident training on communication with families in the intensive care unit. Resident and family outcomes. *Annals of the American Thoracic Society, 13*(4), 512–521.

Thrive. (2020). https://www.sccm.org/Research/Quality/THRIVE

Torres, J., Carvalho, D., Molinos, E., Vales, C., Ferreira, A., Dias, C., . . . Gomes, E. (2017). The impact of the patient post-intensive care syndrome components upon caregiver burden. *Medicina Intensiva, 41*(8), 454–460.

Trotta, R. L., Hermann, R. M., Polomano, R. C., & Happ, M. B. (2020). Improving nonvocal critical care patients' ease of communication using a modified SPEACS-2 Program. *Journal for Healthcare Quality, 42*(1), e1–e9.

van Beusekom, I., Bakhshi-Raiez, F., de Keizer, N. F., Dongelmans, D. A., & van der Schaaf, M. (2015). Reported burden on informal caregivers of ICU survivors: A literature review. *Critical Care, 20*(1), 16.

Velasco, T., Velasco, J. M., Ortega, A., Gómez, D., Lozano, F., & del Barrio, M. (2017). Recomendaciones sobre acogida de familiares en Unidades de Cuidados Intensivos. http://seeiuc.org/wp-content/uploads/2017/10/RECOMENDACIONES-FAMILIAS.pdf

Vincent, J.-L., Shehabi, Y., Walsh, T. S., Pandharipande, P. P., Ball, J. A., Spronk, P., . . . Funk, G.-C. (2016). Comfort and patient-centred care without excessive sedation: The eCASH concept. *Intensive Care Medicine, 42*(6), 962–971.

Weick, K. E. (1995). *Sensemaking in organizations* (Vol. 3). Sage.

World Health Organization. (1948). Preamble to the Constitution of the World Health Organization as adopted by the International Health Conference, New York, 19–22 June, 1946; signed on 22 July 1946 by the representatives of 61 States (Official Records of the World Health Organization, no. 2, p. 100) and entered into force on 7 April 1948. http://www.who.int/governance/eb/who_constitution_en. pdf

Young, A. J., Stephens, E., & Goldsmith, J. V. (2017). Family caregiver communication in the ICU: Toward a relational view of health literacy. *Journal of Family Communication, 17*(2), 137–152.

Zaga, C. J., Berney, S., & Vogel, A. P. (2019). The feasibility, utility, and safety of communication interventions with mechanically ventilated intensive care unit patients: A systematic review. *American Journal of Speech-Language Pathology, 28*(3), 1335–1355.

13 Psychological Treatment Models for Survivors of Critical Illness

AN EARLY OVERVIEW AND REFLECTION ON FUTURE DIRECTIONS

Caroline L. Lassen-Greene, James C. Jackson, and Carla M. Sevin

Introduction

Since the late 1990s, researchers and clinicians have been increasingly aware of a phenomenon now known as postintensive care syndrome (PICS; Hopkins et al., 1999), though the label is less than a decade old (Needham et al., 2012). This condition was first identified in survivors of acute respiratory distress syndrome (ARDS) (Hopkins et al., 1999) but later understood to affect survivors of critical illnesses more broadly. It is marked by the presence of significant deficits—either new or worsened—in one or more of several domains: cognitive, psychological, physical, and functional (Needham et al., 2012). Although a detailed treatment of the origins and pathophysiology of problems after critical illness is beyond the scope of this chapter, the existence of clinically meaningful cognitive difficulties in attention, executive functioning, and memory and—in the psychological arena—depression and posttraumatic stress disorder (PTSD) has been well documented and often copiously described (Davydow et al., 2009; Iwashyna et al., 2010; Jackson et al., 2003; Jackson, Pandharipande et al., 2014; Nickel et al., 2004; Pandharipande et al., 2013).

Caroline L. Lassen-Greene, James C. Jackson, and Carla M. Sevin, *Psychological Treatment Models for Survivors of Critical Illness* In: *Critical Care Psychology and Rehabilitation*. Edited by: Kirk J. Stucky and Jennifer E. Jutte, Oxford University Press. © Oxford University Press 2022. DOI: 10.1093/oso/9780190077013.003.0013

Briefly and very broadly speaking, between 20% and 50% of all intensive care unit (ICU) survivors are adversely affected by vexing issues (cognitive impairment, PTSD, etc.) that did not exist in any meaningful measure prior to the critical illness (Davydow et al., 2009; Pandharipande et al., 2013). These issues often have functional consequences (Jackson, Pandharipande et al., 2014), including persistent problems with instrumental activities of daily living such as managing medications, financial management, shopping, limitations in health care literacy and numeracy, community participation, as well as having difficulties with employment, avoiding or limiting participation in health care, and struggling with relationships (Duggan et al., 2017; Overdorp et al., 2016). Key questions exist regarding how best to prevent PICS and the sequelae of insults to independent functioning and quality of life. Substantial progress has been made in understanding how to mitigate this risk (Morris et al., 2011) through the use of interventions such as the ICU liberation bundle (Pun et al., 2019), a "bundled" approach to care that integrates patient-centered "best practices." Yet there is considerable progress to be made in understanding how to treat the myriad of challenges faced by ICU survivors who develop symptoms of PICS, though nascent efforts are under way to better manage and improve these symptoms so prevalent after critical illness.

In this chapter, we will engage issues related to the management and treatment of PICS though a discussion of the relevant models and approaches to care, focusing on the roles and potential contributions of various disciplines of psychology—including rehabilitation psychology, health psychology, and neuropsychology. Following a general overview of the psychologist's role in addressing the salient needs of ICU survivors, we describe opportunities for the integration of psychology into efforts to promote resilience and thriving in ICU survivors and articulate the aspirational, yet necessary, future directions to promote quality of life in ICU survivors. Our hope is that this chapter may serve as a guide and/or provide a framework through which robust involvement from psychologists can help transform both the landscape of post–critical illness treatment and the lives of survivors.

Difficulties in the ICU: opportunities for psychologists

While the primary focus in this chapter involves models and approaches to the treatment of survivors of ICU hospitalization, we must briefly address issues related to the difficulties encountered by patients during critical illness and the seminal and essential contributions that psychologists can make. Prior to the development of PICS, patients often struggle with cognitive problems while in the ICU: Up to 70% experience delirium at some point during their critical illness and at ICU discharge

(Ely et al., 2001; Young et al., 2010). Many also experience psychological distress and display symptoms of acute stress disorder, depressive symptoms, and existential issues related to death and dying (Wade et al., 2018). Moreover, in our anecdotal experience, many patients with critical illness—particularly in the midst of lengthy ICU stays—grapple with issues of apathy and treatment adherence, though this has largely been unstudied. Historically, few individuals receive psychological consultation, much less treatment, during ICU hospitalization, although in some cases patients are seen by consultation/liaison psychiatrists and neurologists. As such, the integration of psychological services during hospitalization and shortly thereafter is an important goal, as it may improve detection and treatment of difficulties that may develop into PICS following hospitalization by leveraging the skills of the psychologist and the often considerable internal resources of patients. With this being said, few if any data are available comparing the relative effectiveness of inpatient versus outpatient psychological interventions in critically ill patients.

Calibrating expectations about survivorship before discharge

One key function to which we will return throughout this chapter involves education and calibration of expectations; nowhere is this more crucial and truer than in the days immediately prior to discharge from the ICU. This is a time when patients and families sometimes feel a certain euphoria—they now know they are going to survive, sometimes against long odds, and often feel deep relief at the thought of returning home to normalcy. While predicting outcomes is fraught with difficulty and no one wants to "rain on the parade," it is vital to review possible outcomes so that individuals and their care partners are fully apprised of what they might be facing after discharge. It is important that this is done not only with patients but also with their families and care partners, as cognitive impairment, so common and yet often undetected, can hinder meaningful comprehension, particularly when coupled with significant psychological distress (Hatch et al., 2018). We take pains to note that this cognitive impairment is "regularly hidden from view" because patients who are still in the fog of delirium or post-delirium residuals often seem quite "normal" (Girard et al., 2010). Patients may appear to be conversant, respond on cue, and even display a degree of cognitive adroitness, but on closer inspection they are far from cognitively "normal," as they may have problems with orientation, inattention, and executive function and may be intensely confused. This "hidden" cognitive impairment stands in contrast to the aforementioned symptoms of psychological distress and anxiety, which are often more immediately apparent. With this framework in mind, communication with these patients should be adapted to facilitate meaningful comprehension by the patient and care partners.

Outcomes commonly observed among ICU survivors

As patients transition from the ICU to home, leaving critical illness in the "rearview mirror," the life-altering experience of critical illness becomes clearer. Leaving aside for a moment the often monumental physical needs of ICU survivors, the cognitive and psychological difficulties most widely reported after critical illness are deficits in broad-based cognitive functioning as well as depression and PTSD (Jackson et al., 2003). Other less frequently reported issues include a panoply of adjustment-related problems, claustrophobia (often due to being restrained), problems with grief and loss, and, in a small percentage of patients, body image issues (Edinger & Radtke, 1993; Hellgren et al., 2013).

Cognitive impairment in ICU survivors has been variously described using paradigms that in some cases involve "brain injury" and in other cases invoke "dementia." In truth, the neuropsychological deficits observed after critical illness can resemble both of these conditions. As in acquired brain injury, the cognitive changes seen in ICU survivors emerge quickly, tend to be diffuse in nature (i.e., they don't occur first or primarily in memory only but in a range of domains), and may improve over time (Wilcox et al., 2013). Alternatively, some patients experience progressive decline of the sort seen in Alzheimer's disease—perhaps individuals who had preexisting unrecognized mild cognitive impairment that was accelerated by the contributions of critical illness (Janz et al., 2010; Pandharipande et al., 2013). In addition, neuroimaging findings in ICU survivors have shown the presence of pathologic features commonly seen in dementia such as reductions in hippocampal size, recognizing that such changes could have preceded critical illness, even as they could have developed due to the effects of conditions such as sepsis (Gunther et al., 2012; Morandi et al., 2012).

As with cognitive impairment, there are certain distinctive features of the mental health issues affecting individuals with PICS such as depression and PTSD. Depression, occurring in up to one third of all ICU survivors, tends to be somatic in nature (Jackson, Pandharipande et al., 2014). The symptoms typically endorsed (in cohort studies, in clinical trials, and in our experience clinically) tend to reflect a preoccupation with the somatic somewhat more than cognitive symptoms of depression—thoughts of hopelessness, suicidal ideation, and the like. PTSD symptoms are frequently anchored in avoidance and, as Edmondson observed (2014), tend to have a strong "future" orientation—that is, patients are intensely concerned and hypervigilant about the re-emergence of dormant physical symptoms that represent a "ticking time bomb." As with depression, significant symptoms of PTSD are very common (a majority of studies report prevalence rates of between ~10% and ~20%) (Davydow et al., 2009) and are comparable to those observed in other clinical populations such as combat veterans (rates of PTSD among U.S. veterans have been reported to be as high as 17%) (Richardson et al., 2010).

From a functional standpoint, common struggles occur—perhaps not surprisingly—in areas related to work, school, social functioning, and engagement in hobbies and activities (de Rooij et al., 2008; Ferrante et al., 2015; Iwashyna et al., 2010). Cognitive deficits frequently translate rather directly into problems attending, recalling, synthesizing, and retaining information, which is problematic for performance in the classroom, the boardroom, the assembly line, and many other contexts (Overdorp et al., 2016). Social avoidance, often reflecting the presence of PTSD secondary to ICU hospitalization, sometimes becomes the norm, as patients worry about contact with others who could transmit various illnesses to them. They may avoid necessary medical procedures due to the possibility, however remote, that these could be a gateway to a new ICU admission (Edmondson, 2014). Hobbies— previously a source of great joy, connection, and self-esteem—are too often reluctantly abandoned, as they are suddenly too difficult (e.g., mountain biking) or too dangerous (e.g., a patient's partner discourages the patient from going hunting over concerns that the patient's cognitive impairment or mental health issues will lead to deficits in judgment and injury).

Effective models of psychological intervention must, at a minimum, begin with an understanding of the aforementioned issues. Specifically, they must grapple with the particular problems that ICU survivors present and address these problems in a way that can be replicated on a large scale yet are tailored to patients' unique needs. In the next section, we review current models of psychological treatment employed with ICU survivors while offering aspirational goals for the future.

History of treatment of PICS

Critical care specialists of all disciplines care deeply about the outcomes of ICU survivors. Therefore, it seems clear that the historical absence of postdischarge treatment models is a reflection not of apathy but rather a variety of structural realities that are barriers to treatment. Many of these are financial in nature—for example, pharmacists typically play a key role in most clinics devoted to the treatment of PICS, but in many states, they cannot bill or be reimbursed for their services. Others are practical—that is, clinics may require significant office space, and this space may already be designated for other clinical purposes. Certainly, one significant challenge is that a majority of individuals providing care to critically ill patients do not follow them after discharge and have no personal awareness of the difficulties their patients may be experiencing. In many cases, critically ill patients live a great distance from the ICUs where they are treated (they often arrive via helicopter from distant areas), making continuity of care even more difficult. It is not only critical care providers who are frequently in the dark, as primary care providers also often lack a thorough understanding of the trauma their patient may have endured during the ICU stay.

As we have noted, in recent years, an explosion of interest in the topic of PICS has led medical providers—and to a lesser extent mental health clinicians—to increase their familiarity with the issues buffeting and besetting ICU survivors. This development mirrors, albeit in a very small way, survivorship care for other medical populations such as survivors of cancer (Stanton et al., 2005). Treatment programs for cancer survivors have multiplied since the early 2000s. First available only at elite and comprehensive cancer centers, they have rapidly proliferated in the last 20 years. The services they provide are increasingly viewed by patients and leaders in the field as indispensable to excellent cancer care (McCabe et al., 2013), though even in the cancer arena the evidence regarding impact on outcomes is incomplete and sometimes conflicting (Kvale et al., 2016; Mayer et al., 2015; Mays et al., 2011). In contrast to the current state of affairs in the domain of cancer treatment, in the critical care world there are only a handful of programs designed to focus on the unique constellation of needs (including cognitive, psychological, and functional challenges) of medical and surgical ICU survivors. Correspondingly, very few studies have tested their effectiveness, and a majority of these have been negative (Cuthbertson et al., 2009; Petersson et al., 2011; Schandl et al., 2011). As continues to be true in the cancer arena (Monterosso et al., 2019), ongoing questions exist about the effectiveness of such survivorship clinics, and debates persist about not only whether they improve patient outcomes but also whether the models of care they reflect are appropriately designed (Williams & Leslie, 2008).

In a small landmark study that differed from others insofar as there was greater mental health integration, Khan and colleagues (2015) reported results of their newly formed Critical Care Recovery Center, the first such clinic in North America, and described positive outcomes from 53 patients seen at their clinic between July 2011 and May 2012. Patients who had been severely critically ill were seen immediately after hospital discharge by members of an interdisciplinary team that included a physician, a nurse, a case manager, and a mental health professional, among others; when deemed appropriate, patients were followed multiple times after their initial appointment. Among patients who were seen twice ($N = 24$), statistically significant improvements were noted on a symptom checklist (Healthy Aging Brain Center Monitor tool), with a reduction in symptoms reported in cognitive ($p = .04$) and functional ($p = .02$) domains and overall symptoms ($p = .01$); data were analyzed in a simple univariate fashion.

Elsewhere, in a randomized trial conducted at Vanderbilt, investigators explored the impact of an ICU recovery center ($N = 111$) versus usual care ($N = 121$) on a range of outcomes, specifically to include the number of postdischarge interventions received (e.g., medication reconciliation and counseling, psychoeducation, cognitive and mental health screening, which included feedback, multidisciplinary consultation with family, and so forth) as well as mortality and rates of 30-day readmission (Bloom et al., 2019). Patients in the ICU recovery program received twice as many interventions (a median of 2) as did patients in the usual care group ($p < .001$). Although approximately equal numbers of patients were readmitted to the hospital within 30 days, the median time to readmission differed sharply between groups (7 days vs. 21.5 days), favoring those in the treatment group ($p = .03$). The study's composite outcome of death or readmission within 30 days of hospital discharge occurred in 20 patients (18%) in the ICU recovery program group and 36 patients (29.8%) in the usual care group ($p = .04$).

While these studies—limited as they are—point to the possible effectiveness of interdisciplinary-based approaches on a range of outcomes, they of course require replication in larger samples. Of note is the fact that they evaluate the impact of a bundled approach but do little to address specific issues related to the contribution of psychological interventions per se. Nonetheless, there are wide-ranging ways that an interdisciplinary recovery center–based approach could benefit patients, as outlined in Box 13.1.

Current models of PICS treatment

These centers, currently in existence at a few places like the Indiana University Medical Center, Brigham and Women's Hospital, University of Pittsburgh Medical Center, and Vanderbilt Medical Center, reflect a diversity of approaches, but—in their current form at least—they display a number of commonalities. Characteristically, they include providers from disciplines such as critical care medicine, nursing, pharmacy, social work/case management, and psychology. They sometimes include practitioners from physical therapy, occupational therapy, and psychiatry, among others (the selection of the specialties represented is often practical—that is, it reflects the types of professionals available at a given medical center as well as current thinking about the nature of the difficulties experienced following critical illness). Furthermore, they generally focus on individuals in what might be termed the "acute postdischarge phase"—individuals who are within a week to a month of hospital discharge. Finally, they typically take a bundled holistic approach; that is, recovery centers view patients through integrated lenses and treat them in all of their complexity as opposed to in isolation. Figure 13.1 describes one such bundled approach (Critical Illness Recovery and Late Effects [CIRCLE]) that we have used locally in our own work.

BOX 13.1.
BRIEF CLINICAL VIGNETTES FROM A SURVIVORSHIP CLINIC

A. Medication reconciliation and counseling finds the patient to be taking a number of inappropriate medications, including omeprazole and quetiapine, which were prescribed in the ICU. The medications are stopped, decreasing the risk of Clostridium difficile colitis, QT prolongation, and excess somnolence, and freeing the patient from the financial burden of unnecessary medications.

B. Medical evaluation reveals abnormal spirometry, low oxygen saturation, and a hoarse, airy voice. The patient is referred to voice clinic for airway evaluation and started on supplemental oxygen.

C. A patient is seen for a cognitive assessment and displays severe but previously unrecognized cognitive impairment on screening tests of visuospatial and executive ability. He is advised not to drive and is referred for a formal driving evaluation.

D. 6-minute walking distance is severely decreased and the patient is having difficulty caring for her baby due to necrosis of the fingers and toes, a result of high-dose pressors in the ICU. Case management (CM) evaluation reveals the patient never received physical and occupational therapy prescribed at discharge because she did not have a primary care physician (PCP) to receive the paperwork. CM arranges home therapy and assists the patient in finding an in-network PCP.

E. At patient-centered consultation, review of spirometry shows early obstruction concerning for smoking-related lung disease. The patient reveals he stopped smoking in the ICU but has been having cravings. After interdisciplinary review with psychology, pharmacy, and CM, a smoking cessation plan with behavioral and pharmacologic intervention is integrated into a survivorship care plan.

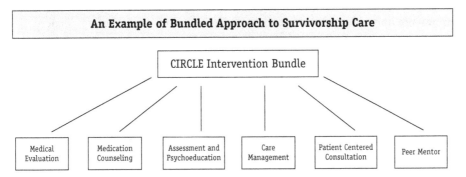

FIGURE 13.1. An example of a bundled approach to survivorship care. The CIRCLE (Critical Illness Recovery and Late Effects) model was used during the development of a ICU recovery clinic.

As for the role that psychologists play in an ICU recovery center, a few goals appear to be primary (these primarily reflect our clinical experience and need to be studied more fully and systematically).

A FOCUS ON ASSESSMENT

As currently designed, most ICU recovery centers emphasize the rapid evaluation of cognitive and psychological problems and view this "early identification" as a key goal, believing that if patients, families, and medical providers become aware that patients are experiencing cognitive impairment, for example, this knowledge can help prevent a range of untoward outcomes. Think for a minute of a college student who experiences cognitive impairment due to severe sepsis; he is planning on returning to his university in 1 month to continue his rigorous academic training in engineering. He sees a psychologist at an ICU follow-up clinic, and this very bright young man earns a score of 21 out of 30 on a Montreal Cognitive Assessment (MoCA), demonstrating major problems with planning and organizing on a clock-drawing task. Armed with this new information (which is supported by additional testing), he and his family decide that he should take a semester off (or perhaps a partial academic load), get assistance to develop effective compensatory strategies, secure accommodations to support his academic efforts, and potentially avert a situation where he would have failed his coursework, forcing him to drop out of the Honors College.

A FOCUS ON PSYCHOEDUCATION

A consistent experience reported by ICU survivors is that they are rarely informed about the many challenges that they may encounter after critical illness. They often experience unfamiliar symptoms not experienced to any degree before (anxiety, disturbing memories of critical illness, problems sleeping, cognitive changes, to name but a few) and have difficulty understanding them and putting them into context. In the absence of any specialized knowledge, they often make negative attributions leading to a range of catastrophic thoughts when difficulties emerge—developments that cause great distress and functional interference. This experience, as described broadly in the psychological literature, stands in marked contrast to the experience of individuals who are told what to potentially expect. For these individuals, having nightmares about the ICU can be upsetting, but the impact is muted to a large degree by their knowledge—aided by a psychologist who normalizes their experience—that this is a frequent outcome after critical illness, that they are not alone in their struggle, and that they are not "going crazy."

USE OF TECHNOLOGY

At many large ICUs across North America, patients often live a great distance from the facilities in which they are treated; thus, receiving regular in-person treatment at an ICU recovery center is not feasible. In this circumstance, psychologists are increasingly relying on tele-technology–based approaches using the HIPAA-compliant versions of platforms such as Skype, Zoom, and more proprietary telehealth platforms so that clinical services can be provided (recognizing that there are limitations to telehealth models, such as the fact that licensed providers can often provide treatment only to individuals residing in the state in which they are licensed). This serves dual purposes: Obviously, it allows for continuation of treatment, but it also allows for the ongoing management of patients experiencing prominent avoidant symptoms of the sort that might preclude them from returning to the medical center that they identify as the source of their trauma.

TAILORED TREATMENT

As with patients living with various other acute or chronic conditions, ICU survivors often experience common cognitive and mental health symptoms but may do so in specific, nuanced, and idiosyncratic ways. As noted previously, patients with depression may report a preponderance of somatic symptoms, and those with PTSD may have avoidant behaviors that translate into anxiety about ongoing medical care, future surgeries, and the like. While standard treatment approaches to these may be effective, tailored approaches that consider the unique challenges, barriers, and goals of individual survivors of critical illness may be appropriate as well.

Even as we strive for the ambitious goals just described, it must be acknowledged that challenges in the treatment of ICU survivors abound—particularly in the early postdischarge period. These challenges are both intensely practical and also conceptual. As a practical matter, the last place many survivors of critical illness want to go is back to the medical center where they nearly died—the facility they may associate with delirium, hallucinations, and any manner of distressing and untoward things. Simply convincing such patients to return for a visit to the clinic is a tall order indeed. Assuming they do arrive, trying to convince individuals who may be physically debilitated or deconditioned to stay engaged over the course of 2 to 3 hours is yet another hurdle. Closely related to this are the clinical difficulties involved in trying to understand whether the cognitive and mental health problems that so commonly exist immediately after discharge are indeed concerning and predictive of worsening problems in the future or whether they are simply vestiges of critical illness that will abate. Yet another challenge is to help patients build on the dynamics that have already ensued during critical illness to help promote healthy lifestyles and behaviors. Finding ways to intervene with such patients to increase the odds that they will not return to previous unhealthy behaviors (e.g., see Chapter 3) is the sort of transformative contribution for which these recovery centers are designed.

Support groups for ICU survivors

Support groups have been one of the primary means of psychological support for survivors of critical illness in the last decade or so. Support groups have proven to be effective in the treatment of a wide range of medical and mental health conditions, including dementia, epilepsy, PTSD, stroke, and many more (Cacciatore, 2007; Christensen et al., 2019; Elafros et al., 2013; Jao et al., 2016). They have much to commend them: They are typically relatively inexpensive to organize, they can easily be "scaled," and they can be delivered by people with relatively little specialized training (whether psychologists or health care professionals from other non–mental health disciplines who typically work as facilitators alongside other patient leaders). Although precise estimates are difficult to ascertain, since the advent of an initiative called THRIVE sponsored by the Society of Critical Care Medicine, approximately 20 support group programs have been formed in North America, with perhaps an equal number of programs operating around the world (www.sccm.org/MyICUCare/THRIVE; Haines et al., 2019). A majority of these are considered "peer support groups"—meaning that while psychologists may facilitate them, they are largely led by patients. As such, they typically provide peer support at no cost to patients.

These groups to date have been marked by a panoply of diverse approaches, with regard to everything from the populations being treated to the context of treatment to the timing of delivery (McPeake et al., 2019). In general, they have targeted patients shortly after their discharge from the ICU, in the belief that many patients are most likely to benefit from treatment in the early postdischarge period. The alternative to this point of view is that many patients are poised to optimally benefit from group therapy long after critical illness, as they have then had sufficient time to process the ordeals they have experienced. Also, a majority of groups have followed a prescribed, time-limited curriculum, though they vary in content. In general, they have been educational in nature and have addressed a circumscribed range of topics such as psychoeducation, stress and coping, issues of adjustment, grieving, and so forth. While the groups are largely attended by ICU survivors, some also integrate family members and care partners.

In the support group model we developed at the ICU recovery center at Vanderbilt, we rely on what might be called a "bottom up" approach, in which topics are largely dictated by group members in the context of an open group that has no fixed termination. Although we have largely attempted to facilitate a peer-led group without any fixed agenda, we have observed that a small number of central themes emerge consistently across groups. These themes relate to the following issues:

1. Identity: Notably, "who am I?" following critical illness in light of physical debility, cognitive difficulties, bodily changes
2. Calibration of expectations: Specifically, what changes and improvements are realistic to expect and what is the natural history of cognitive impairment and PTSD after critical illness
3. Grief and loss: Processing and working through feelings of sadness and loss related to unwanted changes
4. Acceptance: Coming to grips with the persistence and reality of changes after discharge and working to find ways to accept and gradually even embrace them
5. Empowerment: Finding ways to reshape the patient's narrative from one of passivity to one of survivorship and overcoming obstacles and barriers.

Few, if any, support groups for ICU survivors have employed outcome measures to demonstrate efficacy. While anecdotal information buttresses the notion that support groups facilitate change in the context of PICS, perhaps the most significant benefit we have observed relates to the development of rich community and support, both of which are often sorely lacking for individuals after critical illness. As many have described, networks for survivors of conditions such as sepsis and ARDS are few and far between. Although they are members of a fraternity that is numerically very large, they frequently feel intensely isolated and lonely. In our experience, the benefits that individuals with PICS phenotypes experience when they realize they are part of a supportive, understanding "tribe" are palpable and one of the key benefits that prompt our patients to return to the group week after week.

Cognitive rehabilitation

Cognitive rehabilitation is a "systematic, functionally oriented service of therapeutic activities that is based on assessment and understanding of patient's brain-behavioral deficits" (Cicerone et al., 2011). These interventions seek to achieve functional improvements by (1) reinforcing or re-establishing previously learned behavior patterns or (2) establishing new cognitive activity patterns or compensatory mechanisms for impaired neurologic systems. Cognitive rehabilitation is increasingly being applied to patients with medical or psychiatric conditions resulting in cognitive dysfunction such as HIV/AIDS, epilepsy, Parkinson's disease, multiple sclerosis, and schizophrenia. A recent review included 34 studies of cognitive rehabilitation in 11 medical illness groups (Langenbahn et al., 2013). The majority of the studies cited in this review were case series or uncontrolled studies, though 30 of the 34 studies demonstrated positive findings.

In the first investigation of its kind (RETURN-1), survivors of critical illness with executive dysfunction were randomized to either 12 weeks of in-person cognitive rehabilitation (using goal management training [GMT]) and physical rehabilitation via telehealth visits or to a "usual care" condition typically characterized by no formal rehabilitation (Jackson et al., 2012). Over 87% of patients participated in at least one cognitive rehabilitation session; 80% completed all sessions. Despite equivalent executive functioning scores (Tower Test) at baseline, patients receiving the in-home rehabilitation intervention demonstrated significantly improved scores at 3-month follow-up (adjusted $p <$ .01) (Figure 13.2). Patients in the intervention group also reported significantly better daily functioning as measured by the Functional Activities Questionnaire ($p =$ .04) (Pfeffer et al., 1982).

Although to our knowledge exceedingly few ICU survivors receive cognitive rehabilitation, we believe that such an approach may frequently be appropriate in

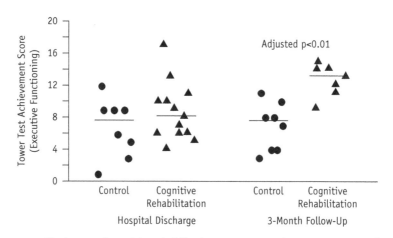

FIGURE 13.2. The impact of cognitive rehabilitation on outcomes. Scores were measured at study enrollment and 3-month follow-up after completion of cognitive rehabilitation intervention. Higher scores reflect better performance on the Tower Test. Baseline scores on the Tower Test were not significantly different between groups.

Jackson, J. C., Santoro, M. J., Ely, T. M., Boehm, L., Kiehl, A. L., Anderson, L. S., & Ely, E. W. (2014). Improving patient care through the prism of psychology: application of Maslow's hierarchy to sedation, delirium, and early mobility in the intensive care unit. *Journal of Critical Care*, *29*(3), 438–444.

certain patient groups or subtypes. While recommending specific approaches is beyond the scope of this chapter—and difficult given limited scientific support for most therapies—one particular method worthy of comment (and referenced in the previous paragraph) is GMT, as it has quite robust empirical support for the treatment of deficits in attention and executive functioning, areas widely reported to be impaired after critical illness (Richard et al., 2019). Based on the theory of "goal neglect," GMT is a stepwise intervention that uses self-awareness and self-monitoring techniques to train patients to "STOP" and monitor ongoing behavior, regaining cognitive control when behavior becomes incompatible with intended goals (Levine et al., 2007). GMT is anchored in "sustained and vigilant attention theory," and it enables patients to actively attend to "higher order" goals critical to functioning (Robertson & Fitzpatrick, 2008). While there may be differences in the spectrum of domains of cognitive impairment due to different types of clinical injury, what these all have in common is greater than the differences, allowing for application of a similar rehabilitation tool such as GMT.

Models of psychological intervention

As discussed, critical illness survivors have significant mental health challenges, particularly in the areas of anxiety, depression, and PTSD. These conditions are commonly treated using established methods and protocols well known to psychologists (e.g., cognitive-behavioral, motivational interviewing, trauma-informed). Key questions do exist, however, regarding "models" of psychological treatment and whether there might be nuances in the ways the aforementioned conditions are treated that could differ from standard approaches.

With respect to treatment models, a majority of approaches employed to date are explicitly interdisciplinary—that is, they occur in a setting in which psychologists are joined by professionals of various specialty areas of practice (occupational and physical therapists, pharmacists, critical care physicians, etc.) due to the multifaceted nature of the difficulties such patients tend to have. In such settings, psychological treatment approaches are informed by the physical limitations patients have, as well as by their cognitive deficits, to ensure that mental health concerns are not treated in isolation. While such approaches have possible advantages, there are also difficulties inherent in these models. A notable one is that clinics, as described earlier in the chapter, typically exist in hospitals or medical centers, places that patients often seek to avoid as they serve as "reminders" of trauma—or, more practically, patients wish to avoid them due to fear of contracting illness that could result in future ICU admissions. In such circumstances, outpatient treatment of mental health conditions in a private-practice context may be recommended and extremely helpful, particularly if the environment in which patients are being treated clearly differs from a hospital setting.

Whether done in a clinic setting or a private practice, one key consideration among psychologists is the ability to competently treat not just one condition (e.g., PTSD) but many. In a recent survey of 4,943 patients, anxiety, depression, and PTSD were common (seen in 46%, 40%, and 22% of patients, respectively), but, crucially, if at least one condition was present, there was a 65% chance that one of the other two would be as well (Hatch et al., 2018). Indeed, not only are multiple mental health conditions present in individuals after critical illness, but these conditions—typically new—have clear social dimensions that must be addressed.

Recent research suggests that nearly one in two individuals who were employed at the time of ICU hospitalization are out of the workforce 12 months after discharge (Kamdar et al., 2020). Financial stress is also common; in one recent study it was identified as one of the top three stressors by up to 48.5% of survivors of critical illness at follow-up, even as it was associated with an increased risk of anxiety and depression (Khandelwal et al., 2018). Therefore, psychologists should thoughtfully consider the role and centrality of external dynamics in the maintenance and worsening of mental health symptoms, even as they should become adept at adopting advocacy roles in assisting survivors of critical illness. These roles may feel unfamiliar, such as writing letters to disability boards, advocating on behalf of patients to employment law attorneys, and helping patients pursue accommodations—employment-related, financial, or otherwise.

Who is the patient? Integrating families into the care of ICU survivors

Whatever else models of psychological treatment of ICU survivors do or don't do, they must recognize the centrality of family in the process of healing (Davidson et al., 2012). Traditionally, ICU care centered exclusively on individual patients, even though it often marginalized families and care partners and overlooked the considerable assistance they could provide. More recently, due to initiatives such as the ABCDEF bundle (i.e., "ICU liberation"), a "bundled" approach to patient care that prioritizes the integration of families into far-reaching aspects of patient care (Ely, 2017), these older orthodoxies are rapidly changing. This trend should be encouraged by psychologists at every turn (recognizing the nuances involved) as familiar support, if available, is typically a "driver" of improved outcomes and enhanced recovery.

The practical expressions of family involvement may necessarily change depending on circumstances, whether patients are actively critically ill and in the hospital versus recovering after discharge. For example, psychological interventions should be provided to family members as readily as they are provided to patients, and exploring the needs of family members should be an explicit priority. Recent literature supports the notion that rates of PTSD are as high or higher among spouses or care partners as they are among patients (Azoulay et al., 2005). Indeed, it is not uncommon for family members to be traumatized even when patients are not. Nevertheless, in our experience, the mental health issues of spouses or children are often ignored. In general, family members and spouses should be encouraged to talk about feelings and concerns related to critical illness and its effects. We often see situations where patients are deeply curious about aspects of their critical illness, but their loved ones are resistant, concerned that patients are unable to handle the stress of such conversations. Challenging these ideas, working through resistances, and helping them understand that growth and intimacy are often achieved in the midst of these conversations are important treatment goals.

Future directions

As we have outlined, survivors of critical illness frequently have serious and wide-ranging difficulties that are likely amenable to psychological and cognitive interventions. Unfortunately, to date, few intervention models have been developed and fewer still have been tested. Moreover, the integration of psychologists in patient care in any kind of programmatic way is far more the exception than the rule, especially in the United States. Our hope is that this chapter and the many chapters in this book represent the beginning of a clarion call to action and mobilization among psychologists of diverse backgrounds to come together and use their considerable talents to improve the lives of individuals living in the shadows of PICS. This effort, to be sure, will be met with challenges—some pedestrian and some herculean—but our bold anticipation is that a decade or two from now, the landscape of post-ICU care, particularly in the psychology arena, will have been transformed and will look considerably different than it does today. In particular, we are optimistic that now-nascent models of treatment—such as ICU recovery centers, which include psychology as a bedrock clinical service—will, if proven effective, be fixtures around the country, whether big or small, providing local resources to survivors of critical illness, wherever they might live, even as we recognize that these recovery center approaches remain somewhat unproven. We further hope for the continued emergence of rigorous research that will help us and our colleagues in other disciplines better understand how to optimally care for individuals after the ICU so as to help avert the public health crisis—still largely unrecognized—that PICS represents.

Finally, we cautiously but excitedly look forward to a day when psychologists will devote careers to the care and management of ICU survivors in the same way that now occurs with primary care patients, individuals with HIV/AIDS, people battling chronic pain, and dozens of other populations, given that the need is great in light of the sheer number of patients who survive critical illnesses. These goals may seem bold and perhaps optimistic, but ICU survivors deserve no less.

Conclusion

Critical illnesses adversely affect a wide range of outcomes in one third to one half of all ICU survivors, including outcomes of high interest to psychologists. Models of treatment for ICU survivors that rely heavily on the contributions of psychologists are increasingly being developed and deployed. Such models of psychological treatment substantially incorporate both individual and group therapy modalities, and these should be tailored, if possible, to fit the nuanced symptoms reported by participants. Few data exist against or in favor of ICU recovery center models as relates to long-term efficacy, but patients widely report psychological services as providing "value" to their experience of survivorship, particularly as it relates to psychoeducation. Although rarely employed to date, cognitive rehabilitation and rehabilitation psychology approaches may play a crucial role in enhancing quality of life and improving long-term functioning in ICU survivors.

References

Azoulay, E., Pochard, F., Kentish-Barnes, N., Chevret, S., Aboab, J., Adrie, C., . . . Schlemmer, B. (2005). Risk of post-traumatic stress symptoms in family members of intensive care unit patients. *American Journal of Respiratory and Critical Care Medicine, 171*(9), 987–994.

Bloom, S. J., Stollings, J. L., Kirkpatrick, O., Wang, L., Byrne, D. W., Sevin, C. M., & Semler, M. W. (2019). Randomized clinical trial of an ICU recovery center pilot program for survivors of critical illness. *Critical Care Medicine, 47*, 1337–1345.

Cacciatore, J. (2007). Effects of support groups on post-traumatic stress responses in women experiencing stillbirth. *Journal of Death and Dying, 55*(1), 71–90.

Christensen, E. R., Golden, S. L., & Gesell, S. B. (2019). Perceived benefits of peer support groups for stroke survivors and caregivers in rural North Carolina. *North Carolina Medical Journal, 80*(3), 143–148.

Cicerone, K. D., Langenbahn, D. M., Braden, C., Malec, J. F., Kalmar, K., Fraas, M., . . . Ashman, T. (2011). Evidence-based cognitive rehabilitation: Updated review of the literature from 2003 through 2008. *Archives of Physical Medicine and Rehabilitation, 92*(4), 519–530.

Cuthbertson, B. H., Rattray, J., Campbell, M. K., Gager, M., Roughton, S., Smith, A., . . . Waldmann, C. (2009). The PRaCTICaL study of nurse led, intensive care follow-up programmes for improving long term outcomes from critical illness: A pragmatic randomised controlled trial. *British Medical Journal, 339,* b3723.

Davidson, J. E., Jones, C., & Bienvenu, O. J. (2012). Family response to critical illness: Postintensive care syndrome—family. *Critical Care Medicine, 40*(2), 618–624.

Davydow, D. S., Gifford, J. M., Desai, S. V., Bienvenu, O. J., & Needham, D. M. (2009). Depression in general intensive care unit survivors: A systematic review. *Intensive Care Medicine, 35*(5), 796–809.

de Rooij, S. E., Govers, A. C., Korevaar, J. C., Giesbers, A. W., Levi, M., & de Jonge, E. (2008). Cognitive, functional, and quality-of-life outcomes of patients aged 80 and older who survived at least 1 year after planned or unplanned surgery or medical intensive care treatment. *Journal of the American Geriatrics Society, 56,* 816–822.

Duggan, M. C., Wang, L., Wilson, J. E., Dittus, R., Ely, E. W., & Jackson, J. C. (2017). Executive dysfunction, depression, and mental health-related quality of life in survivors of critical illness: Results from the BRAIN-ICU Investigation. *Journal of Critical Care, 37,* 72–79.

Edinger, J. D., & Radtke, R. A. (1993). Use of in vivo desensitization to treat a patient's claustrophobic response to nasal CPAP. *Sleep, 16*(7), 678–680.

Edmondson, D. (2014). An enduring somatic threat model of posttraumatic stress disorder due to acute life-threatening medical events. *Social and Personality Psychology Compass, 8,* 118–134.

Elafros, M. A., Mulenga, J., Mbewe, E., Haworth, A., Choma, E., Atadzhanov, M., & Birbeck, G. L. (2013). Peer support groups as an intervention to decrease epilepsy associated stigma. *Epilepsy and Behavior, 21*(1), 188–192.

Ely, E.W. (2017). The ABCDEF bundle: Science and philosophy of how ICU liberation serves patients and families. *Critical Care Medicine, 45*(2), 321–330.

Ely, E. W., Inouye, S. K., Bernard, G. R., Gordon, S., Francis, J., May, L., . . . Dittus, R. (2001). Delirium in mechanically ventilated patients: Validity and reliability of the confusion assessment method for the intensive care unit (CAM-ICU). *Journal of the American Medical Association, 286*(21), 2703–2710.

Ferrante, L. E., Pisani, M. A., Murphy, T. E., Gahbauer, E. A., Leo-Summers, L. S., & Gill, T. M. (2015). Functional trajectories among older persons before and after critical illness. *JAMA Internal Medicine, 175*(4), 523–529.

Girard, T. D., Jackson, J. C., Pandharipande, P. P., Pun, B. T., Thompson, J. L., Shintani, A. K., . . . Ely, E. W. (2010). Delirium as a predictor of long-term cognitive impairment in survivors of critical illness. *Critical Care Medicine, 38,* 1513–20.

Gunther, M. L., Morandi, A., Krauskopf, E., Pandharipande, P., Girard, T. D., Jackson, J. C., . . . Ely, E. W. (2012). The association between brain volumes, delirium duration, and cognitive outcomes in intensive care unit survivors: A prospective exploratory cohort magnetic resonance imaging study. *Critical Care Medicine, 40,* 2022–2032.

Haines, K. J., Sevin, C. M., & McPeake, J. (2019). Key mechanisms by which post-ICU activities can improve in-ICU care: Results of the international THRIVE collaboratives. *Intensive Care Medicine, 45,* 939–947.

Hatch, R., Young, D., Barber, V., Griffiths, J., Harrison, D. A., & Watkinson, P. (2018). Anxiety, depression and post traumatic stress disorder after critical illness: A UK-wide prospective cohort study. *Critical Care, 22*(1), 310–323.

Hellgren, E. M., Lagergren, P., Larsson, A. C., Schandl, A. R., & Sackey, P. V. (2013). Body image and psychological outcome after severe skin and soft tissue infection requiring intensive care. *Acta Anaesthesiologica Scandinavica, 57*(2), 220–228.

Hopkins, R. O., Weaver, L. K., Pope, D., Orme, J. F., Bigler, E. D., & Larson-Lohr, V. (1999). Neuropsychological sequelae and impaired health status in survivors of severe acute respiratory distress syndrome. *American Journal of Respiratory and Critical Care Medicine, 160*(1), 50–56.

Iwashyna, T. J., Ely, E. W., Smith, D. M., & Langa, K. M. (2010). Long-term cognitive impairment and functional disability among survivors of severe sepsis. *Journal of the American Medical Association, 304*(16), 1787–1794.

Jackson, J. C., Ely, E. W., Morey, M. C., Anderson, V. M., Siebert, C. S., Denne, L. B., . . . Hoenig, H. (2012). Cognitive and physical rehabilitation of intensive care unit survivors: Results of the RETURN randomized controlled pilot investigation. *Critical Care Medicine, 40*, 1088–1097.

Jackson, J. C., Hart, R. P., Gordon, S. M., Shintani, A., Truman, B., May, L., & Ely, E. W. (2003). Six-month neuropsychological outcome of medical intensive care unit patients. *Critical Care Medicine, 31*(4), 1226–1234.

Jackson, J. C., Pandharipande, P. P., Girard, T. D., Brummel, N. E., Thompson, J. L., Hughes, C. G., . . . Ely, E. W. (2014). Depression, post-traumatic stress disorder, and functional disability in survivors of critical illness in the BRAIN-ICU study: A longitudinal cohort study. *Lancet Respiratory Medicine, 2*(5), 369–379.

Jackson, J. C., Santoro, M. J., Ely, T. M., Boehm, L., Kiehl, A. L., Anderson, L. S., & Ely, E. W. (2014). Improving patient care through the prism of psychology: Application of Maslow's hierarchy to sedation, delirium, and early mobility in the intensive care unit. *Journal of Critical Care, 29*(3), 438–444.

Janz, D. R., Abel, T. W., Jackson, J. C., Gunther, M. L., Heckers, S., & Ely, E. W. (2010). Brain autopsy findings in intensive care unit patients previously suffering from delirium: A pilot study. *Journal of Critical Care, 25*(538), 7–12.

Jao, Y. L., Epps, F., McDermott, C., Rose, K. M., & Specht, J. K. (2016). Effects of support groups for individuals with early-stage dementia and mild cognitive impairment: An integrative review. *Research in Gerontological Nursing, 10*(1), 1–17.

Kamdar, B. B., Suri, R., Suchyta, M. R., Digrande, K. F., Sherwood, K. D., Colantuoni, E., . . . Hopkins, R. O. (2020). Return to work after critical illness: A systematic review and meta-analysis. *Thorax, 75*(1), 17–27.

Khan, A., Lasiter, S., & Boustani, M. A. (2015). Critical care recovery center: An innovative collaborative care model for ICU survivors. *American Journal of Nursing, 115*(3), 24–46.

Khandelwal, N., Hough, C. L., Downey, L., Engelberg, R. A., Carson, S. S., White, D. B., . . . Cox, C. E. (2018). Prevalence, risk factors, and outcomes of financial stress in survivors of critical illness. *Critical Care Medicine, 46*(6), e530–e539.

Kvale, E. A., Huang, C. S., Meneses, K. M., Demark-Wahnefried, W., Bae, S., Azuero, C. B., . . . Ritchie, C. S. (2016). Patient-centered support in the survivorship care transition: Outcomes from the patient-owned survivorship care plan intervention. *Cancer, 122*, 3232–3242.

Langenbahn, D. M., Ashman, T., Cantor, J., & Trott, C. (2013). An evidence-based review of cognitive rehabilitation in medical conditions affecting cognitive function. *Archives of Physical Medicine and Rehabilitation, 94*, 271–86.

Levine, B., Stuss, D. T., Winocur, G., Binns, M. A., Fahy, L., Mandic, M., . . . Robertson, I. H. (2007). Cognitive rehabilitation in the elderly: Effects on strategic behavior in relation to goal management. *Journal of the International Neuropsychological Society, 13*, 143–152.

Mayer, D. K., Birken, S. A., Check, D. K., & Chen, R. C. (2015). Summing it up: An integrative review of studies of cancer survivorship care plans (2006–2013). *Cancer, 121*, 978–996.

Mays, D., Black, J. D., Mosher, R. B., Heinley, A., Shad, A. T., & Tercyak, K. P. (2011). Efficacy of the Survivor Health And Resilience Education (SHARE) program to improve bone health behaviors among adolescent survivors of childhood cancer. *Annals of Behavioral Medicine, 42*(1), 91–98.

McCabe, M. S., Bhatia, S., Oeffinger, K. C., Reaman, G. H., Tyne, C., Wollins, D. S., & Hudson, M. M. (2013). American Society of Clinical Oncology statement: Achieving high-quality cancer survivorship care. *Journal of Clinical Oncology, 31*(5), 631–640.

McPeake, J., Hirshberg, E. L., Christie, L. M., Drumright, K., Haines, K., Hough, C. L., . . . Iwashyna, T. J. (2019). Models of peer support to remediate post-intensive care syndrome: A report developed by the Society of Critical Care Medicine THRIVE international peer support collaborative. *Critical Care Medicine, 47*(1), e21–e27.

Monterosso, L., Platt, V., Bulsara, M., & Berg, M. (2019). Systematic review and meta-analysis of patient-reported outcomes for nurse led models of survivorship care for adult cancer patients. *Cancer Treatment Reviews, 73*, 62–72.

Morandi, A., Rogers, B. P., Gunther, M. L., Merkle, K., Pandharipande, P., Girard, T. D., . . . Hopkins, R. O. (2012). The relationship between delirium duration, white matter integrity, and cognitive impairment in intensive care unit survivors as determined by diffusion tensor imaging: The VISIONS prospective cohort magnetic resonance imaging study. *Critical Care Medicine, 40*, 2182–2189.

Morris, P. E., Griffin, L., Berry, M., Thompson, C., Hite, R. D., Winkelman, C., . . . Haponik, E. (2011). Receiving early mobility during an ICU admission is a predictor of improved outcomes in acute respiratory failure. *American Journal of the Medical Sciences, 341*(5), 373.

Needham, D. M., Davidson, J., Cohen, H., Hopkins, R. O., Weinert, C., Wunsch, H., . . . Harvey, M. A. (2012). Improving long-term outcomes after discharge from intensive care unit: Report from a stakeholders' conference. *Critical Care Medicine, 40*(2), 502–509.

Nickel, M., Leiberich, P., Nickel, C., Tritt, K., Mitterlehner, F., Rother, W., & Loew, T. (2004). The occurrence of posttraumatic stress disorder in patients following intensive care treatment: A cross-sectional study in a random sample. *Journal of Intensive Care Medicine, 19*(5), 285–290.

Overdorp, E. J., Kressels, R. P. C., Claassen, J. A., & Oosterman, J. M. (2016). The combined effect of neuropsychological and neuropathological deficits on instrumental activities of daily living in older adults: A systematic review. *Neuropsychology Review, 26*, 92–106.

Pandharipande, P. P., Girard, T. D., Jackson, J. C., Morandi, A., Thompson, J. L., Pun, B. T., . . . Ely, E. W. (2013). Long-term cognitive impairment after critical illness. *New England Journal of Medicine, 369*(14), 1306–1316.

Petersson, C. G., Bergbom, I., Brodersen, K., & Ringdal, M. (2011). Patients' participation in and evaluation of a follow-up program following intensive care. *Acta Anaesthesiologica Scandinavica, 55*(7), 827–834.

Pfeffer, R. I., Kurosaki, T. T., Harrah, C. H., Change, J. M., & Filos, S. (1982). Measurement of functional activities in older adults in the community. *Journal of Gerontology, 37*(3), 323–329.

Pun, B. T., Balas, M. C., Barnes-Daly, M. A., Thompson, J. L., Aldrich, J. M., Barr, J. . . . Ely, E. W. (2019). Caring for critically ill patients with the ABCDEF Bundle: Results of the ICU liberation collaborative in over 15,000 adults. *Critical Care Medicine*, *47*(1), 3–14.

Richard, N. M., Bernstein, L. J., Mason, W. P., Laperriere, N., Maurice, C., Millar, B. A., . . . Edelstein, K. (2019). Cognitive rehabilitation for executive dysfunction in brain tumor patients: A pilot randomized controlled trial. *Journal of Neuro-Oncology*, *142*(3), 565–575.

Richardson, L. K., Frueh, C., & Acierno, R. (2010). Prevalence estimates of combat-related post-traumatic stress disorder: Critical review. *Australian and New Zealand Journal of Psychiatry*, *44*(1), 4–19.

Robertson, I. H., & Fitzpatrick, S. M. (2008). The future of cognitive neurorehabilitation. In D. T Stuss, G. Winocur, & I. H. Robertson (Eds.), *Cognitive neurorehabilitation, evidence and application* (pp. 566–574). Cambridge University Press.

Schandl, A. R., Brattstrom, O. R., Svensson-Raskh, A., Hellgren, E. M., Falkenhav, M. D., & Sackey, P. V. (2011). Screening and treatment of problems after intensive care: A descriptive study of multidisciplinary follow-up. *Intensive and Critical Care Nursing*, 27 (2), 94–101.

Stanton, A. L., Ganz, P. A., Kwan, L., Meyerowitz, B. E., Bower, J. E., Krupnick, J. L., . . . Belin, T. R. (2005). Outcomes from the moving beyond cancer psychoeducational, randomized, controlled trial with breast cancer patients. *Journal of Clinical Oncology*, *23*(25), 6009–6018.

Wade, D., Als, N., Bell, V., Brewin, C., D'Antoni, D., Harrison, D. A., . . . POPPI investigators. (2018). Providing psychological support to people in intensive care: Development and feasibility study of a nurse-led intervention to prevent acute stress and long-term morbidity. *BMJ Open*, *8*(7), e021083.

Wilcox, M. E., Brummel, N. E., Archer, K., Ely, E. W., Jackson, J. C., & Hopkins, R. O. (2013). Cognitive dysfunction in ICU patients: Risk factors, predictors, and rehabilitation interventions. *Critical Care Medicine*, *41*(9 Suppl 1), S81–S98.

Williams, T. A., & Leslie, G. D. (2008). Beyond the walls: A review of ICU clinics and their impact on patient outcomes after leaving hospital. *Australian Critical Care*, *21*(1), 6–17.

Young, J., Murthy, L., Westby, M., Akunne, A., & O'Mahony, R. (2010). Diagnosis, prevention, and management of delirium: Summary of NICE guidance. *British Medical Journal*, *341*, c3704.

14 Systemic Factors Impacting Mortality and End-of-Life Issues in Critical Care

Leo C. Mercer, Valerie Canary, and Michelle Maxson

Introduction

The mortality rates in patients admitted to an intensive care unit (ICU) average 10% to 29%, depending on age, comorbidities, and severity of illness. Leading causes of death include multiorgan failure, cardiovascular failure, and sepsis (Barrett et al., 2014). The five most common ICU admission diagnoses are respiratory insufficiency/failure with ventilator support, acute myocardial infarction, intracranial hemorrhage or cerebral infarction, percutaneous cardiovascular procedures, and septicemia or severe sepsis (Barrett et al., 2014). Although a heterogeneous group of patients, they all share the need for more frequent assessment and a greater dependency on technology support, the most common of which is mechanical ventilation, which occurs in nearly 40% of ICU admissions (Wunsch et al., 2013). Within these ICUs exists an interdisciplinary group of caregivers that includes physicians, nurses, advanced practice providers, pharmacists, respiratory therapists, psychologists, social workers, and others, each with unique staffing and workforce challenges.

Despite agreement on its importance, there is a lack of consensus about the implementation of end-of-life care at the bedside. The diversity within patient groups, diseases and conditions, and health care providers results in an environment in which the interplay of a growing number of variables influences the engagement of patients

Leo C. Mercer, Valerie Canary, and Michelle Maxson, *Systemic Factors Impacting Mortality and End-of-Life Issues in Critical Care* In: *Critical Care Psychology and Rehabilitation.* Edited by: Kirk J. Stucky and Jennifer E. Jutte, Oxford University Press. © Oxford University Press 2022. DOI: 10.1093/oso/9780190077013.003.0014 and families in discussions about end-of-life planning and care, futility, palliation, or withdrawal of support.

Scope of the problem

The complexity of end-of-life care is heightened when it involves services in a critical care environment. Admission to an ICU is often described as a "therapeutic trial" of aggressive clinical management occurring in circumstances in which neither the effectiveness of therapy nor the patient's prognosis is known in advance. Only failure of the trial results in consideration of a transition from restorative care to palliative care (Truog et al., 2008). This was described by Mosenthal (2002) as the transition from "cure" to "comfort." It is the decision to initiate this transition that remains a difficult one. This decision is made by critical care practitioners, many of whom view the death of a patient as a personal failure and discussions about palliation or withdrawal of care as merely evidencing that in advance. Unfortunately, this dynamic often forecloses meaningful dialogue about the subject. Observations of the behaviors among intensivists when engaging with families and decision-makers in discussions about end-of-life care have confirmed the significant variation in messaging about prognosis, pain and suffering, and limits on aggressive care and interventions. This variability remains even when these discussions are contextualized by the patient's preference for a "good death." It is not surprising, then, that, in a setting in which the discussions about futility and withdrawal of care, prognosis, and palliative management are largely unstructured, the resulting decisions are quite variable.

In addition to factors unique to critical care practitioners, which make discussions and decisions regarding end-of-life care difficult, patient and family beliefs and expectations play a significant role in these critical interactions. The degree to which patient and family expectations will hamper any consideration of a transition from cure to comfort is described by Finucane (1999):

> For most patients, two fundamental facts ensure that the transition to death will remain difficult. First is the widespread and deeply held desire not to be dead. This is not only existential angst, or the dread of ultimate insignificance, it is also the struggle to avoid annihilation. Second is medicine's inability to predict the future, and to give patients a precise, reliable prognosis about when death will come. When death is the alternative, many patients who have only a small amount of hope will pay a high price to continue the struggle. Several other factors, such as certain societal values or family dynamics, also may make it difficult for a patient to make the transition to dying. (p. 1670)

Furthermore, systematic changes in the reporting of physician-specific outcomes, both publicly and to specialty society registries, have the potential to impose even greater complexity in making decisions regarding end-of-life care and their timing. The proliferation of models that grade or score hospital performance and safety, and that include mortality rates unadjusted for the effects of hospice or palliative care within them, are likely to have measurable effects on the involvement of either.

Second-order effects of unmanaged ICU-related end-of-life issues

Despite widespread acceptance of the importance of end-of-life planning and management in the care of critically ill patients, it is frequently deprecated by seemingly more urgent clinical concerns in the individual patient while influenced by an erroneous perception among stakeholders of the limitless nature of critical care resources (Crippen & Whetstine, 1999). However, an evolving body of evidence has developed that, despite improved palliative care services in the ICU, implicates the failure to manage both end-of-life aspects of care and nontherapeutic interventions in limiting access to critical care (Khandelwal et al., 2015; Roczen et al., 2016). In other words, there are real-world consequences of failing to address end-of-life issues in the critical care environment. When units are deemed fully occupied but are caring for patients who are receiving nontherapeutic and/or potentially inappropriate care, this effectively limits access to other patients with conditions in whom care in an ICU is definably both therapeutic and appropriate. If such patients are required to wait for an ICU bed, the effect on mortality is quantifiably higher. This is one of several "second-order" or derivative effects of unmanaged end-of-life issues in critical care.

In the rare circumstances in which there is a relative abundance of critical care beds, these second-order impacts are limited. However, in most large hospitals, the demand for critical care resources frequently exceeds their ready availability, with significant detrimental impact on critically ill patients forced to wait for care. This occurs despite an increase in the number of new ICU beds within this group of hospitals created between 2000 and 2010 (Wallace et al., 2015). More than 5 million patients are admitted annually to the available 104,000 adult critical care beds in the United States (Barrett et al., 2014). Critical care beds account for approximately 16% of the total bed capacity in American hospitals (Society of Critical Care Medicine, 2020), and the mean occupancy rate within these units averages 70% in larger hospitals, although this rate is frequently higher when "staffed capacity" is considered (Halpern & Pastores, 2006). The term "staffed capacity" describes the capacity of a unit not in terms of the number of physical beds but rather the number of beds for which there is staff to care for patients within them. It is a dynamic metric that more accurately describes a unit's capacity to admit and care for critically ill patients than one in which occupancy is expressed relative to the fixed number of physical beds. Although more critical care capacity continues to be built, resulting in an increase in the aggregate number of critical care beds, the additional capacity is unlikely to produce significantly or sustainably improved access to the ICU for those who require admission. High occupancy and prolonged lengths of stay due to unaddressed end-of-life and palliative care service improvements, and the continued provision of nonbeneficial care, represent opportunities for improvements that would effectively increase ICU capacity without adding expensive space. Absent these efforts, scenarios will continue in which there exists little equipoise between those patients fortunate enough to already be admitted to the ICU who may not need to be, and those with conditions awaiting admission who clearly do.

Several studies have shown a direct impact on mortality associated with delays in admission to the ICU (Hall et al., 2018; Huang et al., 2010; Ofoma et al., 2020). Although multiple reasons were identified for admission delay, a consistent finding in each of these studies was that critical care units were at full capacity. The association of delayed admission to the ICU with increased mortality has also been shown across multiple specialties. In patients with respiratory failure, delays in admission to the ICU exceeding 1 hour were associated with increased mortality, length of stay, and duration of mechanical ventilation (Hsieh et al., 2017). Delays in admission to a critical care unit of as little as 6 hours have been associated with significantly increased mortality in critically ill surgical patients (Bing-Hua, 2014). In addition, the practice of "boarding" patients in the emergency department (ED) while awaiting an ICU bed yields significantly worse outcomes (e.g., including hospital mortality) across all patients and specialties (Boulain et al., 2020; Mohr et al., 2020). For patients on medical-surgical units who deteriorate and require transfer to an ICU, delays are also associated with adverse outcomes (Mardini et al., 2012; Young et al., 2003).

There are multiple reasons for delays in the availability of ICU beds, such as:

Inadequate numbers of ICU beds

Increases in demand (Mullins et al., 2013), such as those encountered in the ongoing pandemic of coronavirus disease of 2019 (COVID-19)

Staffing shortages across the interdisciplinary workforce of the ICU (Khanna et al., 2019)

Inefficiencies in the management of critical care resources

Lack of defined admission and discharge criteria (Kim et al., 2015)

Critical care units not directed by trained intensivists (Kim et al., 2018; Logani et al., 2011)

Critical care units in which capacity is affected by patients receiving nonbeneficial or potentially inappropriate care.

However, without regard to the specific causes of limited critical care capacity, there is little doubt that delays in access for patients who require the monitoring and treatment strategies uniquely available in an ICU are associated with increased risk for adverse outcomes, including death.

Nonbeneficial care

The term "futile care" is controversial, and much has been written about its meaning, assessment, and even the appropriateness of its use (Armstrong et al., 2014; Kon, 2018; Kon et al., 2016; Schneiderman, 2011; Truog & White, 2013). The terms "nonbeneficial care" and "potentially inappropriate treatment" are used in the context of this discussion only to note that the care of at least some patients in an ICU is, in the view of their physicians, care that prolongs life but does not achieve a meaningful benefit. It is in this group of patients that the failure to engage in end-of-life planning has direct and adverse second-order effects on those for whom timely admission to the ICU is foreclosed by unit occupancy.

In a study of 1,136 patients in which a total of 6,916 assessments were undertaken by 36 critical care specialists, 11% were perceived as receiving nonbeneficial treatment and a further 6.7% as probably receiving nonbeneficial treatment. It was further noted that of those perceived to be receiving nonbeneficial treatment, approximately 70% did not survive their hospital admission, 85% died within 6 months of discharge, and the survivors remained in severely compromised health states (e.g., placed in a long-term acute care facility and maintained on life-sustaining treatment; Huynh et al., 2013). A subsequent study of the incidence and duration of nonbeneficial care in end-of-life admissions in three Australian hospitals revealed that 12.1% of these patients received nonbeneficial care for a mean of 15 days, with 5.25 of these days in the ICU (Carter et al., 2017).

A seminal article, "The Opportunity Cost of Futile Treatment in the ICU," published in *Critical Care Medicine* in 2014 (Huynh et al., 2014), reported research that was the first to show that when nonbeneficial care is provided in an ICU, harm results in patients who might benefit from ICU care but whose admission is delayed because of the lack of beds. The study specifically examined the role that nonbeneficial care plays in the unavailability of beds to quantify the "opportunity costs" (i.e., the costs expressed in terms of measurably higher risks of complications and death) imposed on those critically ill patients whose opportunity for admission to an ICU was foreclosed by the lack of an available bed. The research was conducted across five ICUs in a single institution. Using a survey instrument, critical care clinicians identified patients receiving treatment that, in their opinion, would not result in benefit. The authors found that on 16% of days when an ICU was full, at least one patient was receiving nonbeneficial care. During those days, 33 patients were boarded in the ED for more than 4 hours, and nine patients waited more than 1 day to be transferred from an outside hospital, two of whom died while waiting for an available ICU bed. The authors described this as an unjust system in which patient access to intensive care is limited because ICU beds are occupied by patients receiving nonbeneficial care (Huynh et al., 2014): "The ethic of 'first come, first served' is not only inefficient and wasteful but it is also contrary to Medicine's responsibility to provide healthcare resources to best serve society" (Huynh et al., 2014, p. 1981).

Although the study had several limitations, it created a framework by which the second-order impacts of nonbeneficial care could be better understood. It is clear from this study that there is a group of patients, albeit difficult to objectively quantify, to whom care is being provided in the ICU that is viewed on clinical grounds as being nonbeneficial and whose contribution to ICU occupancy has a direct impact on the availability of critical care resources, often with adverse effect on the care of those waiting for a bed.

Factors with adverse effects on family/surrogate decision-makers

An essential skill critical to effective engagement with patients, families, and surrogate decision-makers in the ICU is the ability to communicate fluidly with them using verbal and nonverbal means. For example, identifying nonverbal cues during a conversation can be useful for directing an interaction, while at other times nonverbal cues can signal the need to end the conversation. One study revealed that half of the families of patients in the ICU experience inadequate communication with critical care physicians (Azoulay et al., 2000). Most family members and surrogates wish to discuss patient prognosis when discussing end-of-life issues with a physician (Apatira et al., 2008; Curtis & White, 2008). It is indeed concerning that one study reported that, after reviewing the content of discussions with families about end-of-life care, physicians failed to discuss prognosis for survival in over one third of the physician–family conferences and instead centered the conversation on limiting life support (White et al., 2007).

Communication skills, both verbal and nonverbal, are critical to providing comprehensive palliative care services. Poor communication skills, or the unwillingness to communicate with surrogates or families, effectively forecloses the provision of services designed to (1) minimize patient discomfort, (2) provide families with solace, (3) mitigate "optimism bias," and (4) lessen the likelihood of prolonged ICU stays and nonbeneficial care. Despite the importance of discussions with families about prognosis, functional outcomes, withdrawal of care, and palliative management, efforts at improvement employing a variety of methodologies have failed to yield consistent success. Neither (1) interventions using a quality improvement framework targeting clinicians, a well-proven and effective change methodology in the clinical setting (Curtis et al., 2011), nor (2) those that enlisted the support of palliative care teams (clinicians ostensibly well trained in communication skills appropriate to this setting) in providing informational and emotional support meetings for family surrogate decision-makers (Carson et al., 2016), yielded significant improvements in length of stay, time to withdrawal of mechanical ventilation, quality of death and dying assessments by families and nurses, or symptoms of anxiety and depression in family surrogate decision-makers.

Unfortunately, but not surprisingly, the two major predictors of failed efforts to provide appropriate end-of-life services to patients/families in the critical care environment—namely infrequent or inadequate discussion with surrogate decision-makers about patient prognosis and excessive optimism associated with recovery—have common causes but also common solutions (Schenker et al., 2012). The cause of both is the failure to effectively communicate with patients and surrogate decision-makers across all expected domains; the solution is to do it better.

The persistence of excessive optimism or "optimism bias" by surrogates has become a significant predictor and driver of failed efforts to involve palliative care early in a patient's management (Zier et al., 2012). White and colleagues (2016) described the prevalence and nature of factors resulting in discordance about prognosis between physicians and surrogate decision-makers, the most common source of which was a combination of misunderstanding and hopefulness. Excessive optimism is characterized by persistent and rigidly held beliefs that the patient will "fight" to survive, that the omnipotence of modern critical care practice will prevail (therapeutic optimism bias), or that having survived their previous near-death event, in some mystical fashion the patient will prevail in the current near-death rematch. The line between what is viewed as an "appropriate" amount of hope (and no less, lest one be accused of "giving up" too soon) and excessive optimism is vanishingly thin. Surrogate decision-makers possessed of optimism bias are entrenched in their belief in a patient's recovery and insist that "everything" be done (including invasive procedures) to ensure this outcome. This position may be maintained even at the cost of continued pain, fear, anxiety, and hopelessness in those for whom they are expected to advocate and despite the concordant assessment of multiple physicians that it is unethical to continue to perform painful interventions without counterbalancing benefit.

Not surprisingly, influences contributing to optimism bias include religion, faith, pre-illness quality of life, distrust of experts, and reliance on sources of information other than physicians. A recent report describing the causes of overly optimistic expectations with respect to prognosis by surrogate decision-makers and their consequences describes direct effects, including (1) significantly longer duration of ICU treatment among nonsurvivors before death, resulting in a 56% longer ICU length of stay and (2) a significantly longer time to withdrawal of life support among dying patients whose surrogates had unrealistically optimistic prognostic expectations compared with those who did not (White et al., 2019). It should be emphasized that although hope for recovery of a seriously ill or injured patient by families and surrogates is an appropriate and important coping behavior, when hope is transformed into a bias through which every care decision is interpreted, patients and their surrogate decision-makers may face dire consequences, including prolongation of invasive procedures without realistic prospects for recovery (Siegel, 2019).

Conversely, people who are disabled often experience the reverse effect: Rather than an "optimism bias," they may experience a "disability paradox." The "disability paradox" refers to the discrepancy between a higher self-reported quality of life by a disabled person and a lower quality of life perceived by their health care providers or supports. Historically, people with disabilities have experienced disparities in access to health care services, including lifesaving efforts (Lund & Ayers, 2020). This may be heightened during a time of medical rationing when personnel and equipment are both scarce and in high demand—such as during the COVID-19 pandemic. Systems of care, especially critical care, should be designed in a manner that is attentive to and has built-in safeguards to minimize the impact of these biases, which carry a very real risk of discrimination and potentially unethical decisions, especially during high-stress events (Andrews et al., 2021; Lund & Ayers, 2020).

The effects of unmanaged end-of-life issues on ICU occupancy are well described, and many of the challenges associated with their mitigation are well known (Gruenberg et al., 2006; Schwarze et al., 2014). However, an emerging barrier to engaging with patients and families in these decisions is the development of patient registries that report physician-specific outcomes, both publicly and to a variety of third-party entities. Many of these registries use 30-day mortality as the principal, and sometimes only, quality benchmark. A well-described consequence of its use as a proxy for quality, however, is that surgeons will recalibrate their threshold for performing all but emergent procedures based on their assessment of the postoperative mortality risk (Joynt et al., 2012). An excellent viewpoint article offers a short but compelling summary of likely effects associated with the use of this metric (Kupfer, 2013). Using 30-day mortality as the sole "goalpost" in defining quality of care and the single outcome measure for which surgeons were held accountable had immediate and significant impacts on the care of patients in the ICU. In patients whose postoperative course was complicated by clinical adversity, critical care management transitioned, in most cases without discussion, to one with a single-minded focus on this metric. An early casualty of this management paradigm is the preemption of do-not-resuscitate orders and consultation requests for palliative care services without the consent of certain surgeons or clinical services (D'Amico et al., 2009; Grant et al., 2014; Katz, 2018). The actions directed at reducing 30-day mortality following surgery were not limited to those undertaken in the postoperative period. Indeed, the willingness of some surgeons to perform higher-risk surgical procedures was conditioned on an "informal" agreement that the patient and family would not limit aggressive postoperative care or withdraw care in the event of postoperative complications (Schwarze et al., 2013). The proliferation of models that grade hospital performance and/or safety and that include mortality rates unadjusted for the effects of comorbidities, complications unrelated to a surgical procedure, and hospice or palliative care are likely to have both known and unknown effects on the role of palliative care in the critical care environment (Cassel et al., 2010).

Implications of end-of-life management on organ procurement

End-of-life concerns as they affect the care of patients considered candidates for organ procurement are, with several important exceptions, quite similar to those seen in patients who are not candidates. It is important to stress that end-of-life matters should not unduly influence or play an undesirable role in the initial management, ongoing resuscitation, and care of patients who later become candidates for organ procurement. Active care of the patient continues until a diagnosis of brain death is made or the legal next of kin requests a withdrawal of support. In those patients in whom injuries—frequently traumatic brain injuries—are catastrophic and progress to declaration of neurologic death, their potential for organ procurement and authorization to donate requires that any concerns should be prioritized for resolution as they arise. Intensivists caring for patients who are organ donors function within a compressed care timeline as it pertains to laboratory, diagnostic, and required medical procedures. Delays in care that unnecessarily extend the period of time between brain death determination and organ recovery risk interval hemodynamic instability, pneumonia, and other conditions that render some or all organs unsuitable for recovery and eventual transplant.

The Joint Commission and U.S. Department of Health and Human Services Centers for Medicare & Medicaid Services (CMS) have developed requirements for hospitals regarding identification of potential donors, evaluation of medical suitability, and approach for donation. Current Conditions of Participation require hospitals to notify in a timely manner the regional organ procurement organization (OPO) of all imminent and actual hospital deaths (Conditions of Participation for Hospitals, 1998). With respect to imminent death, this operationally translates into notification within 1 hour about patients who meet the hospital's clinical triggers indicating death is likely in those with severe neurologic injury. The regulation reserves solely to the OPO the determination of the medical suitability of any organ and, in the absence of alternative arrangement, the OPO will also determine medical suitability of potential tissue or eye donors (Conditions of Participation for Hospitals, 1998). It is important to note that the CMS Conditions of Participation explicitly state that only an OPO representative or designated requestor may approach the family of a potential donor for consent for organ, tissue, or eye donation (Conditions of Participation for Hospitals, 1998). The practical result of this section of the regulation is to remove physicians from the potential ethical conflict arising from the duality of roles—that is, as both a caregiver whose principal role is providing lifesaving interventions and that of an advocate for organ donation when that effort is seen to fail. Furthermore, although loved ones often have important questions and imminent psychological needs once a decision for organ donation is made, these are often addressed by social work or pastoral service providers working for the OPO as opposed to hospital-affiliated mental health professionals.

Lastly, the question of the intent of the patient upon death concerning organ donation is settled if they are registered or designated organ donors. How this is communicated following an incapacitating illness or injury varies from state to state, but it is commonly noted on an individual's driver's license, an advance directive, or via inquiry of a state's donor registry. The revocability of such a designation is also determined by applicable state law.

End-of-life considerations due to pandemic or disaster events

The recent SARS-CoV-2 pandemic has occasioned much discussion about the allocation of care to patients with COVID-19 in the face of resource constraints. Considerations arose mainly in response to concerns for surges in demand for ICU beds and ventilators exceeding the capacity to meet them.

Although the discussion about their implementation is recent, recognition of the need and planning for such a scenario has been ongoing for some time. Since Hurricane Katrina in 2005, 36 states have developed or are developing crisis standards of care (CSC) plans and the protocols underpinning their implementation in the event that restricted allocations of care are required by disasters or pandemic events.

In 2009, following the review of state-based plans for enacting CSC plans, the Institute of Medicine published the report "Guidance for Establishing Crisis Standards of Care for Use in Disaster Situations," which described the ethical framework upon which they relied as well as the essential elements required for successful implementation and acceptance. The American Medical Association endorsed these principles in the 2016 publication "Allocating Limited Health Care Resources: Code of Medical Ethics Opinion 11.1.3."

In broad terms, features common to most CSC plans include efforts to ensure that triage decisions and other modifications to clinical practice are not imposed upon individual clinicians, including triage and allocation processes that incorporate current evidence-based severity-of-illness scoring tools; shared decision-making by a "triage committee" or an equivalent body with representative membership; and limited scope for appeals of triage decisions.

The essential ethical elements applicable to all such plans or protocols include (1) a duty to care, (2) a duty to steward resources, (3) consistency in application, (4) demonstration of fairness, (5) transparency, (6) proportionality in their execution, and, finally, (7) provision of accountability of individual decisions and implementation of standards, as well as accountability of government entities. On June 12, 2020, in response to concerns for critical limitations in critical care capacity statewide due to a surge in the number of patients with COVID-19, statewide triage protocols for acute care facilities were implemented based on the Arizona Crisis Standards of Care Plan, 3rd edition (with addendum specific to COVID-19). At the time of writing this chapter, only Arizona had executed a CSC plan.

Impact of end-of-life issues in the ICU: problems or polarities

The manner in which end-of-life concerns are addressed in the complex critical care environment has remained a seemingly unsolvable feature of critical care practice for decades. Indeed, for an event that is foretold at birth and that will befall every inhabitant of the planet at some point, that consensus remains elusive is, at times, perplexing. More perplexing, however, is the persistence of efforts to mitigate the impact on critical care unit operations by using traditional problem-solving techniques in pursuit of a singular or best solution. The fact that there are no durable and broadly applicable interventions that result in the consistent mitigation of the impact of caring for the dying patient in the ICU, despite years of research and a voluminous body of scholarly publications on the subject, invites an alternative approach.

Mortality and end-of-life issues in the ICU are, quite simply, not problems for which there are singular or even best solutions. Rather, end-of-life issues in the ICU are best seen as "polarities," a characteristic of complex systems in which interdependent but opposing pairs of points of view or means of addressing a problem exist. An example of a polarity in contemporary critical care practice is that of ensuring that ICU resources are available to those who need them while respecting the right of autonomy of current patients or their surrogates who continue to hope for recovery even when unlikely, if not irrational. A system of care in which the benefits of admission to a critical care unit for patients whose recovery is likely, but for whom critical care is foreclosed by a full ICU, in part due to the provision of nonbeneficial or potentially inappropriate care to those whose improvement is vanishingly improbable, represent diametrically opposing positions. Polarities such as the one described and their means of mitigation are generally well known, affect patients and caregivers alike, and have persisted despite multiple well-intentioned efforts at remediation, the failure of which has rendered them even more resistant to subsequent improvement efforts.

Idealized proposed elements of an alternative model

Improvements in mitigating the impact of end-of-life issues in critical care have proven to be particularly difficult to devise, implement, and sustain. Reasons for this include the fact that they must occur in a setting of what is in effect a collision between two highly complex systems with frequently polarized perspectives regarding the role of the ICU. However, notwithstanding the challenges associated with efforts to improve the delivery of palliative and end-of-life services across the U.S. health care system, the impacts associated with not doing it well are far greater when they occur in a critical care unit than in less-intensive areas of the hospital. It is against this backdrop, and because of greater urgency in facilitating an alternative approach to the status quo occasioned by the recent COVID-19 pandemic, that the proposals are briefly outlined in Box 14.1. These ideas represent actionable improvements in renewed efforts to better manage the polarities at the core of palliative and end-of-life care in the ICU.

BOX 14.1.
ACTIONABLE SUGGESTIONS FOR IMPROVEMENT IN PALLIATIVE AND
END-OF-LIFE CARE ON THE ICU

Procedural and policy change
- Development of critical care/ICU policies that create procedures to deal more effectively with end-of-life care
- Trigger-directed proscriptive consultation and engagement of palliative care teams
- More integrated use of ethics committees and risk management
- Implementation of standards- and evidence-based approaches to communication for all members of the care team

Staffing
- Appropriate staffing of palliative care teams and processes
- Interdisciplinary and multicultural providers integrated on palliative care teams
- Recognition that an interdisciplinary approach is required that includes all stakeholders, especially psychologists and physicians working in collaboration

Prognosis-related issues
- Improved prospective prognostic toolsets
- Acceptance of imprecision but with more standardized communication of the real-world implications

Family/collateral/staff support
- Development of supportive care "step-down" capabilities within hospitals that, in the case of prognostic uncertainty, allow for continued though less aggressive care rather than the "all-or-nothing" approach currently typified by ICU discharge following end-of-life decisions
- Better and more humane management of biases in families, surrogates, and providers
- Better understanding and mitigation of the effects of outcome-based scorecard reporting on behaviors affecting determinations of surgical candidacy based on a priori assessments of the risk of complications or mortality
- More comprehensive and organized education and support for patients, providers, and families and surrogates

Conclusion

Identifying, understanding, and implementing measures to mitigate the impact of unmanaged end-of-life issues have been constant features of critical care practice for several decades. Most of the implemented improvements were developed and incorporated into the ICU workflow in a manner and over a period lacking a perception of urgency. By contrast, in the current critical care environment, a greater understanding of the direct adverse impacts that unit occupancy has on those patients who require specialty critical care but cannot access it has led to the need for practical and ethically appropriate solutions. These solutions must simultaneously address the role of unmanaged end-of-life care and nontherapeutic interventions in the availability of critical care resources. In the future, we hope that solutions will efficiently and effectively mobilize multiple resources within the interdisciplinary team while also advancing educational initiatives and psychological support for loved ones and staff members dealing with end-of-life issues.

References

American Medical Association. (2016). Allocating limited health care resources: Code of medical ethics opinion 11.1.3. https://www.ama-assn.org/delivering-care/ethics/allocating-limited-health-care-resources

Andrews, E. E., Ayers, K. B., Brown, K. S., Dunn, D. S., & Pilarski, C. R. (2021). No body is expendable: Medical rationing and disability justice during the COVID-19 pandemic. *American Psychologist, 76*(3), 451–461. http://dx.doi.org/10.1037/amp0000709

Apatira, L., Boyd, E. A., Malvar, G., Evans, L. R., Luce, J. M., Lo, B., & White, D. B. (2008). Hope, truth, and preparing for death: Perspectives of surrogate decision makers. *Annals of Internal Medicine, 149*(12), 861–868. https://doi.org/10.7326/0003-4819-149-12-200812160-00005

Armstrong, M. H., Poku, J. K., & Burkle, C. M. (2014). Medical futility and nonbeneficial interventions: An algorithm to aid clinicians. *Mayo Clinic Proceedings, 89*(12), 1599. doi:10.1016/j.mayocp.2014.08.017

Azoulay, E., Chevret, S., Leleu, G., Pochard, F., Barboteu, M., Adrie, C., & Schlemmer, B. (2000). Half the families of intensive care unit patients experience inadequate communication with physicians. *Critical Care Medicine, 28*(8), 3044–3049. doi:10.1097/00003246-200008000-00061

Barrett, M. L., Smith, M. W., Elixhauser, A., Honigman, L. S., & Pines, J. M. (2014). Utilization of intensive care services, 2011. Statistical Brief #185. Healthcare Cost and Utilization Project. Agency for Healthcare Research and Quality. November 2014. http://hcup-us.ahrq.gov/reports/statbriefs/sb185-Hospital-Intensive-Care-Units-2011.jsp. Accessed 19 March 2020. *Association, 308*(14), 1460–1468.

Bing-Hua, Y. U. (2014). Delayed admission to the intensive care unit for critically surgical patients is associated with increased mortality. *American Journal of Surgery, 208*(2), 268–274. https://doi.org/10.1016/j.amjsurg.2013.08.044

Boulain, T., Malet, A., & Maitre, O. (2020). Association between long boarding time in the emergency department and hospital mortality: A single-center propensity score-based analysis. *Internal Emergency Medicine, 15*(3), 479–489. doi:10.1007/s11739-019-02231-z

Carson, S. S., Cox, C. E., Wallenstein, S., Hanson, L. C., Danis, M., Tulsky, J. A., . . . Nelson, J. E. (2016). Effect of palliative care–led meetings for families of patients with chronic critical illness: A randomized clinical trial. *Journal of the American Medical Association, 316*(1), 51–62. doi:10.1001/jama.2016.8474

Carter, H. E., Winch, S., Barnett, A. G., Parker, M., Gallois, C., Willmott, L., . . . Graves, N. (2017). Incidence, duration and cost of futile treatment in end-of-life hospital admissions to three Australian public-sector tertiary hospitals: A retrospective multicentre cohort study. *BMJ Open, 7*(10), e017661. doi:10.1136/bmjopen-2017-017661

Cassel, J. B., Jones, A. B., Meier, D. E., Smith, T. J., Spragens, L. H., & Weissman, D. (2010). Hospital mortality rates: How is palliative care taken into account? *Journal of Pain and Symptom Management, 40*(6), 914–925. https://doi.org/10.1016/j.jpainsymman.2010.07.005

Conditions of Participation for Hospitals, 42 CFR § 482.45 (1998). https://www.govinfo.gov/app/details/CFR-2010-title42-vol5/CFR-2010-title42-vol5-sec482-45

Crippen, D., & Whetstine, L. (1999). ICU resource allocation: Life in the fast lane. *Critical Care, 3*(4), R47–R51. doi:10.1186/cc354

Curtis, J. R., Nielsen, E. L., Treece, P. D., Downey, L., Dotolo, D., Shannon, S. E., . . . Engelberg, R. A. (2011). Effect of a quality-improvement intervention on end-of-life care in the intensive care unit: A randomized trial. *American Journal of Respiratory and Critical Care Medicine, 183*(3), 348–355. doi:10.1164/rccm.201006-1004OC

Curtis, J. R., & White, D. B. (2008). Practical guidance for evidence-based ICU family conferences. *Chest, 134*(4), 835–843. doi:10.1378/chest.08-0235

D'Amico, T., Krasna, M., Krasna, D., & Sade, R., (2009). No heroic measures: How soon is too soon to stop? *Annals of Thoracic Surgery, 87*(1), 11–18. doi:10.1016/j.athoracsur.2008.09.075

Finucane, T. E. (1999). How gravely ill becomes dying: A key to end-of-life care. *Journal of the American Medical Association, 282*(17), 1670–1672. doi:10.1001/jama.282.17.1670

Grant, S. B., Modi, P. K., & Singer, E. A. (2014). Futility and the care of surgical patients: Ethical dilemmas. *World Journal of Surgery, 38*(7), 1631–1637. doi:10.1007/s00268-014-2592-1

Gruenberg, D. A., Shelton, W., Rose, S. L., Rutter, A. E., Socaris, S., & McGee, G. (2006). Factors influencing length of stay in the intensive care unit. *American Journal of Critical Care, 15*(5), 502–509. doi:10.4037/ajcc2006.15.5.502

Hall, A. M., Stelfox, H. T., Wang, X., Chen, G., Zuege, D. J., Dodek, P., . . . Bagshaw, S. M. (2018). Association between afterhours admission to the intensive care unit, strained capacity, and mortality: A retrospective cohort study. *Critical Care, 22*(1), 97. doi:10.1186/s13054-018-2027-8

Halpern, N. A., Pastores, S. M., Thaler, H. T., & Greenstein, R. J. (2006). Changes in critical care beds and occupancy in the United States 1985–2000: Differences attributable to hospital size. *Critical Care Medicine, 34*(8), 2105–2112.

Hsieh, C., Lee, C-C, Hsu, H., Shih, H-I, Lu, C., & Lin, C. (2017). Impact of delayed admission to intensive care units on patients with acute respiratory failure. *American Journal of Emergency Medicine, 35*(1), 39–44. doi:10.1016/j.ajem.2016.09.066

Huang, Q., Thind, A., Dreyer, J. F., & Zaric, G. S. (2010). The impact of delays to admission from the emergency department on inpatient outcomes. *BMC Emergency Medicine, 10*, 16. doi:0.1186/1471-227X-10-16

Huynh, T. N., Kleerup, E. C., Raj, P. P., & Wenger, N. S. (2014). The opportunity cost of futile treatment in the ICU. *Critical Care Medicine, 42*(9), 1977–1982. 10.1097/CCM.0000000000000402

Huynh, T. N., Kleerup, E. C., Wiley, J. F., Savitsky, T. D., Guse, D., Garber, B. J., & Wenger, N. S. (2013). The frequency and cost of treatment perceived to be futile in critical care. *JAMA Internal Medicine, 173*(20), 1887. doi:10.1001/jamainternmed.2013.10261

Institute of Medicine. (2009). *Guidance for establishing crisis standards of care for use in disaster situations: A letter report.* National Academies Press. doi:10.17226/12749

Joynt, K., Blumenthal, D. M., John Orav, E., Resnic, F. S., & Jha, A. K. (2012). Association of Public Reporting for Percutaneous Coronary Intervention With Utilization and Outcomes Among Medicare Beneficiaries With Acute Myocardial Infarction. *JAMA, the Journal of the American Medical Association, 308*(14), 1460–1468.

Katz, N. M. (2018). The term "supportive care" is preferable to "palliative care" for consults in the cardiothoracic intensive care unit. *Journal of Thoracic and Cardiovascular Surgery, 155*(5), 2030–2031. https://doi.org/10.1016/j.jtcvs.2017.12.117

Khandelwal, N., Kross, E. K., Engelberg, R. A., Coe, N. B., Long, A. C. & Curtis, J. R. (2015). Estimating the effect of palliative care interventions and advance care planning on ICU utilization. *Critical Care Medicine, 43*(5), 1102–1111. https://doi.org/10.1097/ccm.0000000000000852

Khanna, A. K., Majesko, A. A., Johansson, M. K., Rappold, J. F., Meissen, H. H., & Pastores, S. M. (2019). The multidisciplinary critical care workforce: An update from SCCM. https://www.sccm.org/Communications/Critical-Connections/Archives/2019/The-Multidisciplinary-Critical-Care-Workforce-An

Kim, J. E., Lee, S., Jeong, J., Lee, D. H., & Jeong, J. (2018). Intensive care unit admission protocol controlled by intensivists can reduce transfer delays from the emergency department in critically ill patients. *Hong Kong Journal of Emergency Medicine, 26*(2), 84–90. doi:10.1177/1024907918789284

Kim, S., Chan, C. W., Olivares, M., & Escobar, G. (2015). ICU admission control: An empirical study of capacity allocation and its implication for patient outcomes. *Management Science, 61*(1), 19–38. doi:10.1287/mnsc.2014.2057

Kon, A. A. (2018). Futile and potentially inappropriate interventions: Semantics matter. *Perspectives in Biology and Medicine, 60*(3), 383–389. doi:10.1353/pbm.2018.0012

Kon, A. A., Shepard, E. K., Sederstrom, N. O., Swoboda, S. M., Marshall, M. F., Birriel, B., & Rincon, F. (2016). Defining futile and potentially inappropriate interventions: A policy statement from the Society of Critical Care Medicine ethics committee. *Critical Care Medicine, 44*(9), 1769–1774. doi:10.1097/CCM.0000000000001965

Kupfer, J. M. (2013). The morality of using mortality as a financial incentive: Unintended consequences and implications for acute hospital care. *Journal of the American Medical Association, 309*(21), 2213–2214. doi:10.1001/jama.2013.5009

Logani, S., Green, A., & Gasperino, J. (2011). Benefits of high-intensity intensive care unit physician staffing under the Affordable Care Act. *Critical Care Research and Practice, 2011*, 170814. doi:10.1155/2011/170814

Lund, E. M., & Ayers, K. B. (2020). Raising awareness of disabled lives and healthcare rationing during the COVID-19 pandemic. *Psychological Trauma: Theory, Research, Practice, and Policy, 12*(S1), S210–S211. https://doi.org/10.1037/tra0000673

Mardini, L., Lipes, J., & Jayaraman, D. (2012). Adverse outcomes associated with delayed intensive care consultation in medical and surgical inpatients. *Journal of Critical Care, 27*(6), 688–693. doi:10.1016/j.jcrc.2012.04.011

Mohr, N., Wessman, B., Bassin, B., Elie-Turenne, M., Ellender, T., Emlet, L., Ginsberg, Z., Gunnerson, K., Jones, K., Kram, B., Marcolini, E., & Rudy, S.(2020). Boarding of critically Ill patients in the emergency department. *Journal of the American College of Emergency Physicians Open, 1*(4), 423–431. https://doi-org.proxy1.cl.msu.edu/10.1002/emp2.12107

Mosenthal, A. C. (2002). Managing death in the intensive care unit: The transition from cure to comfort. *Journal of Pain and Symptom Management, 23*(1), 83–84. doi:10.1016/S0885-3924(01)00382-7

Mullins, P. M., Goyal, M., Pines, J. M., & Gerson, L. (2013). National growth in intensive care unit admissions from emergency departments in the United States from 2002 to 2009. *Academic Emergency Medicine, 20*(5), 479–486. https://doi.org/10.1111/acem.12134

Ofoma, U. R., Montoya, J., Saha, D., Berger, A., Kirchner, H. L., McIlwaine, J. K., & Kethireddy, S. (2020). Associations between hospital occupancy, intensive care unit transfer delay and hospital mortality. *Journal of Critical Care, 58*, 48–55. doi:10.1016/j.jcrc.2020.04.009

Roczen, M. L., White, K. R., & Epstein, E. G. (2016). Palliative care and intensive care units. *Journal of Hospice & Palliative Nursing, 18*(3), 201–211. doi:10.1097/NJH.0000000000000218

Schenker, Y., Tiver, G. A., Hong, S. Y., & White, D. B. (2012). Association between physicians' beliefs and the option of comfort care for critically ill patients. *Intensive Care Medicine, 38*(10), 1607–1615. doi:10.1007/s00134-012-2671-4

Schneiderman, L. J. (2011). Defining medical futility and improving medical care. *Journal of Bioethical Inquiry, 8*(2), 123–131. doi:10.1007/s11673-011-9293-3

Schwarze, M. L., Brasel, K. J., & Mosenthal, A. C. (2014). Beyond 30-day mortality: Aligning surgical quality with outcomes that patients value. *JAMA Surgery, 149*(7), 631–632. https://doi.org/10.1001/jamasurg.2013.5143

Schwarze, M. L., Redmann, A. J., Alexander, G. C., & Brasel, K. J. (2013). Surgeons expect patients to buy in to postoperative life support preoperatively: Results of a national survey. *Critical Care Medicine, 41*(1), 1–8. https://doi.org/10.1097/CCM.0b013e31826a4650

Siegel, M. D. (2019). The unintended consequences of hope. *Critical Care Medicine, 47*(9), 1267–1268. https://doi.org/10.1097/CCM.0000000000003878

Society of Critical Care Medicine. (2020, May 12). United States resource availability for COVID-19. https://www.sccm.org/Blog/March-2020/United-States-Resource-Availability-for-COVID-19

Truog, R. D., Campbell, M. L., Curtis, J. R., Haas, C. E., Luce, J. M., Rubenfeld, G. D., & Kaufman, D. C. (2008). Recommendations for end-of-life care in the intensive care unit: A consensus statement by the American College of Critical Care Medicine. *Critical Care Medicine, 36*(3), 953–963. https://doi.org/10.1097/ccm.0b013e3181659096

Truog, R. D., & White, D. B. (2013). Futile treatments in intensive care units. *JAMA Internal Medicine, 173*(20), 1894. doi:10.1001/jamainternmed.2013.7098

Wallace, D. J., Angus, D. C., Seymour, C. W., Barnato, A. E., & Kahn, J. M. (2015). Critical care bed growth in the United States: A comparison of regional and national trends. *American Journal of Respiratory and Critical Care Medicine, 191*(4), 410–416. doi:10.1164/rccm.201409-1746oc

White, D. B., Carson, S., Anderson, W., Steingrub, J., Bird, G., Curtis, J. R., . . . Hough, C. L. (2019). A multicenter study of the causes and consequences of optimistic expectations about prognosis by surrogate decision-makers in ICUs. *Critical Care Medicine, 47*(9), 1184–1193. https://doi.org/10.1097/CCM.0000000000003807

White, D. B., Engelberg, R. A., Wenrich, M. D., Lo, B., & Curtis, J. R. (2007). Prognostication during physician–family discussions about limiting life support in intensive care units. *Critical Care Medicine, 35*(2), 442–448. https://doi.org/10.1097/01.ccm.0000254723.28270.14

White, D. B., Ernecoff, N., Buddadhumaruk, P., Hong, S., Weissfeld, L., Curtis, J. R., . . . Lo, B. (2016). Prevalence of and factors related to discordance about prognosis between physicians and surrogate decision makers of critically ill patients. *Journal of the American Medical Association, 315*(19), 2086–2094. https://doi.org/10.1001/jama.2016.5351

Wunsch, H., Wagner, J., Herlim, M., Chong, D. H., Kramer, A. A., & Halpern, S. D. (2013). ICU occupancy and mechanical ventilator use in the United States. *Critical Care Medicine, 41*(12), 2712–2719. https://doi.org/10.1097/CCM.0b013e318298a139

Young, M. P., Gooder, V. J., McBride, K., James, B., & Fisher, E. S. (2003). Inpatient transfers to the intensive care unit: Delays are associated with increased mortality and morbidity. *Journal of General Internal Medicine, 18*(2), 77–83. doi:10.1046/j.1525-1497.2003.20441.x

Zier, L. S., Sottile, P. D., Hong, S. Y., Weissfield, L. A., & White, D. B. (2012). Surrogate decision makers' interpretation of prognostic information: A mixed methods study. *Annals of Internal Medicine, 156*(5), 360–366.

15 Ethical Considerations in Psychological Consultation to Critical Care Settings

Alan Lewandowski, Brighid Fronapfel, Jack Spector,
Kirk Szczepkowski, and Scott Davidson

Introduction

This chapter discusses the role of the specialist psychologist with interdisciplinary consultation and treatment teams on critical and intensive care units. In particular, the focus is on the ethical quandaries faced by psychologists in such settings and a mechanism for approaching what ethical conflicts may occur. Case examples are provided, each exemplifying one of the American Psychological Association (APA) ethical standards, and a model for ethical psychological consultation in critical care settings is proposed.

The dynamic and complex nature of a critical care unit (CCU), intensive care unit (ICU), or trauma care unit (TCU) can constitute a challenging environment for psychologists, especially if they have not had prior exposure and formal training in hospital consultation and liaison work. Unfortunately, most training programs in psychology do not typically include rotations in intensive care settings. As a result, patient consultations to a critical, intensive, or trauma care unit may be intimidating or confusing, particularly when ethical dilemmas arise (Self et al.,

Alan Lewandowski, Brighid Fronapfel, Jack Spector, Kirk Szczepkowski, and Scott Davidson, *Ethical Considerations in Psychological Consultation to Critical Care Settings* In: *Critical Care Psychology and Rehabilitation*. Edited by: Kirk J. Stucky and Jennifer E. Jutte, Oxford University Press. © Oxford University Press 2022. DOI: 10.1093/oso/9780190077013.003.0015

2018). Nevertheless, it is our position that by the nature of their training in interpersonal and behavioral interventions and their understanding of psychopathology, psychology specialists (e.g., rehabilitation psychologists, health psychologists, and neuropsychologists) can offer both clinical and ethical assistance in the highly stressful CCU environment.

Given the patient population and medical factors requiring hospitalization, the ethical dilemmas that occur when providing psychological consultation to the CCU are quite different compared to those arising in traditional outpatient medical clinics or inpatient psychiatric settings (Bibler & Miller, 2019; Moon & Kim, 2015). Injury from trauma is the fifth leading cause of mortality in the United States and the leading cause of death for those 45 years old or younger (Rhee et al., 2014; Søreide, 2009). Multiple critical care injuries (polytrauma) represent approximately 40% of admissions to hospitals (Bach et al., 2017). Further, critical care hospitalizations for patients older than age 65 presenting with heart failure, cardiac disorders, diabetes complications, pulmonary disease, and liver failure account for approximately 46% of ICU admissions. Not surprisingly, the preexisting medical comorbidities of advanced age are a considerable risk factor, particularly in those older than 75 years of age (Fuchs et al., 2012). However, as the patient population ages, geriatric trauma has grown significantly and now makes up greater than 20% of trauma admissions to the CCU (Llompart-Pou et al., 2017).

Compared to traditional areas of clinical service, psychological practice with patients who have life-threatening conditions and who are hospitalized on a CCU, ICU, or TCU can be very stressful, requiring time-sensitive decisions that can produce distinct ethical concerns challenging one's knowledge of prevailing ethical standards (Firn et al., 2020). As a result, psychologists need to be mindful that ethical practice (rather than the practice of ethics) is not a static process and that ethics are shaped over time by social and societal changes, technological and medical treatment advances, and modifications to state regulations and statutes.

The ethical practice of psychology is also complicated by the fact that ethical dilemmas in critical care settings are not always clear-cut, especially in an interdisciplinary environment that requires interdependent collaboration instead of autonomy as well as varying professional expertise and levels of responsibility for patient care (Rose, 2011). Further complicating factors include the complexity of patient illnesses, injuries, and comorbidities; rapidly changing medical demands in response to patient status; interprofessional collaboration; varying technical skills among health care specialists; institutional procedures and guidelines; and potential conflicting demands from patients' families or between caregivers. Additional, but no less important, variables include personal, cultural, and religious beliefs.

Psychology consultation in critical care

The primary focus of critical care is the emergent medical stabilization of the patient. As a result, the cognitive, emotional, and psychological needs of the patient and family members are understandably a secondary consideration and may not be immediately addressed, if at all (Turner-Cobb et al., 2016). Ethically, this is of concern, as the impact of trauma or critical illness on a patient's mental status can be more disabling than the residual physical deficits associated with the injury or illness in question. This is particularly true when considering that cognitive and emotional recovery from many diseases, illnesses, and injuries can continue for years after the primary symptoms have been addressed (Azoulay et al., 2017; Khan et al., 2003). Consequently, the impact of long-term medical and psychological consequences can significantly decrease the probability of returning to one's pre-injury status (da Costa et al., 2019; Griffith et al., 2020; Richmond et al., 2009).

Providing competent psychological care to patients in a critical care setting is a privilege that can offer a great deal of personal and professional satisfaction. Consulting to a critical care team offers the opportunity to work closely with professionals of different health care disciplines and apply the principles of behavior to medically complex cases, assisting with patient diagnosis, treatment, and disposition within a relatively short period of time (Ervin et al., 2018). More than practice building, the interdisciplinary collaboration available in a critical care setting allows for the kind of professional fulfillment and collegial bonding that one can only experience in similar high-intensity environments that challenge ethical practice (e.g., the U.S. military's command consultation process) (Howe & Jones, 1994; Hunter & Goodie, 2010; Williams & Kennedy, 2011).

Unlike many clinical and academic settings, the intensity in any critical care setting naturally leads to a mutually wary and perhaps prolonged process of integrating into the interdisciplinary team (Donovan et al., 2018). Over a period of time and through participating in daily rounds, formal and informal consultations, providing pressing examinations, expediting clinical referrals, and assisting in urgent dispositions, psychologists joining a critical care team can expect challenges to their clinical skills, sensitivity to group structure, commitment to the highest level of patient care, and willingness to commit to the team and the process.

In the early stages of integration, it is not unusual for a clinician to be tested with difficult and complex cases complicated by diagnostic dilemmas, overinvolved family members, and demanding disposition requirements. In these situations, psychologists are judged by how well they solve problems as much as by their diagnostic acumen and clinical skills. Over time, once they have consistently demonstrated their value and have been accepted by the team, psychologists may be afforded a high level of status commensurate with the medical providers, and therefore accorded a high level of trust that can include the discernment of ethical dilemmas. However, with this trust comes a high level of responsibility.

For many critical care teams, the psychologist may be the only specialist with both cognitive and emotional-behavioral expertise. The psychologist's involvement can increase treatment success by improving intensivists' ability to address a patient's physical and psychological needs (Torrence et al., 2014). Unlike neurologists, physiatrists, and psychiatrists, who have frequent interactions and conjoint training or teaching with psychologists and neuropsychologists, intensivists and trauma surgeons may have little past experience with psychological evaluations or neuropsychological consultations (Tremont et al., 2002). Therefore, physicians may have difficulty accurately appreciating and discerning the quality of the psychologist's prior training and the accuracy of the psychologist's diagnoses, clinical skills, or treatment recommendations.

In such an environment, undertrained, inexperienced, or incompetent (if well-meaning) clinicians can unintentionally do a great deal of harm (McDaniel et al., 2014). It is not uncommon for a psychologist to join a team of other clinicians and allied health professionals with varying levels of expertise (e.g., speech and language pathologists, social workers, occupational and physical therapists, counselors, or even art or recreation therapists) who have already gone through the acculturation process with respect to joining the critical care team. Dealing with scientifically questionable interpretations, recommendations, or interventions from other clinicians, including other psychologists, can pose a hazard to the psychologist's own place on the team. The degree of sensitivity and tact that a psychologist must exercise in navigating team dynamics under such circumstances cannot be underestimated.

Psychological care as part of an interdisciplinary team

Most psychologists are familiar with primary care providers and secondary care physician specialists who practice in outpatient and local or community hospital settings. However, unless they have had specific training, they are likely unacquainted with the highly specialized procedures, treatments, medical equipment, protocols, and clinician expertise provided by interdisciplinary clinical teams in a tertiary care setting such as a level 1 or 2 trauma center that monitors and treats the most severely injured or ill patients with life-threatening conditions.

While there is no standard template, the interdisciplinary composition of a critical care or trauma health care team includes intensivist and non-intensivist physicians or surgeons; residents in training; advanced practice providers, such as a nurse practitioner and physician assistant; critical care nurses; and clinicians from pharmacy, medical social work, dietetics, occupational and/or physical therapy, and spiritual care (Ervin et al., 2018; Strasser et al., 2008). As opposed to an outside consultant, a psychologist integrated into the fabric of the critical care team is involved in the day-to-day responsibilities of the ICU and the patients whose rapidly changing status and complex care they are tasked to manage (Donovan et al., 2018). Even though there is some degree of overlap between disciplines, the collaborative communication and clinical observations between team members result in reduced mortality and improved patient outcome (Costa et al., 2018; Fleisher, 2010; Kim et al., 2010; Yoo et al., 2016).

Professional ethics and critical care consultation

Why, then, is it so important to consider ethics when consulting in a critical care setting?

First, regardless of the setting, adherence to sound ethical practice is fundamental to psychological service delivery; professional standards provide direction when resolving clinical questions with conflicting values (Fisher, 2017). However, more than just a set of guidelines for clinical practice, ethical thinking and behavior in critical care reflect a process of discernment that balances a patient's personal needs, self-determination, privacy, and decisional capacity with that which is judged medically best for the person and their caregivers while protecting the patient from unnecessary or ineffective psychological treatment. Given the acute and urgent nature of hospital-based trauma and critical care medicine—in particular the daily consideration of matters literally involving life and death—perhaps no other medical setting presents more pressing ethical challenges for psychologists.

Second, as members of a hospital interdisciplinary team, psychologists must not only know their own ethical code of conduct but must demonstrate that knowledge and skillset in everyday practice with allied health professionals and both medical and administrative colleagues (Dobmeyer & Rowan, 2014). Psychological ethics in critical care are not simply a matter of how one thinks; rather, they encompass interpersonal skills, commitment to a team, acting professionally and within the scope of one's training, assessing clinical data objectively, and contributing in a conscientious manner to the team's overall care of patients in life-threatening circumstances.

Lastly, ethics are fundamental to psychological treatment in critical care because of the impact of critical illness or injuries on patients and their families (Meunier-Beillard et al., 2017; Rose et al., 2019). When patients are admitted to an intensive care setting, they are, by definition, in a helpless state (Quenot et al., 2017), and it is incumbent on the psychologist to remain mindful of this vulnerability. Consider this high-intensity medical environment from a psychological perspective. Regardless of the cause of the injury or illness, patients are admitted because they are generally in a perilous and unstable physical state with an uncertain medical outcome. Whether patients are conscious or unconscious, their family members are likely experiencing significant emotional distress (Goldberg et al., 2020; Johnson et al., 2019; Pochard et al., 2005). Because of varying levels of incapacity, family members often become the patient's representatives for medical care, and both the patient and the caregivers are quickly confronted with an enormous amount of information (Beesley & Brown, 2020). The abrupt loss of the patient's autonomy enhances a caregiver's sense of vulnerability as questions are posed and information is provided about changing medical status, technical procedures, medications, surgical interventions, and even life support. This proxy medical decision-making often occurs with limited time for discernment and is complicated by worry and fear, despair, and food and sleep deprivation (de Jong et al., 2020). The shifting array of specialists from multiple medical teams representing wide-ranging levels of expertise and speaking in unfamiliar technical language makes circumstances even more confusing, particularly if families receive conflicting reports from clinicians or have different perceptions of the information provided to them.

The complexity of an ICU requires that patients and their family members relinquish control, surrender a certain level of critical judgment, make decisions quickly, and interact with care providers who have limited time in hopes of making the correct decision about matters that are serious at best and that have life-and-death implications at worst (Shannon, 2001; Wendler, 2019). This unfamiliar environment, which is highly emotionally charged and where the consequences can be dire, can create unanticipated ethical dilemmas outside those of a typical outpatient clinical practice (Stucky & Warren, 2019). Thus, while psychologists should always strive to engage in ethical practice, this is particularly important when dealing with vulnerable populations such as those encountered in critical care settings (Pittaway et al., 2010; Quest & Marco, 2003).

Codes of ethics

Ethical standards guiding patient care are not unique to psychology. Ethical codes have been established by multiple mental health, medical, and medically related disciplines and specialties that include osteopathic and allopathic medicine, nursing, psychiatry, physical and occupational therapy, speech therapy and audiology, social work, and pharmacy (American Academy of Physicians Assistants [AAPA], 2013; American Medical Association [AMA], 2001, 2016; American Nurses Association

[ANA], 2015; American Occupational Therapy Association [AOTA], 2015; American Osteopathic Association [AOA], 2016a, 2016b; American Pharmacists Association, 1994; American Physical Therapy Association, 2019; American Psychiatric Association, 2013; American Speech-Language-Hearing Association [ASHA], 2016; National Association of Social Workers [NASW], 2017).

Most medical and allied medical professions address the difference between principles and standards and endorse common themes that include beneficence, nonmaleficence, integrity, responsibility, fidelity, respect of patient's dignity and rights, competence, human relations or interactions, confidentiality or privacy issues, training or education, and research. Although there are differences among disciplines, the common theme is one of responsible behavior consistent with the respective profession's standards (Baum et al., 2009).

Physicians of the AMA and the AOA share the same ethical principles and emphasize patient–physician relationships, consent, communication and decision-making, privacy, confidentiality and medical recordkeeping, self-regulation, and research. Similar to psychology, in their shared codes, the AMA and AOA address conceptual ethical issues such as confidentiality, honesty, trust, respect, nondiscrimination, abandonment of care, promotion of scientific knowledge and competence, self-regulation, advertisement and designation of credentials, resolution of disputes, adherence to the law, and misconduct regarding sexual contact, harassment, and misrepresentation of research. Dissimilar to psychology, but not surprisingly given the obligations of physical medicine, the AMA and AOA also provide supplemental guidance on medical innovations, reproductive medicine, end-of-life issues, organ procurement and transplantation, and influence from the medical industry, as well as recognizing that circumstances may occur in which physicians must act in the absence of complete information (AMA, 2016; AOA, 2016a, 2016b).

With respect to allied health professionals, the ANA's ethics principles endorse justice, beneficence, nonmaleficence, accountability, fidelity, autonomy, and veracity (ANA, 2015), whereas the AOTA emphasizes altruism, equality, freedom, justice, dignity, truth, and prudence (AOTA, 2015). ASHA endorses four primary principles under the areas of competence and responsibility (ASHA, 2016, p. 2). The AAPA, ANA, and NASW also include the importance of recognizing cultural and social diversity (AAPA, 2013; ANA, 2015; NASW, 2017).

Regardless of the profession or medical specialty, the purpose of ethical standards across professions is generally the same. Codes of conduct establish agreed-upon standards among members of that discipline that serve as the basis to guide behavior toward sound decision-making. Ethical guidelines establish clear parameters by which a discipline defines its values and principles, associates them with professional conduct, and thereby holds members of that profession accountable for their conduct (Baum et al., 2009; Firn et al., 2020).

Ethical behavior is a manifestation of moral character and mindful deliberation (Hogan, 1973; Lewandowski, 2012). The importance of ethical standards rests in their ability to provide clarification of moral action by defining constraints and boundaries of behavior for members of a particular discipline. Ethical guidelines not only provide a basis for the standards of care of one's patients but also extend to their families and interactions with other clinical professionals, allied health providers, and those involved in medical administration and management. As principles that guide one's decision-making, they encompass more complex and higher-order issues that often arise in an ICU such as clinical competency, accuracy in recording clinical observations, timeliness in recordkeeping, confidentiality, and supervision.

Psychological ethics in critical care consultation

For psychologists, the APA's Ethical Principles of Psychologists and Code of Conduct (EPPCC) is the primary source for ethical guidance, whether one is engaged in clinical practice, academics, consultation, or administration (APA, 2017). Compared to the ethical codes of other disciplines, the 1953 code was data-driven in that it was based on an analysis of the content of actual ethical vignettes (e.g., publication credits, misrepresentation of findings) submitted by over 2,000 psychologists (Smith, 2003). Having been revised several times and continually updated, it is the one document that provides definitions of ethical behavior pertaining to the contemporary practice of psychology. By embracing the EPPCC, psychologists demonstrate a commitment to practicing the science of psychology in a manner that requires critical thinking and behavioral self-discernment.

The EPPCC provides psychologists with a framework that guides professional decision-making and encompasses both aspirational values and standards of behavior. At times it overlaps with individual state laws that regulate psychology practice, but more so, it serves as a tool that informs and educates psychologists, other medical or nonmedical professionals, students in training, and the public. The EPPCC has undergone several revisions, each of which set the highest standards for professional psychology based on research and practice as well as consensus among clinicians and providers, and with respect to professional and social norms and mores. In short, the ethics code establishes psychology's integrity as a profession (Fisher, 2017).

General principles of the APA ethics code

Prior to defining enforceable standards, the APA ethics code first describes five general principles from which enforceable standards are derived. Consistent with other ethics codes (AAPA, 2013; AMA, 2016; ANA, 2015; NASW, 2017), these principles serve as an aspirational guide for psychological decision-making based on moral values; their intent is to guide psychologists toward the very highest ethical ideals of the profession (APA, 2017). The five general principles are:

A. Beneficence and Nonmaleficence
B. Fidelity and Responsibility
C. Integrity
D. Justice
E. Respect for People's Rights and Dignity (APA, 2017, pp. 3–4).

Principle A, Beneficence and Nonmaleficence, emphasizes a psychologist's obligation to behave responsibly and competently to promote others' welfare and to do no harm, while Principle B, Fidelity and Responsibility, gives prominence to establishing trust, maintaining professional standards, and accepting responsibility for one's actions. Principle C, Integrity, requires demonstrating one's commitment through honest and unbiased practice, particularly with vulnerable populations, whereas Principle D, Justice, encourages recognition of social, cultural, religious, or financial variables that affect impartiality. Lastly, Principle E, Respect for People's Rights and Dignity, emphasizes the importance of privacy, decisional capacity, role differences, and autonomy of diverse groups helped by psychologists.

Ethical standards of the APA ethics code

In contrast to the five aspirational general principles, the 10 ethical standards of the EPPCC are prescriptive—that is, they are directives intended to protect patients or clients by providing specific guidance as to what a psychologist is required to do (or avoid) in the course of practice. Violating these can result in formal complaints, educational or administrative actions, sanctions, or even losing one's license to practice.

STANDARD 1: RESOLVING ETHICAL ISSUES

Standard 1 addresses the misuse or misrepresentation of a psychologist's work, disagreements with legal regulations and authorities, conflicts with organizations, pursuing informal resolutions referring to state or national ethics panels or state licensing agencies, cooperating with ethics investigations, addressing reckless complaints, and discrimination from filing or being a person of interest in an ethical complaint (APA, 2017, pp. 4–5).

Given the variety of ethical codes and standards of practice pertaining to the different professionals involved in critical care settings, psychologists may be required to address questions regarding their own conduct or to confront questions about the ethical practices of other members of the treatment team. For example, a psychologist's work could be misused by other team members or misrepresented by hospital administration. Accordingly, psychologists should ensure that the critical care team and hospital administration understand the role of the psychologist as a member of the treatment team and the limits on their scope of practice. Psychologists must be alert to colleagues within their own profession and other professions who overstep the boundaries imposed by limitations in their own education, training, and credentialing, and thus engage in unethical practice. Conflicts can also occur as a result of the interdisciplinary nature of the trauma team. This aspect of work in such settings may lead to conflicts, as various team members see their scope of practice and ethical boundaries differently than do psychologists. Nonetheless, informal or formal resolution of such conflicts is essential to maintaining a smoothly running and effective team.

Case 1: A clinical psychologist joins a neurotrauma team, one of whose members is an art therapist. The psychologist is asked to evaluate a young male with a tibia fracture, multiple rib fractures, and a minor concussion. He has no recall of his accident. Nonetheless, he has been identified by the art therapist as likely having posttraumatic stress disorder (PTSD) because his drawings reflect "a lot of psychological 'stuff' suggesting childhood emotional trauma." On his part, the patient reports no psychiatric history, symptoms, or concerns.

In this case, the art therapist overstepped the scope of her professional practice by wandering into matters of psychological diagnosis and intervention. She was creating treatment and disposition problems for the patient and for the team that did not actually exist. In response, the psychologist noted in the chart that there was no evidence of emotional distress in general nor an acquired stress disorder in particular, and thus no psychological barriers to discharge, once medically cleared.

In an ideal team environment the psychologist would also find a professional way in which to discuss the situation with the art therapist and work toward solutions in the best interest of patient care and effective team collaboration. Psychologists should also strive to model ethical behavior and professionalism and maintain awareness of, and respect for, personal and professional boundaries. Credibility is measured by one's interpersonal skills, social intelligence, and professional conduct. Negative behaviors such as tardiness, condescension, entitlement, engaging in gossip, or squabbling with staff will damage the team's opinion of a psychologist's professionalism. A psychologist's credibility on the critical care team can be jeopardized by their conduct in a single case or their handling of a single ethical quandary.

Behaving in a knowledgeable, respectful, professional, and ethical manner will result in positive appraisals of the psychologist's competence. Psychologists on critical care teams should take advantage of opportunities to demonstrate sound judgment and diagnostic acumen as well as innovative assessment techniques and treatment plans, be a cooperative and supportive member of the treatment team, and display empathy and understanding with the patient and their family. Psychologists on critical care teams will often see patients and their families coping poorly and performing at their worst. Ethical psychologists will respect the process and appreciate that there will be times when they may not feel particularly validated, or even liked, by the very persons they are trying to help.

STANDARD 2: COMPETENCE

Standard 2 addresses practicing within one's scope of education and training, delivering emergency services, maintaining clinical proficiency, establishing clinical judgments based on scientifically supported information, assigning work to others, and being self-aware of personal issues that might interfere with professional duties (APA, 2017, p. 5).

Psychologists are ethically required to practice in a competent manner and to do so within the limits imposed by their education, training, and credentialing (APA, 2013). In this sense, Standard 2 is particularly important, as it is likely that psychologists working in a critical care setting will encounter patients and problems with which they have had limited training and experience. The ethical psychologist's inclination to approach such cases with caution, carefully research the problem at hand, and/or seek peer consultation may be at odds with the time pressure inherent to critical care settings and the expectations of the treatment team. At the same time, and under the same conditions, psychologists may be confronted with colleagues who are practicing well out of their professional depth and are treating patients or providing information or recommendations that fall far short of the prevailing standard of care. Complicating matters, the patient self-selection process that naturally occurs in routine clinical practice can be absent in critical care settings, where location and circumstance may dictate who appears for treatment. Under such circumstances, psychologists must be prepared to work with patients and families from different cultures who may not be fluent in the psychologist's language. In these situations, ethical psychologists must recognize their own limitations with respect to interacting with such patients, caregivers, and their loved ones.

Case 2: A board-certified neuropsychologist is made aware that a counseling psychologist has begun providing assessments for a neurotrauma team. She wears a white coat that simply says "Dr. Smith" but does not distinguish herself as a non-physician. She identifies herself verbally and with printed material as a "licensed clinical psychologist" who is "self-educated" in neuropsychology through continuing education workshops and membership in a national organization. She routinely over-diagnoses brain injury in mildly concussed patients; makes inaccurately dire prognoses to patients, family members, and medical staff; and routinely recommends referral of such patients to her spouse's psychotherapy practice.

In this situation, the counseling psychologist is practicing well beyond her professional education, training, and experience and is misrepresenting her credentials (see also Standard 5: Advertising and Other Public Statements). In so doing, she places patients, team members, and the hospital at risk. Consistent with APA guidance regarding informal resolutions, a decision was made to have a face-to-face discussion regarding these ethical problems in the presence of a mutual colleague; this was felt to be preferable to simply reporting Dr. Smith to the state licensing board. After the meeting, a memorandum for record was generated detailing the specific ethical concerns and recommended courses of action, which included accurately identifying herself as a counseling psychologist, seeking training and supervision in patient matters pertaining to neuropsychology, and refraining from referring to her spouse's practice without first disclosing the potential conflict of interest. She was encouraged to review the EPPCC and to pursue fellowship training toward board certification in neuropsychology. The memo was sent to Dr. Smith and to the physician directing the neurotrauma team.

STANDARD 3: HUMAN RELATIONS

Standard 3 addresses discrimination, sexual harassment, belittling or harassing others, avoiding or minimizing harm, engaging in multiple relationships, avoiding conflicts of interest, providing service through third parties, using one's authority to exploit others, interprofessional cooperation, obtaining informed consent, providing treatment as an agent of an organization, and planning for interruptions in service.

First and foremost, psychologists must work to avoid doing emotional harm directly or recommending treatments that have the capacity to do physical or emotional harm. They must be wary of interactions that split the interests of patients, their families, and staff, and be wary when such conflicting relationships are affecting the treatment team's ability to provide optimal care. Careful attention must be paid in situations such as shared decision-making, discussions about life-prolonging interventions, or end-of-life issues. In these instances, psychologists must clearly define their role within the treatment team. Issues also arise when psychologists or other team members use initial interactions on the ICU to refer the patient or their family for other services or to their own practice. Not all such referrals are unethical, but psychologists must be mindful not to take advantage of the intense and dependent relationships that can form in ICU settings as a lever to providing treatment in other contexts. Psychologists must be mindful of the potential contributions and expertise of other professionals and refer when appropriate.

Case 3: A patient with asthma and type 2 diabetes mellitus is admitted to the emergency department for shortness of breath and is placed on oxygen with a nasal cannula. He becomes tachypneic and hypoxic and is ultimately diagnosed with COVID-19. Because he cannot maintain his airway, he is transferred to the ICU, where he is intubated, given steroids, and placed in a medical coma. A worsening condition leads to maximum ventilator support, and despite subsequent chemical paralysis and intermittent pronation, over time he continues to decline and progresses to multisystem organ failure. After an extended meeting with an academic internist, the intensivist, pastoral care staff, and the family, all possible outcomes and contingencies are addressed. There is consensus about discontinuing life support the next day. The following morning, the team psychologist neglects to read the medical notes and instead reviews only the overnight nursing observations of slight (but insignificant) improvement. He arrives before the treatment team and provides encouragement to the family, who are advised that while the patient is gravely ill, his illness may be survivable. The family members are confused; they change their minds regarding the discontinuation of life support, rescind the patient's do-not-attempt-resuscitation/advance directive orders, and demand full ongoing care.

This case highlights the complexity of shared decision-making in the ICU, given the fluid nature of complex critical illness. Even when looking at similar clinical scenarios, interdisciplinary team members may differ on prognosis or simply present the same information in different lights (more vs. less optimistic). In this case, the psychologist has not only practiced outside his area of competence, but the decision to communicate medically insignificant improvement to the family prior to consultation with the treatment team undercuts the previous day's consensus and could result in undue harm. The psychologist should have fully reviewed the medical record before consulting with the family. The psychologist must take responsibility for the error, report it to the treatment team, jointly formulate a plan to mitigate the harm, and resolve to be more diligent in the future.

In the event a psychologist on an ICU faces a resolvable ethical dilemma due to their own faulty judgment or clinical error, it is best to admit the error and take responsibility where appropriate, apologize, make restitution, and change their behavior in order to prevent similar ethical lapses in the future (Leibovich & Zilcha-Mano, 2016; Wu et al., 1991). After engaging in this self-examination and mitigation process, the psychologist should move on from the dilemma and continue to provide quality care to the patient and critical care team (Fischer et al., 2006). While taking responsibility for a mistake is always difficult, it demonstrates integrity, and ethically it can be a defining moment in a psychologist's career.

STANDARD 4: PRIVACY AND CONFIDENTIALITY

Standard 4 addresses protecting confidential information, confidentiality limits, recording voices and images, minimizing intrusion on private information, releasing private information, collegial consultations, and disclosing information through oral or written public formats (APA, 2017, pp. 7–8).

The intensity and close working relationships on an interdisciplinary trauma or critical care team have the potential to create situations that interfere with a psychologist's (and other team members') ability to comply with HIPAA standards with respect to patient privacy and security of records. In a critical care setting, psychologists must be aware of all applicable standards of confidentiality, especially if the psychologist is a consultant to that service and not an employee of the hospital itself. Given this, challenges may arise due to the number of physicians, residents, and allied medical professionals involved who represent a broad range of disciplines and who often rotate between different hospital services or because of shift work (e.g., days vs. nights vs. weekends). This can be further complicated by ongoing interactions and conversations with immediate and distant family members or close friends, all of whom may have a genuine interest but nonetheless do not necessarily represent the patient or have a right to the patient's private health information. Also, by virtue of being in an ICU, patients often lack at least some level of orientation or are minimally responsive, although many are medically sedated or otherwise incapacitated. Therefore, they are unable to grant informed consent for psychological procedures or treatment, or even give permission to speak with family members and convey findings to third parties.

Case 4: An unmarried 20-year-old with no partner or children, and with a chronic psychiatric history, leaves a suicide note with a no-code request and signs their organ donor card. The patient attempts to commit suicide by driving their car into a bridge abutment; the crash results in what is unquestionably a non-survivable traumatic brain injury that will progress to brain death over the next 24 hours. There are no medical directives, and the trauma surgeon asks the psychologist to contact the patient's parents, who are out of the country, to establish needed communication. In the ensuing conversation, the psychologist agrees to honor the parents' request that the patient remain on life support until they return in 5 days. The psychologist conveys this commitment to the treatment team, who are upset that the patient will be occupying an ICU bed for 5 days, while their condition deteriorates and the window for organ transplantation closes.

One of the pillars of ethics is informed consent for treatment. This case demonstrates the complexities of end-of-life situations when no legal documentation is available, especially when laws regarding consent vary from state to state. The patient's suicide note and "no-code" request are not inherently legal testaments, as they were signed only by the patient, whose cognitive state and competence at the time of signing are unknown. The psychologist should consult with the hospital's ethics committee and legal office for advice and direction. In this case, the parents will likely be considered the patient's next of kin. Their decision to keep the patient on life support until they return may have to be honored, despite the potential negative impact on organ donation. The psychologist should be aware that the parents' request may affect the collaborative workings of the interdisciplinary treatment team, as some members will urge termination of care so as to maintain organ viability while others will agree to support the patient until the parents return. The psychologist can function as an intermediary between the interdisciplinary team and the patient's family, working toward a resolution that honors the patient and the family while adhering to ethical standards and best medical practice.

STANDARD 5: ADVERTISING AND OTHER PUBLIC STATEMENTS

Standard 5 addresses deceiving others through misleading, fraudulent, or false claims; responsibility for self-promotional statements of oneself or supervisees; accuracy in announcements or describing workshops and seminars; public comments through electronic transmissions; solicitation of patient testimonials; and using influence to solicit business from patients/clients (APA, 2017, pp. 8–9).

Psychologists are responsible for presenting their credentials in an honest and accurate fashion and ensuring that their education, training, and credentialing are conveyed accurately by others. As medical institutions engage in marketing and advertising of trauma and critical care services, psychologists must be alert and proactive as to how their professional expertise is presented to the public. Psychologists should consider the ethical implications related to presentations made at professional activities or via the media. Psychologists must consider the impact and level of appropriateness of their public statements and scrutinize such statements thoroughly and ethically.

> *Case 5*: A recently graduated general psychologist is hired by a large multi-clinic mental health organization and assigned by the psychiatry department to assist in their contracted care to a local ICU. The critical care nurse administrator describes the psychologist on their website as "board eligible in neuropsychology" and a "fully credentialed clinical psychologist" with a listing that reads "Dr. Smith, Psy.D., FLP" (meaning "fully licensed psychologist"). Before the psychologist has an opportunity to correct the record with respect to their credentials, they are scheduled for a group presentation at a national meeting on psychological consultation in critical care settings.

The psychologist is ethically obligated to correct the misstatements even if they are not responsible for the error. In this situation, the inaccuracies need to be brought to the attention of the nurse administrator and the website administrator. The presentation materials that wrongly refer to the psychologist's credentials need to be corrected, and the psychologist should address this point prior to beginning the presentation.

STANDARD 6: RECORDKEEPING AND FEES

Standard 6 addresses the generation and retention of records; maintaining confidentiality when storing, transferring, or disposing of electronic or written records; refusing to release records for non-receipt of payment; specifying compensation and reimbursement arrangements for professional services; being accurate with services, research, fees, diagnoses, and clinical findings; and avoiding fees for referrals (APA, 2017, pp. 9–10).

Psychologists are required to keep records of their interactions with patients, their family, staff, and outside entities. As previously noted, the critical care environment can be so time-intense, fluctuating, and complex that it may be difficult to thoroughly document patient, family, and staff interactions in real time. Under such conditions, it can be equally difficult to complete notes in the electronic health record in a timely manner or to discuss the implications of fees and confidentiality with persons who have limited capacity to absorb such details, or who may (mistakenly) assume that all services provided in the ICU will be reimbursed by their insurance carrier.

Case 6: A psychologist rounding with a critical care team is tasked with providing cognitive evaluations for an unusually large number of patients whose care is complicated by psychosocial or emotional concerns. Pressure for diagnoses and disposition necessitates consecutive abbreviated bedside examinations, sometimes while training neuropsychology residents or fellows. Over the course of 3 hours, numerous patients are assessed and responses are recorded on smartphones, personal laptops, notepads, test forms, or paper, including the back of a file folder. Later, when the psychologist attempts to recall and consolidate data for his reports, individual patient information and recollections of the separate examinations become conflated. To make matters worse, after entering his reports into the electronic health record, the psychologist loses the non–password-protected laptop. It is later revealed that the laptop contained hundreds of patients' data and reports.

The first issue is the size of the psychologist's caseload. Unfortunately, productivity is sometimes emphasized over quality in certain hospital systems, sections, units, or clinics. Psychologists should be aware of their ability to effectively monitor their caseload and the number of patients they can safely treat. In this case, the psychologist is both training and mentoring students, and thus is obliged to be mindful of his duty to ensure quality care as well as proper supervision and trainee oversight. In addition to the size of the psychologist's case load, patient information and data should only be recorded and stored in accordance with HIPAA guidelines. The haphazard recording of data on multiple personal devices is a violation of HIPAA policies and most hospitals' regulations. Steps should be taken to ensure the collection, storage, and distribution of protected patient information according to HIPAA guidelines. In this case, the psychologist must reliably reconstruct that day's examinations, where possible, or reexamine those patients where he cannot. The loss of the personal laptop containing unprotected patient medical information represents a gross violation of professional ethics and an egregious breach of HIPAA security rules. The psychologist is obliged to inform the hospital's compliance office and contact each patient whose privacy was violated in accordance with HIPAA and hospital requirements. It would also be advisable to contact one's liability carrier in anticipation of formal ethics and malpractice complaints.

STANDARD 7: EDUCATION AND TRAINING

Standard 7 addresses responsibilities for supervisors of training and education programs, accuracy in describing and advertising training programs, ensuring accuracy in teaching, protecting students' personal information, requiring psychotherapy as part of a course or program condition, evaluating students and supervisees, and having sexual relationships with students or supervisees (APA, 2017, p. 10).

Psychologists in teaching hospitals will often be in contact with physician trainees in the form of medical students, interns, residents, and fellows, and will frequently be accompanied by trainees in other disciplines, including their own graduate students, interns, and postdoctoral fellows. Professional duties typically include teaching bedside evaluations, modeling psychotherapeutic interventions, and consulting for behavioral problems with patients and family members. Psychological and neurocognitive findings may be presented at daily rounds, and one may be asked to lecture at teaching and grand rounds. Psychologists have an ethical obligation to provide supervision in a respectful manner consistent with trainees' levels of experience and to maintain the quality of their teaching activities to reflect best practices and current standards of care with respect to their particular areas of clinical expertise.

Case 7: A critical care team psychologist successfully supervises and trains graduate students, interns, and postdoctoral fellows who demonstrate skill at bedside neurocognitive examinations. The psychologist usually provides "eyes on" supervision of trainees' work, but occasionally it is necessary to attend to more pressing clinical demands, requiring students to conduct the evaluation independently. An intern with limited clinical experience who is questioned by family members about a patient's prognosis is unsuccessful in deferring their inquiries. Feeling pressured, the intern unintentionally provides incorrect information based on a misunderstanding of the parameters of the injury and data gleaned from several inaccurately scored tests.

Psychologists are liable for the work of their supervisees and must make sure they are adhering to all pertinent laws and professional ethical guidelines. Psychologists should also regularly assess supervisees' development, as individuals in training may not have a sufficiently accurate understanding of their boundaries of competence. In this case, the psychologist should have permitted clinical activities in the absence of direct supervision only when the supervisee had clearly demonstrated sufficient competence. The psychologist should have been more accessible to the supervisee for direction and support, particularly as the patient's family pressed for information. The psychologist should meet with the family, address their concerns, correct the misinformation, and model appropriate consultation behaviors for their trainee. The psychologist should later debrief the intern, provide education, and develop a plan for dealing with similar situations.

On a related note, as an emerging area of specialization in the United States, critical care psychology is not a recognized specialty by the APA. Furthermore, specific training standards and competency requirements have yet to be formally established. In the future it is the hope that such developments occur in the interest of improving patient care and advancing the specialty.

STANDARD 8: RESEARCH AND PUBLICATION

Standard 8 addresses obtaining institutional approval prior to conducting research; obtaining agreement from research participants regarding risks, adverse consequences, benefits, and incentives; obtaining consent for recording voices and images; situations in which informed research consent may not be necessary; avoiding inappropriate or coercive inducements for research participation; use of deceptive methods; providing participants with research conclusions; ensuring appropriate animal care; accurately reporting findings; plagiarizing; ensuring authorship credit; duplicating published work; withholding data to preclude confirmation of findings; and respecting authors' proprietary rights (APA, 2017, pp. 10–12).

One of the factors that distinguishes level 1 trauma centers from levels 2 and 3 is the requirement to engage in research toward publication (American Trauma Society, n.d.). Psychologists practicing in such settings are frequently called upon to collect data related to the cognitive and emotional functioning of trauma patients or to assist in data collection and analysis for team members in other disciplines. Given the complex and time-sensitive environment of an ICU, the likelihood of some diminishment in cognitive capacity of the patient, and the varying research objectives between the specialties of the interdisciplinary team, a number of ethical challenges can develop for a psychologist hoping to conduct and publish research based upon data collected on a critical care service.

Case 8: An intensivist initiates a research protocol correlating early posttraumatic amnesia while in the emergency room and on the ICU with measures of impairment toward improving prognosis of functional outcome. Most patients, although not all, are fully oriented and administered serial evaluations until their critical status resolves. All patients or their legal representative provide consent upon admission. Later, after the study is published, counsel for one of the patients lodges a formal complaint to the hospital's ombudsman and the state board of psychology, arguing that their client was forced to participate in a research study detrimental to their legal claims, and without having capacity to consent.

Before collecting data, this research protocol should have been submitted to an institutional review board (IRB) to ensure that it met necessary ethical standards for methods and potential risks. A part of this process likely would have established how capacity to consent would be determined, whether a legal representative could consent on the patient's behalf, what information must be included on the consent form, and how the patients' identities would be obscured. Assuming that this study was approved by the institution's IRB, the psychologist should contact the IRB, disclose this situation, and seek guidance on how to proceed. The psychologist should also speak with the hospital's legal counsel and with their own liability carrier.

STANDARD 9: ASSESSMENT

Standard 9 addresses the foundations used for demonstrating assessment findings; the appropriate administration, scoring, and interpretation of tests that are reliable and valid; informed consent and patient capacity to submit for evaluation; the release of test data and compliance with the law and court orders; the development, validation, and standardization of new tests; the influence of situational, ethnic, spiritual, and cultural variables in test interpretation; the prohibition of individuals who are unqualified to conduct assessments; excluding the use of obsolete or outdated tests for clinical decision-making; the use of automated or test-scoring services for diagnostic and interpretive purposes; providing explanations of test findings; and preserving legal and contractual obligations for maintaining the security of test instruments, protocols, and manuals (APA, 2017, pp. 12–14).

Diagnostic interviewing and psychometric assessment are among the skills that define psychology and separate psychologists from other disciplines. However, the demanding nature of an ICU frequently limits the type and extent of the assessments and interviews conducted. Psychologists are often required to perform testing rapidly and under less than standardized conditions, with patients who have altered mental status and limited response capabilities. Bedside screening, truncated tests, and abridged case histories are more common than not. Under such conditions, psychologists must be aware of the limitations of the evaluations they are performing and be careful not to draw conclusions or make prognoses beyond the limited power of the techniques employed.

Case 9: A psychologist is tasked by the chief of service on a trauma unit to screen neurocognitive functioning in patients prior to discharge. Because they do not have time to see every patient prior to discharge, the psychologist engages an occupational therapist, speech-language pathologist, and social worker to administer and score a cognitive screening test and conduct a brief interview. The psychologist then enters the patient's responses and test scores into a computerized scoring and interpretive program. The report generated by the scoring system is directly excerpted and pasted into the patient's electronic medical record. The psychologist then provides the diagnosis, signs the assessment note, and bills for the examination.

Psychologists are obligated to use assessment methods that are reliable, valid, and applicable to the patients or settings where they are employed. When using technicians or other extenders, they are required to competently train others in assessment techniques for those procedures they are qualified to administer, supervise appropriately, and maintain quality control. Similarly, psychologists use computerized scoring or diagnostic procedures that have established reliability, validity, and sensitivity in a manner that is appropriate for the setting and patient population. In addition, psychologists do not offer diagnoses on ICU patients they have not directly examined, and they bill accurately and only for those services they have completed or that have been performed under their direct supervision. In doing so, they avoid submitting claims that may be considered fraudulent by the hospital and third-party payers.

In this case, the psychologist was so far removed from the assessment process and was using procedures that were inadequately validated that they should not have provided diagnoses, signed the chart, or billed for services. While using extenders of different disciplines on an ICU is not ideal, no one health profession "owns" the assessment of cognition in acute care and inpatient rehabilitation settings, and many hospital staffing policies dictate the use of allied health professionals to assess similar cognitive or emotional functions. Consistent with their hospital privileges and responsibilities, psychologists strive to take responsibility for the quality of cognitive and emotional assessments that occur on their units, to supervise allied professionals and trainees in a competent and respectful manner, and to directly address differences in professional orientation, goals, and contributions when disagreements occur.

STANDARD 10: THERAPY

Standard 10 addresses informed consent and its limitations in the delivery of psychotherapy to include fees and the nature and course of treatment; providing therapeutic services to families and persons in relationships; cooperation with other therapists and recognition of their potential contributions, responsibilities, and confidentiality limits in group psychotherapy; delivering professional services in possible competing treatment situations; sexual intimacies with patients, their partners or family members, former sexual partners, or former patients/clients; disruption of professional services; and termination of psychotherapy (APA, 2017, pp. 14–15).

In the wake of potentially catastrophic injuries or illness, psychologists on an ICU frequently provide emotional care to patients and their families. This requires navigating between supporting and encouraging positive outcomes and giving false hope or obliterating hope altogether. Under these stressful conditions, caregivers are inclined to misinterpret or over-interpret a psychologist's contributions as a way of coping with the uncertain medical outcomes and rapidly changing consequences of injuries. In addition, patients may be sedated and families in shock and sleep-deprived, hence overwhelmed or inattentive when the first psychological contact is made. Psychologists should be aware that the therapeutic connection they establish in the ICU may not continue as the patient and their family make their way to secondary care facilities or home. They must also remain mindful that the tentative connection made in the ICU may serve as the basis for a much more powerful therapeutic alliance as the patient recovers. It should be clear that the ICU is fraught with the potential for the blurring of emotional boundaries and psychotherapeutic mishap; the ethical psychologist is aware of these pressures on the therapeutic process and takes them into account.

Case 10: A psychologist on an ICU is involved in the care of a patient with sepsis and critical illness myopathy (CIM) following prolonged high-dose steroid treatment. Although the psychologist has no experience treating CIM, the initial depression, suicidal thoughts, and predicted impact on the spouse and their marriage are addressed and the patient is discharged. As part of ongoing rehabilitation, the couple receives outpatient psychotherapy from the psychologist that emphasizes accepting the "new normal." While in therapy, the patient expresses an interest in ongoing individual sessions with a chaplain who provided a spiritual consultation in the ICU. This chaplain is experienced with this type of treatment and knowledgeable about interventions to resume some type of sexual intimacy in the context of CIM-related erectile dysfunction. The psychologist is aware that the chaplain has no formal mental health license. The patient and his spouse ask that the psychologist coordinate their treatment with that of the chaplain. The psychologist conveys to the patient that his depression is insufficiently controlled to benefit from any conjoint treatment at the present time, dismisses his request, and restructures this as false optimism.

Psychologists in the ICU are ethically required to be familiar with the common diseases or injuries that present in such settings and to familiarize themselves when they are confronted with more unusual conditions. They strive to take the patient's desires into consideration and to cooperate with other professionals on the interdisciplinary team who may have specialty training or greater expertise than they do. They are sensitive to issues of cross-professional cooperation and strive to minimize conflicts when they occur. In the present case, the psychologist should have conferred with the chaplain, discussed and considered issues of sexual intimacy and its importance to the client's marriage instead of dismissing them outright, and attempted to work conjointly with the chaplain while explaining what reservations they might have.

Psychological ethics and decision-making

While knowing and following ethical guidelines are essential to psychological practice in critical care settings, understanding the process of making ethical decisions is of even greater value (Canter et al., 1994). Psychologists in critical care settings face moral complexities and contextual factors that can influence the decision-making process (Rogerson et al., 2011). Many of these variables are encapsulated in Jones's (1991) moral intensity model as discussed in Lincoln and Holmes (2011). Of the six dimensions that make up this model, the authors found that four had a significant impact on ethical decision-making:

1. Magnitude of consequence (the degree of potential harm or benefit)
2. Social consensus (level of agreement among a social group when appraising a proposed action)
3. Probability of effect (the likelihood of anticipated consequences, benefit, and/ or harm)
4. Proximity (the degree of physical, cultural, social, or psychological closeness one feels to a given situation).

While each of these variables influences ethical decisions, the magnitude of consequences in an ICU is often quite high (Gopalan & Pershad, 2019). In addition, the interdisciplinary nature of this environment requires input from many disciplines as well as individuals from the patient's support system, increasing the potential for further complications. Some decisions truly address life-or-death situations while others have potential for long-term physical, cognitive, and psychological complications. As a result, the complexity and acutely stressful nature of a critical care setting can generate dilemmas of moral intensity that influence one's awareness, judgement, and, ultimately, ethical action. Not surprisingly, the acutely stressful nature of critical care may lead a psychologist to overly identify with a patient or provider, or excessively distance oneself as an emotionally protective measure. For psychologists practicing in critical care, ongoing efforts to increase awareness of these influences will help minimize their impact on ethical decision-making.

A consolidated model for ethical decision-making in critical care

There are several sound models relating to theoretical and practical ethical decision-making in the professional literature. Most come from medical, mental health, legal, and military sources. While some emphasize values, character, and principles, others are more pragmatic. Regardless of the particular model or guide, all support careful reasoning and provide some type of conceptual framework to deliberate and resolve moral dilemmas (Beauchamp, 1984; Bush, 2018; Bush et al., 2020; Fisher, 2017; Han, 2015; Jones, 1991; Knapp et al., 2015; Lincoln & Holmes, 2011; Meyer-Zehnder et al., 2017; Pryzwansky & Wendt, 1999; Williams & Kennedy, 2011). The following model is therefore not unique but rather an integration of several approaches, offering a commonsense framework by which to reason through an ethical concern in an orderly and methodical manner.

STEP 1: IDENTIFY AND DEFINE THE PROBLEM

Regardless of the circumstances, it is incumbent on the psychologist to recognize an ethical dilemma as a potential conflict between one's values and beliefs (at least as they pertain to potential behavioral choices involving the needs of critically ill patients) and the institution for which they work (Braunack-Mayer, 2001). Identifying an obvious ethical problem such as falsely documenting a patient visit (when a patient encounter did not occur) does not require a great deal of discernment.

In contrast, the ethical issues distinct to psychology in critical care are likely to be more subtle, such as (1) resolving conflicts with colleagues regarding patient capacity; (2) termination of life support; (3) obtaining informed consent when there is no designated guardian; (3) failing to appreciate religious or cultural differences when using normed tests to make diagnoses; (4) not documenting the effect of interpreters, third-party observers, or nonstandardized test administration; and (5) making diagnoses based upon others' observations in lieu of one's own examination.

The first step when faced with a potential ethical quandary is to trust your instincts and initial reaction. Collect the pertinent facts by listening to all relevant parties and verify specific and essential information (APA, 2014; Beckman et al., 2016; Beesley & Brown, 2020; Belitz, 2020; Erstad et al., 2011; McDaniel et al., 2014; Self et al., 2018; Willemse et al., 2020).

STEP 2: CONSULT

Resolving an ethical dilemma requires time to discern the relevant EPPCC standard(s) and to develop an initial strategy. In addition to reviewing the ethics code, the process of resolution sometimes requires consultation with other medical professionals on the critical care team as well as exploring resources (e.g., one's state or hospital ethics committee, the institution's or unit's policies and procedures) and/or seeking peer consultation from colleagues whose opinions you trust.

Psychologists should consider both the immediate and longer-term effects of their ethical decisions and the implications for the patient, family members, treatment team, and institution. They should try to determine the impact on others who might be affected by their decisions and understand others' perspectives. Where possible, psychologists should reach out to colleagues and mentors who also consult in hospitals or have experience with similar concerns. Time and situation permitting, psychologists should also consider reaching out to colleagues not practicing in critical care settings to obtain perspectives outside of the framework of critical care, which may aid in generating alternative ideas, actions, or outcomes. Peer consultation is an essential component of the ethical problem-solving process. Psychologists working in critical care should also participate in continuing education regarding professional ethics. They should maintain memberships in national and state organizations, and they may wish to volunteer for ethics, human subjects, or other committee memberships in the institutions in which they practice.

STEP 3: DECIDE

After deliberating possible outcomes, the psychologist must decide on a course of action. Since the choices one makes may affect a number of individuals, psychologists may need to discuss their decision with the physician ultimately responsible for the patient's care. If one's initial emotional response to a decision is one of discomfort or ambivalence, the intended action may be in error. Under such circumstances, the psychologist might imagine having to defend their decision to a mentor, colleague, or family member to help determine whether they are content with the decision they have made.

STEP 4: IMPLEMENT AND EVALUATE

Even after deciding upon a solution to an ethical quandary, it can be difficult to execute the resolution. The time spent considering a solution is of no benefit if the plan is not carried out. Resolving an ethical concern requires the psychologist to execute the plan. When the action is implemented, it is equally important to evaluate its consequences. In doing so, the psychologist (as well as other team members) needs to evaluate the action's effectiveness as well as any possible unintended consequences. In doing so, one may help set a standard or strategy for future or similar ethical situations.

Conclusion

Psychological consultation in critical care settings is similar to that in other areas of psychological practice with regard to the need for an appreciation of relationships, confidentiality, patient autonomy, supervisory responsibilities, professional boundaries, role clarification, documentation, competency, evidence-based decision-making, and diagnostic acumen. However, in an interdisciplinary critical care setting, psychologists must also have a greater sense of their role on the team as it pertains to the patient, the medical staff, allied health providers, trainees, and the institution.

Ethics are not static, and solutions to ethical dilemmas may not always be clear-cut; thus, psychologists may be forced to choose from the least undesirable of several options. At times, psychologists may exhibit lapses in ethical judgment due to inadequate training, poor awareness of practice standards, a lack of familiarity with relevant laws and regulations, or deficient knowledge regarding hospital policy and procedures. Psychologists can also succumb to unethical behavior as a result of personal financial strain, alcohol or substance abuse, diminished cognitive capacity, or situational stress. Potential ethical problems in critical care settings can often be avoided by maintaining *ethical situational awareness*, defined as constant vigilance for potential ethical quandaries, particularly in complex, stressful, and/or time-sensitive environments such as the ICU (Lewandowski, 2015). Moreover, psychologists should be aware of their personal values and professional strengths and weaknesses and how each may affect their ethical decision-making.

In summary, ethical dilemmas are best avoided or managed by being proactive rather than reactive. Ethical predicaments do not typically develop in an abrupt or unanticipated manner. Rather, they often begin with seemingly insignificant or unintentional errors of judgment that might appear harmless at the time but eventually develop into something more insidious. It is incumbent on the psychologist in the critical care setting to anticipate problems before they develop by being vigilant about the interactions that might progress into misunderstandings or dilemmas. However, rather than focusing on the mitigation of potential negative outcomes or the avoidance of ethical complaints, psychologists are better served by thinking about professional ethics as a guide to good practice. Simply put, psychologists should know their (ethical) code, exercise good judgment, and seek peer consultation early in the ethical decision-making process. One's first and last priority is to strive to do good and do no harm.

References

American Academy of Physician Assistants. (2013). Guidelines for ethical conduct for the PA profession (adopted 2000, amended 2004, 2006, 2007, 2008, reaffirmed 2013). https://www.aapa.org/wp-content/uploads/2017/02/16-EthicalConduct.pdf

American Medical Association. (2016). *AMA code of medical ethics.* https://www.ama-assn.org/delivering-care/ethics/code-medical-ethics-overview

American Nurses Association. (2015). *Code of ethics for nurses with interpretive statements.* https://www.nursingworld.org/coe-view-only

American Occupational Therapy Association. (2015). Occupational therapy code of ethics. *American Journal of Occupational Therapy, 69*(3), 1–8.

American Osteopathic Association. (2016a). *Code of ethics.* https://osteopathic.org/about/leadership/aoa-governance-documents/code-of-ethics

American Osteopathic Association. (2016b). AOA rules and guidelines on physicians' professional conduct. https://osteopathic.org/about/leadership/aoa-governance-documents/aoa-rules-and-guidelines-on-physicians-professional-conduct/

American Pharmacists Association. (1994). *Code of ethics.* https://www.pharmacist.com/code-ethics

American Physical Therapy Association. (2019). *Code of ethics for the physical therapist.* www.apta.org/ethics/core

American Psychological Association. (2013). Guidelines for psychological practice in health care delivery systems. *American Psychologist, 68*(1), 1–6. https://doi.org/10.1037/a0029890

American Psychological Association. (2014). *Guidelines for clinical supervision in health service psychology.* https://www.apa.org/about/policy/guidelines-supervision.pdf

American Psychological Association. (2017). Ethical principles of psychologists and code of conduct (2002, amended effective June 1, 2010, and January 1, 2017). https://www.apa.org/ethics/code/

American Speech-Language-Hearing Association. (2016). *Code of ethics.* https://www.asha.org/Code-of-Ethics/

American Trauma Society (n.d.). *Trauma center levels explained.* https://www.amtrauma.org/page/traumalevels

Azoulay, E., Vincent, J., Angus, D., Arabi, Y., Brochard, L., Brett, S., . . . Herridge, M. (2017). Recovery after critical illness: Putting the puzzle together—a consensus of 29. *Critical Care, 21*(1), Article 296. https://doi.org/10.1186/s13054-017-1887-7

Bach, J., Leskovan, J., Scharschmidt, T., Boulger, C., Papadimos, T., Russell, S., . . . Stawicki, S. (2017). The right team at the right time: Multidisciplinary approach to multi-trauma patients with orthopedic injuries. *International Journal of Critical Illness and Injury Science, 7*(1), 32. https://doi.org/10.4103/IJCIIS.IJCIIS_5_17

Baum, N., Gollust, S., Goold, S., & Jacobson, P. (2009). Ethical issues in public health practice in Michigan. *American Journal of Public Health, 99*(2), 369–374. https://doi.org/10.2105/AJPH.2008.137588

Beauchamp, T. (1984). *Medical ethics: The moral responsibilities of physicians.* Prentice-Hall.

Beckman, M., Weigelt, J., Ali, J., & Bell, R. (2016). Ethical issues in the surgical ICU. In J. Ali (Ed.), *Surgical critical care handbook* (pp. 251–262). World Scientific Publishing. https://doi.org/10.1142/9519

Beesley, S., & Brown, S. (2020). Family involvement in ICU. In R. C. Hyzy & J. McSparron (Eds.), *Evidence-based critical care* (pp. 805–812). Springer. https://doi.org/10.1007/978-3-030-26710-0_108

Belitz, J. (2020) How to intervene with unethical and unprofessional colleagues. In L. Roberts (Ed.), *Roberts academic medicine handbook* (pp. 243–252). Springer.

Bibler, T., & Miller, S. (2019). "What if she was your mother?" Toward better responses. *Journal of Critical Care, 49*, 155–157. https://doi.org/10.1016/j.jcrc.2018.10.031

Braunack-Mayer, A. J. (2001). What makes a problem an ethical problem? An empirical perspective on the nature of ethical problems in general practice. *Journal of Medical Ethics, 27*(2), 98–103. https://doi.org/10.1136/jme.27.2.98

Bush, S. (2018). *Ethical decision making in clinical neuropsychology* (2nd ed.). Oxford University Press.

Bush, S., Connell, M., & Denney, R. (2020). *Ethical practice in forensic psychology: A guide for mental health professionals* (2nd ed.). American Psychological Association. https://doi.org/10.1037/0000164-000

Canter, M., Bennett, B., Jones, S., & Nagy, T. (1994). *Ethics for psychologists: A commentary on the APA Ethics Code.* American Psychological Association.

Costa, D., Valley, T., Miller, M., Manojlovich, M., Watson, S., McLellan, P., . . . Iwashyna, T. (2018). ICU team composition and its association with ABCDE implementation in a quality collaborative. *Journal of Critical Care, 44*, 1–6. https://doi.org/10.1016/j.jcrc.2017.09.180

Cour, M., Turc, J., Madelaine, T., & Argaud, L. (2019). Risk factors for progression toward brain death after out-of-hospital cardiac arrest. *Annals of Intensive Care, 9*(1), Article 45. https://doi.org/10.1186/s13613-019-0520-0

da Costa, J. B., Taba, S., Scherer, J. R., Oliveira, L. L. F., Luzzi, K. C. B., Gund, D. P., . . . Duarte, P. A. D. (2019). Psychological disorders in post-ICU survivors and impairment in quality of life. *Psychology & Neuroscience, 12*(3), 391–406. https://doi.org/10.1037/pne0000170

de Jong, A., Kentish, N., Souppart, V., Jaber, S., & Azoulay, E. (2020). Post-intensive care syndrome in relatives of critically injured patients. In J. Preiser, M. Herridge, & E. Azoulay (Eds.), *Post-intensive care syndrome: Lessons from the ICU (under the auspices of the European Society of Intensive Care Medicine)* (pp. 247–259). Springer.

Dobmeyer, A., & Rowan, A. (2014). Core competencies for psychologists: How to succeed in medical settings. In C. M. Hunter, C. L. Hunter, & R. Kessler (Eds.), *Handbook of clinical psychology in medical settings* (pp. 77–98). Springer.

Donovan, A., Aldrich, J., Gross, A., Barchas, D., Thornton, K., Schell-Chaple, H., . . . Lipshutz, A. (2018). Interprofessional care and teamwork in the ICU. *Critical Care Medicine, 46*(6), 980–990. https://doi.org/10.1097/CCM.0000000000003067

Erstad, B., Haas, C., O'Keeffe, T., Hokula, C., Parrinello, K., & Theodorou, A. (2011). Interdisciplinary patient care in the intensive care unit: Focus on the pharmacist. *Pharmacotherapy, 31*(2), 128–137. https://doi.org/10.1592/phco.31.2.128

Ervin, J., Khan, J., Cohen, T., & Weingart, L. (2018). Teamwork in the intensive care unit. *American Psychologist, 73*(4), 468–477. https://doi.org/10.1037/amp0000247

Firn, J., Rui, C., Vercler, C., De Vries, R., & Shuman, A. (2020). Identification of core ethical topics for interprofessional education in the intensive care unit: A thematic analysis. *Journal of Interprofessional Care, 34*(4), 453–460. doi:10.1080/13561820.2019.1632814

Fischer, M. A., Mazor, K. M., Baril, J., Alper, E., DeMarco, D., & Pugnaire, M. (2006). Learning from mistakes: Factors that influence how students and residents learn from medical errors. *Journal of General Internal Medicine, 21*(5), 419–423. https://doi.org/10.1111/j.1525-1497.2006.00420.x

Fisher, C. B. (2017). *Decoding the ethics code: A practical guide for psychologists* (4th ed.). Sage.

Fleisher, L. (2010). The effect of multidisciplinary care teams on intensive care unit mortality. *Archives of Internal Medicine, 170*(10), 369–376. https://doi.org/10.1001/archinternmed.2010.124

Fornan, C., Clark, D., Henry, R., Lalchandani, P., Kim, D., Putnam, B., . . . Demetriades, D. (2019). Current burden of gunshot wound injuries at two Los Angeles County level 1 trauma centers. *Journal of the American College of Surgeons, 229*(2), 141–149.

Fuchs, L., Chronaki, C. E., Parks, S., Novak, V., Baumfeld, Y., Scott, D., . . . Celi, L. (2012). ICU admission characteristics and mortality rates among elderly and very elderly patients. *Intensive Care Medicine, 38*(10), 1654–1661. https://doi.org/10.1007/s00134-012-2629-6

Gacouin, A., Maamar, A., Fillatre, P., Sylvestre, E., Dolan, M., Le Tulzo, Y. & Tadie, J. (2017). Patients with preexisting psychiatric disorders admitted to ICU: A descriptive and retrospective cohort study. *Annals of Intensive Care, 7*(1), 1–9. https://doi.org/10.1186/s13613-016-0221-x

Goldberg, R., Mays, M., & Halpern, N. A. (2020). Mitigating post-intensive care syndrome—family: A new possibility. *Critical Care Medicine, 48*(2), 260–261. https://doi.org/10.1097/CCM.0000000000004152

Gopalan, P., & Pershad, S. (2019). Decision-making in ICU: A systematic review of factors considered important by IUC clinician decision makers with regard to ICU triage decisions. *Journal of Critical Care, 50*(2), 99–110.

Griffith, D., Merriweather, J., & Walsh, T. (2020). Coordinating rehabilitation in hospital after ICU discharge: Priorities and pitfalls. In J. C. Preiser, M. Herridge, & E. Azoulay (Eds.), *Post-intensive care syndrome: Lessons from the ICU* (pp. 343–357). Springer.

Han, H. (2015). Virtue ethics, positive psychology, and a new model of science and engineering ethics education. *Science and Engineering Ethics, 21*(2), 441–460. https://doi.org/10.1007/s11948-014-9539-7

Hogan, R. (1973). Moral conduct and moral character: A psychological perspective. *Psychological Bulletin, 79*(4), 217–232. https://doi.org/10.1037/h0033956

Howe, E., & Jones, F. (1994). Ethical issues in combat psychiatry. In F. D. Jones, L. R. Sparacino, V. L. Wilcox, & J. M. Rothberg (Eds.), *Military psychiatry: Preparing in peace for war* (pp. 115–131). Office of the Surgeon General.

Hunter, C., & Goodie, J. (2010). Operational and clinical components for integrated-collaborative behavioral healthcare in the patient-centered medical home. *Families, Systems, & Health*, *28*(4), 308–321. https://doi.org/10.1037/a0021761

Johnson, C. C., Suchyta, M. R., Darowski, E. S., Collar, E. M., Kiehl, A. L., Van, J., . . . Hopkins, R. O. (2019). Psychological sequelae in family caregivers of critically ill intensive care unit patients: A systematic review. *Annals of the American Thoracic Society*, *16*(7), 894–909.

Jones, T. M. (1991). Ethical Decision Making by Individuals in Organizations: An Issue-Contingent Model. *The Academy of Management Review*, *16*(2), 366. https://doi.org/10.2307/258867

Khan, F., Baguley, I., & Cameron, I. (2003). Rehabilitation after traumatic brain injury. *Medical Journal of Australia*, *178*(6), 290–295. https://doi.org/10.5694/j.1326-5377.2003.tb05199.x

Kim, M., Barnato, A., Angus, D., Fleisher, L., Fleisher, L., & Kahn, J. (2010). The effect of multidisciplinary care teams on intensive care unit mortality. *Archives of Internal Medicine*, *170*(4), 369–376. https://doi.org/10.1001/archinternmed.2009.521

Knapp, S., Gottlieb, M., & Handelsman, M. (2015). *Ethical dilemmas in psychotherapy: Positive approaches to decision making*. American Psychological Association. https://doi.org/10.1037/14670-000

Lee, J., & Ward, N. (2019). Emerging ethical challenges in critical care for the 21st century: A case-based discussion. *Seminars in Respiratory and Critical Care Medicine*, *40*(5), 655–661. https://doi.org/10.1055/s-0039-1698408

Leibovich, L., & Zilcha-Mano, S. (2016). What is the right time for supportive versus expressive interventions in supervision? An illustration based on a clinical mistake. *Psychotherapy*, *53*(3), 297–301. https://doi.org/10.1037/pst0000078

Lewandowski, A. (2012). *Establishing ethical guidelines and standards of practice for the Michigan Psychological Association*. https://www.michiganpsychologicalassociation.org/ethics_committee.php

Lewandowski, A. (2015). Supervision requirements for psychologists licensed in the State of Michigan. https://www.michiganpsychologicalassociation.org/ethics_committee.php

Lincoln, S. H., & Holmes, E. K. (2011). Ethical decision making: A process influenced by moral intensity. *Journal of Healthcare, Science and the Humanities*, *1*(1), 55–69.

Llompart-Pou, J. A., Pérez-Bárcena, J., Chico-Fernández, M., Sánchez-Casado, M., & Raurich, J. M. (2017). Severe trauma in the geriatric population. *World Journal of Critical Care Medicine*, *6*(2), 99–106. https://doi.org/10.5492/wjccm.v6.i2.99

McDaniel, S., Grus, C., Cubic, B., Hunter, C., Kearney, L., Schuman, C., . . . Johnson, S. (2014). Competencies for psychology practice in primary care. *American Psychologist*, *69*(4), 409–429. https://doi.org/10.1037/a0036072

Meunier-Beillard, N., Dargent, A., Ecarnot, F., Rigaud, J. P., Andreu, P., Large, A., & Quenot, J. P. (2017). Intersecting vulnerabilities in professionals and patients in intensive care. *Annals of Translational Medicine*, *5*(4), S39. https://doi.org/10.21037/atm.2017.09.01

Meyer-Zehnder, B., Albisser Schleger, H., Tanner, S., Schnurrer, V., Vogt, D. R., Reiter-Theil, S., & Pargger, H. (2017). How to introduce medical ethics at the bedside: Factors influencing the implementation of an ethical decision-making model. *BMC Medical Ethics, 18*(1), Article 16. https://doi.org/10.1186/s12910-017-0174-0

Moon, J. Y., & Kim, J.-O. (2015). Ethics in the intensive care unit. *Tuberculosis and Respiratory Diseases, 78*(3), 175. https://doi.org/10.4046/trd.2015.78.3.175

Mulvey, H., Haslam, R., Laytin, A., Diamond, C., & Sims, C. (2020). Unplanned ICU admission is associated with worse clinical outcomes in geriatric trauma patients. *Journal of Surgical Research, 245*, 13–21. https://doi.org/10.1016/j.jss.2019.06.059

National Association of Social Workers. (2017). *Code of ethics of the national association of social workers.* https://www.socialworkers.org/About/Ethics/Code-of-Ethics/Code-of-Ethics-English

Pittaway, E., Bartolomei, L., & Hugman, R. (2010). "Stop stealing our stories": The ethics of research with vulnerable groups. *Journal of Human Rights Practice, 2*(2), 229–251. https://doi.org/10.1093/jhuman/huq004

Pochard, F., Darmon, M., Fassier, T., Bollaert, P. E., Cheval, C., Coloigner, M., Merouani, A., Moulront, S., Pigne, E., Pingat, J., Zahar, J. R., Schlemmer, B., Azoulay, E., & French FAMIREA study group (2005). Symptoms of anxiety and depression in family members of intensive care unit patients before discharge or death: A prospective multicenter study. *Journal of Critical Care, 20*(1), 90–96. https://doi.org/10.1016/j.jcrc.2004.11.004

Pryzwansky, W., & Wendt, R. (1999). *Professional and ethical issues in psychology: Foundations of practice.* W.W. Norton & Co.

Quenot, J., Ecarnot, F., Meunier-Beillard, N., Dargent, A., Large, A., Andreu, P., & Rigaud, J. (2017). What are the ethical issues in relation to the role of the family in intensive care? *Annals of Translational Medicine, 5*(Suppl 4), S40. doi:10.21037/atm.2017.04.44

Quest, T., & Marco, C. (2003). Ethics seminars: Vulnerable populations in emergency medicine research. *Academic Emergency Medicine, 10*(11), 1294–1298. https://doi.org/10.1111/j.1553-2712.2003.tb00616.x

Rhee, P., Joseph, B., Pandit, V., Aziz, H., Vercruysse, G., Kulvatunyou, N., & Friese, R. (2014). Increasing trauma deaths in the United States. *Annals of Surgery, 260*(1), 13–21.

Richmond, T., Amsterdam, J., Guo, W., Ackerson, T., Gracias, V., Robinson, K., & Hollander, J. (2009). The effect of post-injury depression on return to pre-injury function: A prospective cohort study. *Psychological Medicine, 39*(10), 1709–1720. doi:10.1017/S0033291709005376

Rogerson, M. D., Gottlieb, M. C., Handelsman, M. M., Knapp, S., & Younggren, J. (2011). Nonrational processes in ethical decision making. *American Psychologist, 66*(7), 614–623. https://doi.org/10.1037/a0025215

Rose, L. (2011). Interprofessional collaboration in the ICU: How to define? *Nursing in Critical Care, 16*(1), 5–10. https://doi.org/10.1111/j.1478-5153.2010.00398.x

Rose, L., Muttalib, F., & Adhikari, N. (2019). Psychological consequences of admission to the ICU. *Journal of the American Medical Association, 322*(3), 213–215.

Self, M., Wise, E., Beauvais, J., & Molinari, V. (2018). Ethics in training and training in ethics: Special considerations for postdoctoral fellowships in health service psychology. *Training and Education in Professional Psychology, 12*(2), 105–112. https://doi.org/10.1037/tep0000178

Shannon, S. E. (2001). Helping families prepare for and cope with death in the ICU. In J. R. Curtis & G. D. Rubenfeld (Eds.), *Managing death on the ICU: The transition from cure to comfort* (pp. 165–182). Oxford University Press.

Smith, D. (2003). The first code. *Monitor on Psychology, 34*(1), 63. http://www.apa.org/monitor/jan03/firstcode

Søreide, K. (2009). Epidemiology of major trauma. *British Journal of Surgery, 96*(7), 697–698. https://doi.org/10.1002/bjs.6643

Strasser, D., Uomoto, J., & Smits, S. (2008). The interdisciplinary team and polytrauma rehabilitation: Prescription for partnership. *Archives of Physical Medicine and Rehabilitation, 89*(1), 179–181. https://doi.org/10.1016/j.apmr.2007.06.774

Stucky, K., & Warren, A. M. (2019). Rehabilitation psychologists in critical care settings. In L. A. Brenner, S. A. Reid-Arndt, T. R. Elliott, R. G. Frank, & B. Caplan (Eds.), *Handbook of rehabilitation psychology* (3rd ed., pp. 483–496). American Psychological Association. https://doi.org/10.1037/0000129-029

Torrence, N., Mueller, A., Ilem, A., Renn, B., DeSantis, B., & Segal, D. L. (2014). Medical provider attitudes about behavioral health consultants in integrated primary care: A preliminary study. *Families, Systems, & Health, 32*(4), 426–432. https://doi.org/10.1037/fsh0000007

Tremont, G., Westervelt, H. J., Javorsky, D. J., Podolanczuk, A., & Stern, R. A. (2002). Referring physicians' perceptions of the neuropsychological evaluation: How are we doing? *Clinical Neuropsychologist, 16*(4), 551–554. https://doi.org/10.1076/clin.16.4.551.13902

Turner-Cobb, J., Smith, P., Ramchandani, P., Begen, F., & Padkin, A. (2016). The acute psychobiological impact of the intensive care experience on relatives. *Psychology, Health & Medicine, 21*(1), 20–26. https://doi.org/10.1080/13548506.2014.997763

Wendler, D. (2019). The value in doing something. *Critical Care Medicine, 47*(2), 149–151. doi:10.1097/CCM.0000000000003503

Willemse, S., Smeets, W., van Leeuwen, E., Nielen-Rosier, T., Janssen, L., & Foudraine, N. (2020). Spiritual care in the intensive care unit: An integrative literature research. *Journal of Critical Care, 57*, 55–78. https://doi.org/10.1016/j.jcrc.2020.01.026

Williams, T., & Kennedy, C. (2011). Operational psychology: Proactive ethics in a challenging world. In C. H. Kennedy & T. J. Williams (Eds.), *Ethical practice in operational psychology: Military and national intelligence applications* (pp. 125–140). American Psychological Association. https://doi.org/10.1037/12342-000

Wu, A., Folkman, S., McPhee, S., & Lo, B. (1991). Do house officers learn from their mistakes? *Journal of the American Medical Association, 265*(16), 2089–2094.

Yoo, E., Edwards, J., Dean, M., & Dudley, R. (2016). Multidisciplinary critical care and intensivist staffing: Results of a statewide survey and association with mortality. *Journal of Intensive Care Medicine, 31*(5), 325–332. https://doi.org/10.1177/0885066614534605

16 Research in the Critical Care Environment
Dorothy Wade, Deborah Smyth, and David C. J. Howell

Introduction

For the past 20 years, research into the psychological impact of critical care has burgeoned, from early studies uncovering patients' experience of hallucinations, delusions, and posttraumatic stress disorder (PTSD; Granberg et al., 1999; Jones et al., 2001, 2007) to recent publications reporting large randomized clinical trials (RCTs) of psychological interventions such as patient diaries on the critical care unit (Garrouste-Orgeas et al., 2019) and a complex nurse-led intervention to reduce acute critical care stress (Wade et al., 2019). The earliest research was conducted by critical care nurses or doctors, and nurse-led research in particular continues. However, more recently, psychologists have also been involved in studying critical care psychological risk factors and outcomes (e.g., Jackson et al., 2007) and in developing psychological interventions that could benefit patients, families, and staff (e.g., Wade et al., 2018; Wilson et al., 2018).

In this chapter we outline the major areas of psychological and rehabilitation research being conducted in critical care as well as gaps that remain. We also review research areas corresponding to (1) the early acute critical care phase, (2) the in-hospital rehabilitation phase, and (3) the post-hospital recovery period. The focus is on patient-centered research. We then discuss how critical care psychologists or others can initiate psychological research, what kind of teams they need to assemble,

Dorothy Wade, Deborah Smyth, and David C. J. Howell, *Research in the Critical Care Environment* In: *Critical Care Psychology and Rehabilitation*. Edited by: Kirk J. Stucky and Jennifer E. Jutte, Oxford University Press. © Oxford University Press 2022. DOI: 10.1093/oso/9780190077013.003.0016 and the challenges they could face working in critical care environments. We draw on our team's experience conducting linked, critical care psychology research studies, each building on the previous work, that have spanned more than a decade and compare this to methods used by other researchers in multidisciplinary rehabilitation including psychological aspects in critical care settings.

Major areas of study in critical care psychology

Research studies about psychological aspects of critical care admission have investigated outcomes, risk factors, and the assessments and interventions relevant to three phases: in the critical care unit, in-hospital rehabilitation, and post-hospital discharge.

PSYCHOLOGICAL OUTCOMES

Psychological research about critical care has addressed the prevalence of adverse psychosocial outcomes such as anxiety, depression, PTSD, poor health-related quality of life, or cognitive impairment in the months or years after hospital discharge. Furthermore, studies have endeavored to identify risk factors, whether psychological, clinical, or sociodemographic, for these outcomes (e.g., Davydow et al., 2008; Wade et al., 2012). Large prospective cohort studies indicate that approximately 50% of patients in critical care develop clinically significant symptoms of anxiety, depression, or PTSD following hospital discharge (Hatch et al., 2018). Patients with posttraumatic stress symptoms may experience flashbacks and intrusive memories of delusional/hallucinatory episodes from delirium, which is common in critical care patients, as well as from actual events within the ICU (Jones et al., 2001; Wade et al., 2014). Significant postdischarge problems with cognition in domains such as attention, memory, and executive function have been reported but are not yet well quantified (Wilcox et al., 2013). Quality of life, both physical and mental, remains lower for ICU survivors than for the general population. Mental health issues and cognitive impairment are important domains of postintensive care syndrome (PICS; Figure 16.1), along with the third domain of physical difficulties (Needham et al., 2012).

RISK FACTORS FOR ADVERSE PSYCHOLOGICAL OUTCOMES

Research into the acute phase of critical care admission has explored the range of patient experiences and investigated modifiable and nonmodifiable risk factors

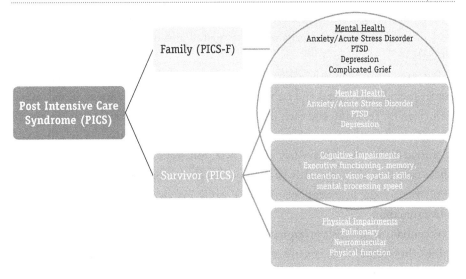

FIGURE 16.1. Psychological domains of PICS
Needham et al., 2012

for adverse psychological and cognitive outcomes. From 45% to 80% of patients experience acute stress symptoms (e.g., panic, fear, anxiety, depressed mood, anger, irritability), which may be associated with stressors frequently identified by critical care patients such as pain, thirst, hunger, nausea, fatigue, invasive procedures and monitoring (Novaes et al., 1997; Puntillo et al., 2010; Wade, 2010). As many patients have multiple morbidities, treatments, and setbacks, they may be traumatized more than once in the ICU setting. Mechanical ventilation has been identified as a particularly stressful experience: "I suppose the misery is worth it. But I would offer this as a good torture for Guantanamo" (Carruthers et al., 2018, p. 68). Further stressors include loud noise and limited access to daylight, windows, or clocks, leading to sensory overload and/or deprivation, circadian rhythm dysregulation, and sleep disruption. Patients can feel isolated and alienated, unable to communicate, yet painfully aware of their and other people's suffering (Alonso-Ovies & Heras, 2016).

Patients in critical care units often receive a cocktail of psychoactive drugs including opioids for pain, benzodiazepines for anxiety, hypnotics for sleep, and sedatives/anesthetics to help them tolerate mechanical ventilation. Studies have shown that iatrogenic coma and immobilization are common in critical care, yet can be harmful, leading to delirium, long-term cognitive impairment, and ICU-acquired weakness (Jackson, Santoro, et al., 2014). The environment, stress, and illness factors may also contribute to delirium in critical care, a syndrome that often features terrifying hallucinations and delusions. Consisting of the five domains of cognitive deficits, attentional deficits, psychomotor disturbance, circadian rhythm disturbance, and emotional dysregulation (Maldonaldo, 2017; Figure 16.2), delirium affects up to 80% of patients who are mechanically ventilated and up to 50% of nonventilated patients (Ely et al., 2001).

Potentially modifiable precipitating risk factors for long-term psychological outcomes include emotional and behavioral factors such as acute stress, mood, agitation, need for restraint, and early intrusive memories in the critical care unit, as well as cognitive disturbances such as hallucinations, delusions, duration of delirium, and cognitive dysfunction (Davydow et al., 2008; Jones et al., 2007; Wade et al., 2012). These factors could potentially be modified by psychological, behavioral, cognitive, or pharmacologic interventions to reduce stress, manage delirium, or improve cognitive function.

Potentially modifiable precipitating clinical risk factors include use of benzodiazepines, duration of sedation, use of vasopressors and inotropes, type of illness (acute respiratory distress syndrome/sepsis), and increasing numbers of organ support interventions such as mechanical ventilation (Pandharipande et al., 2006; Wade et al., 2012). Patients also have predisposing risk factors that cannot be modified yet nevertheless could be taken into account or used to predict those who are more likely to be at risk of poor outcomes. They include demographic factors such as

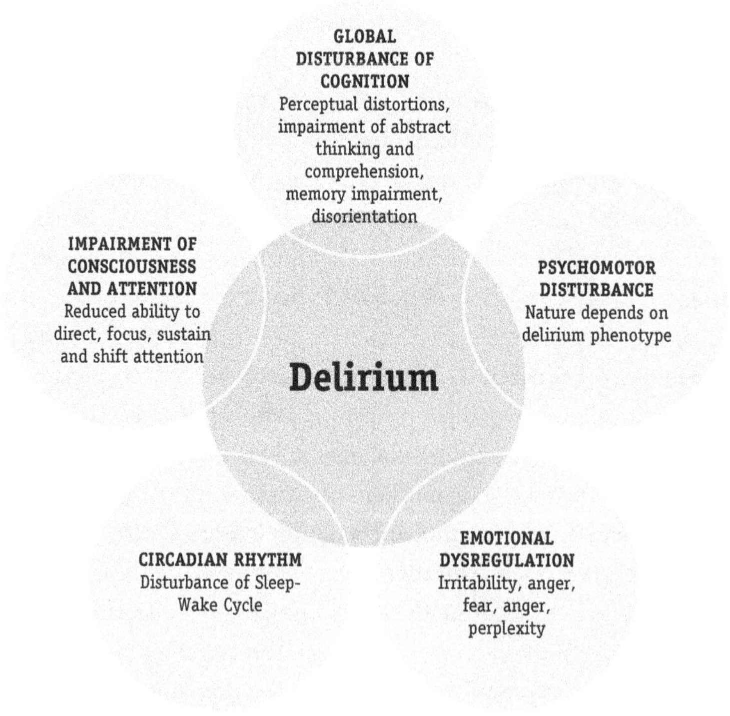

FIGURE 16.2. The five core domains of delirium
Maldonaldo, 2017

TABLE 16.1.

Risk factors for psychological and cognitive morbidities following critical illness

Precipitating/modifiable risk factors	Predisposing risk factors
Acute stress in the ICU	Comorbid psychopathology
Longer duration of sedation	Type of illness (acute respiratory distress syndrome/sepsis)
Longer period of delirium	Younger age
Use of inotropes or vasopressors	Lower education level
Use of benzodiazepines	Premorbid history of psychological health difficulties
Mood in the ICU	Female sex
Early intrusive memories of the ICU	Lower socioeconomic status
Agitation and need for restraint	

Davydow et al., 2008; Jackson, Pandharipande, et al., 2014; Pandharipande et al., 2013; Wade et al., 2012, 2013.

younger age, female gender, lower socioeconomic status, and lower education level as well as a history of chronic health problems or psychopathology (e.g., Davydow et al., 2008; Wade et al., 2013; Table 16.1).

PSYCHOLOGICAL ASSESSMENT AND INTERVENTIONS

Assessment

Psychological research has also led to the development and validation of screening tools to detect risk factors such as acute stress and delirium among patients in critical care environments. The Intensive Care Psychological Assessment Tool (IPAT), a valid measure of acute stress now used in the United Kingdom and international critical care units, consists of 10 items assessing sleep, communication, anxiety, low mood, hallucinations, delusions, and traumatic memories (Wade et al., 2014). Scores above 7 (range 0–20) indicate a need for further psychological assessment and/or interventions. The Confusion Assessment Method for the Intensive Care Unit (CAM-ICU), which assesses mental status, inattention, altered consciousness, and disorganized thinking, is the most researched tool to detect delirium in critical care, but other measures are being developed and tested (Ely et al., 2001; Ouimet et al., 2006).

Psychologist researchers are particularly interested in the development of psychological interventions that target risk factors and could reduce adverse psychosocial outcomes. Such interventions could be introduced in the acute critical care phase, the in-hospital rehabilitation phase, or the post-hospital recovery phase (Box 16.1).

BOX 16.1.
POTENTIAL PSYCHOLOGICAL INTERVENTIONS REQUIRING FURTHER
DEVELOPMENT AND RESEARCH

In-ICU

Cognitive-behavioral therapy (CBT) for ventilated patients

Combined cognitive rehabilitation (goal management training) and physical therapy
for ventilated patients

Psychologist-led management of delirium and agitation

Music therapy and complementary therapies to reduce acute stress in the ICU

Psychologist-led relational approaches (e.g., being present, acknowledging distress,
exploring meaning, reducing isolation)

Use of clinical psychologists in the ICU to tackle distress and early trauma symptoms

Nurse-led psychological support in the ICU

Protocol-driven family support in the ICU

Occupational therapy-led behavioral activation to address symptoms of depression and
physical function

Patient-friendly written information ICU discharge pack to improve early rehabilitation

Post-ICU

Post-ICU mindfulness program via telephone or mobile phone appTelephone-based
coping skills training program delivered by clinical psychologistICU patient dia-
riesEye movement desensitization and reprocessing therapy for post-ICU patients
with PTSD*

General practitioner–led, psychologist-supervised narrative therapy for post-
ICU PTSD

Psychologist-led intervention for PTSD combining CBT and narrative exposure
therapy5-week MDT rehabilitation program

---

*This is now a "conditionally recommended" rather than "strongly recommended" therapy by the American
Psychological Association (https://www.apa.org/ptsd-guideline/ptsd.pdf).

Interventions in the acute phase

A systematic review of psychological, pharmacologic, and behavioral interventions
suggested preliminary, albeit limited, evidence that the onset of PTSD could be prevented in acute medical patients (Birk et al., 2019). Nine interventions trialed in critical care included cognitive-behavioral therapy (CBT), mindfulness, earplugs and
eye masks, ICU diaries, a rehabilitation workbook, evidence-based sedation practices, and an enhanced rehabilitation program delivered immediately after the critical care stay. The enhanced rehabilitation program included mobilization, exercise,

diet therapy, occupational therapy, and speech and language therapy. Another systematic review identified 23 studies of interventions designed to reduce acute critical care stress; 12 of them were found beneficial, although evidence was deemed weak to moderate. These promising interventions included music and nature sounds therapy for ventilated patients and mind–body therapies such as acupressure (Wade et al., 2016).

Environmental interventions have been considered to reduce triggers of fear in critical care, such as inability to communicate, noise, unnatural light, crowding, shapes and shadows at nighttime, and missing one's family. Psychological first aid (PFA) is an evidence-informed approach for helping people affected by a traumatic incident to reduce distress and foster coping. PFA provides key actions to help people feel safe, including reassurance through normalizing the experience, helping people reunite with loved ones, and enabling voluntary sharing of experiences (World Health Organization, 2011). The five principles of PFA aim to create a sense of safety, calm, connectedness, confidence/control, and hope after a traumatic event (Box 16.2).

Environmental improvements and elements from PFA and CBT were combined in an intervention to reduce acute stress in a cluster-randomized clinical trial (Provision of Psychological Support to People in Intensive Care [POPPI]) with 1,453 patients (Wade et al., 2019). Participants screened as having acute stress in units randomized to the intervention received three nurse-led stress support sessions based on elements of CBT for psychosis (Fowler et al., 1995) that aimed to reduce stress, including distress related to hallucinations and delusions. The primary outcome was self-reported PTSD severity at 6 months, while secondary outcomes included depression and anxiety. No significant differences in outcomes were found. Suggested explanations for this result include the possibility that the intervention was delivered at the wrong time—whether too early or too late. Perhaps a wider group of multidisciplinary staff should be given more intensive training and supervision than was provided in the POPPI trial in managing delirious, stressed, and traumatized patients during the earliest acute critical care phase. Alternatively, practitioner psychologists could deliver more intensive interventions including trauma-focused therapy at a later timepoint when patients may be more ready and able to receive it.

Adding clinical psychologists to the critical care team was associated with a significant reduction in later PTSD and need for psychiatric medication in one study (Peris et al., 2011). Each patient received five or six clinical psychology interventions. However, the study used a historical control rather than a randomized design, and the authors did not provide detailed information about which interventions were given. Other studies have claimed that a psychologist working with individuals

BOX 16.2.

FIVE PRINCIPLES OF PSYCHOLOGICAL FIRST AID FOR CRITICAL
CARE PATIENTS

When people suffer a frightening experience such as admission to critical care, they have five main needs: safety, calm, connectedness, confidence, and hope. The following tips help staff to deliver the five principles of psychological first aid.

Safety

All critical care patients need to hear messages of safety, whether they are on CPAP (continuous positive airway pressure) or other NIV (noninvasive ventilation); about to be ventilated; are already ventilated and sedated; have a tracheostomy; after extubation/decannulation. Tell them:

- You are a nurse (etc.) and wearing a mask (etc.) to prevent infection
- They have been ill, but they are in a safe place
- This is a hospital; the people around them are doctors and nurses
- Acknowledge that they may feel upset or frightened.
- If patients are delirious or agitated, speak in a gentle, soothing voice; use open visible body language; do not crowd them; move slowly; use short sentences, speak to them little and often; do not either argue or agree with them about strange beliefs they may express; just emphasize your aim is to keep them comfortable and safe.

Calm

Information, distraction, and relaxation can help lower anxiety.

- Give clear, simple information about illness and treatment and reassuring news about their family where possible. Continue to repeat key information as they may not retain it.
- Hold their hand, ask them about themselves, talk to them calmly about what they see around them, offer small gestures such as combing hair, play music.
- Teach slow breathing/relaxation/calm place exercises. Use relaxation apps.

Connectedness

You are very busy, but it makes a real difference to patients and their recovery if you:

- Find time to talk to them
- Find ways to help them communicate
- Help them to use a phone to text or FaceTime family/friends
- Offer and help to organize a family video call
- Ask if they have any messages for loved ones before being ventilated

Confidence/control

As soon as possible, give patients a sense of control and confidence that they can start to look after themselves.

- Start by finding small ways they can do some self-care, such as having a wash/eating/ brushing teeth/rehab routine.
- Help them to find out any information they want to know.
- Help them communicate about their feelings and worries.

Hope

Encourage hope and realistic optimism wherever possible.

- Point out any signs of progress, as patients often don't notice these.

Find out what is important to them and help them achieve steps toward them, such as get off ventilator, sit up, eat and drink, get out of bed, walk to the toilet, leave critical care, go home.

Based on Wade, D., Howell, D., & Phillips, A. (2020). Psychological care of Covid-19 critical care patients: Staff guide 2/1. www.ics.ac.uk/ICS/COVID-19/COVID-19_patient_and_relative/Patient_and_Relative_Resources.aspx

in critical care, should help to reduce social isolation; establish a day/night cycle; treat anxiety, hallucinations, and delusions with cognitive-behavioral approaches (Bennun, 2001); and provide positive suggestions for ventilated, sedated patients (Varga et al., 2013). Psychotherapy sessions have also been proposed to explore the meanings of hallucinations and delusions. In a case series study, ventilator-dependent patients were reported to have successfully weaned with the help of CBT (Cohen et al., 2019).

The use of cognitive rehabilitation to improve cognitive outcomes from critical care has been proposed, and a small feasibility study providing cognitive and physical rehabilitation for mechanically ventilated patients was carried out (Brummel et al., 2014). However, more research is needed to determine the efficacy and feasibility of cognitive rehabilitation in critical care (see Chapter 6 for additional discussion).

Family well-being in critical care has also been the subject of research. In a recent RCT, flexible visitation did not reduce the incidence of delirium but did increase family satisfaction and reduce family psychological distress (Rosa et al., 2019). A systematic review showed that interventions consisting of the provision of medical information and/or emotional support to enhance communication and shared decision-making between family members and medical teams were effective in reducing length of stay (mean difference = −0.89; 95% confidence interval [CI] = −1.50 to −0.27). Mortality rates were not affected, suggesting that appropriate lifesaving treatments for those likely to survive were not hindered, but inappropriate or ineffective life-sustaining treatments may have been reduced. Interventions such as providing leaflets and educational materials were ineffective unless combined with offering family members time to ask questions and develop trusting relationships (Lee et al., 2019) (see Chapter 12 for additional discussion).

Interventions after leaving critical care (in-hospital rehabilitation)

The UK's National Institute of Care and Health Excellence (NICE) quality standard (2017) emphasizes the importance of patients leaving the critical care unit armed with an individualized rehabilitation plan. The effect of provision of postdischarge information has not been widely researched, but a feasibility study of 158 patients given a written critical care discharge information packet based on a psychological self-regulation theory provided preliminary data that the intervention could help to optimize early rehabilitation (Bench et al., 2015).

Interventions in the post-hospital recovery period

With increased awareness of PICS, there is a growing literature on post-critical care interventions, including follow-up clinics, peer support groups, group psychological interventions, and individual psychological interventions. To date, there is very limited evidence to support the effectiveness of follow-up clinics. A nonblinded multicenter RCT of nurse-led follow-up clinics across three hospitals recruiting 286 patients (192 at 1-year follow-up) found no difference at 12 months in health-related quality of life (as measured by the SF-36) (Cuthbertson et al., 2009). The clinics were found to be significantly more costly than standard care and not cost-effective.

In a study of 40 patients from one hospital in Scotland, participants took part in a 5-week peer-supported rehabilitation program including pharmacy, physiotherapy, nursing, medical, and psychology input. There was improvement in quality of life at 12 months for patients in the intervention group compared to historical controls. Self-efficacy improved during the program and at 1 year after the intervention. The authors reported that 88% of participants returned to employment or volunteering compared to 46% of the control group (McPeake et al., 2017).

One function of follow-up clinics can be to return the critical care diary that staff and relatives had completed in layman's terms during the patient's critical care stay; the original rationale was to fill a memory gap pertaining to the ICU admission as a preventive intervention for posttraumatic stress. An RCT to assess the impact of diaries on the psychological well-being of patients and families at 3 months after discharge in 367 patients found no difference between control and intervention groups; therefore, the findings did not support the use of a diary as a preventive measure for PTSD (Garrouste-Orgeas et al., 2019). However, there seemed to be a diverse range of opinions from survivors and their families about the utility of the diary, suggesting that other potential mechanisms to aid recovery exist and that some patients benefit while others do not.

Another way of providing support to critical care survivors is via peer support groups. A review of support groups found six models of peer support: community-based, psychologist-led outpatient, models within follow-up clinics, groups within the unit, peer mentorships, and online. These groups experience common barriers to sustainability, including limited funding and recruitment (McPeake et al., 2019). However, a survey with a 56% response rate by the UK Intensive Care Society (Groves et al., 2020) found that 46 (48%) of UK critical care units ran peer support groups, with attendees describing overwhelmingly positive experiences in the groups.

A number of RCTs of psychological interventions in the post-hospital period have been conducted. One RCT, the Rapit study, in 10 hospitals evaluated a nurse-led post-hospital recovery program in which patients were given a journal of their stay and three follow-up consultations. There was no difference in quality of life, depression, PTSD, or service use, but there was some reduction in anxiety (Jensen et al., 2016). A 3-month-long mindfulness program was found to be feasible and acceptable to post-critical care patients, whether delivered by phone (with a therapist) or by a mobile telephone application. The same team developed a 6-week psychologist-delivered telephone-based coping skills training program based on CBT principles. In an RCT, the coping skills program did not improve psychological distress symptoms compared with an education program; however, it did alleviate symptoms of distress at 6 months among patients with high baseline distress 2 weeks after their discharge home (Cox et al., 2018). This may suggest that psychological interventions should be delivered to those who have specific risk factors (e.g., higher baseline distress) rather than to all patients.

Only small studies have been published regarding interventions designed to improve or prevent post-critical care cognitive impairment. A study of 21 patients showed that a cognitive, physical, and functional rehabilitation intervention that included goal management training improved executive and cognitive functioning (Jackson et al., 2012). A proof-of-concept study of 24 patients that used 18 computerized brain-training exercises to aid cognitive rehabilitation found improvement in attention, processing speed, memory, and executive function (Wilson et al., 2018).

Gaps in the literature

GAPS IN THE LITERATURE ON PSYCHOLOGY AND CRITICAL CARE

This survey reveals many gaps in the literature, particularly regarding the efficacy of psychological interventions that could reduce distress in the acute critical care, hospital, or post-hospital settings. This could reflect the lack of certainty regarding risk factors for undesirable psychological outcomes following critical illness. The finding that acute stress in critical care predicts adverse long-term outcomes has been repeated in several studies; however, in the POPPI trial, reducing acute stress did not lead to a reduction in subsequent PTSD. Hallucinations and delusions appear to be associated with the early formation of traumatic memories from critical care. However, cohort studies have not consistently found an association between delirium and PTSD (Svenningsen et al., 2015; Wolters et al., 2016). The role of psychoactive drugs in the genesis of PTSD, depression, and other unfavorable outcomes remains under-researched, with continuing uncertainty regarding identity, dose, and duration of drugs and the outcomes with which they are associated. The role of other clinical factors such as invasive medical interventions and sociodemographic risk factors is also under-researched. Finally, research may have focused too exclusively on psychiatric outcomes such as PTSD and depression, whereas other outcomes such as poor psychological adjustment to illness may be equally or more relevant and common.

GAPS IN RESEARCH ON INTERVENTIONS IN THE ICU SETTING

Delirium is a highly distressing experience for many patients (Wade et al., 2014) that leads to dangerous outcomes; treating it is a clear goal for interdisciplinary teams including psychologists. The treatment of choice in many critical care units remains the use of antipsychotics such as haloperidol or quetiapine, even though evidence is lacking to support this practice (e.g., Girard et al., 2018). In a prospective study of more than 15,000 adults, use of the "ICU liberation" bundle of care (including elements such as earlier awakening, de-sedation, and mobilization) was associated with reduced likelihood of delirium (Pun et al., 2019). However, a recent systematic review found no evidence that nonpharmacologic interventions can reduce the incidence, duration, or severity of delirium in critical care. The authors hypothesized that their finding may be due to the lack of large, well-conducted studies of those types of intervention. Certainly, the expert consensus is that nonpharmacologic interventions are preferable for both prevention and treatment of delirium (Scottish Intercollegiate Guidelines Network [SIGN], 2019; Box 16.3).

BOX 16.3.
NONPHARMACOLOGIC DELIRIUM RISK REDUCTION AND TREATMENT

Risk reduction

The following components should be considered as part of care for patients at risk of developing delirium

- *Orientation and ensuring patients have their glasses and hearing aids*
- *Promoting sleep hygiene (including use of ear plugs)*
- Early mobilization
- Pain control
- Prevention, early identification and treatment of postoperative complications
- Maintaining optimal hydration and nutrition
- Regulation of bladder and bowel function
- Provision of supplementary oxygen, if appropriate
- *Ward moves should be avoided wherever possible for patients at risk of delirium*
- *Prior to surgery, patients and carers should be advised of the risk of developing delirium, to alleviate distress and help with management if it does occur*
- *Where possible, assistance should be sought from a patient's relatives and carers to deliver care to reduce the risk of delirium developing*
- Anaesthetic management: Depth of anaesthesia should be monitored in all patients aged over 60 years under general anaesthesia for surgery expected to last more than one hour, with the aim of avoiding excessively deep anaesthesia

Treatment

Healthcare professionals should follow established pathways of good care to manage patients with delirium

- First consider acute, life-threatening causes of delirium, including low oxygen level, low blood pressure, low glucose level, and drug intoxication or withdrawal
- Systematically identify and treat potential causes (medications, acute illness, etc) noting that multiple causes are common
- Optimize physiology, management of concurrent conditions, environment *(reduce noise), medications, and natural sleep, to promote brain recover*
- *Specifically detect, assess causes of, and treat agitation and/or distress, using non-pharmacological means only, if possible*
- *Communicate the diagnosis to patients and carers, encourage involvement of carers, and provide ongoing engagement and support*
- Aim to prevent complications of delirium such as immobility, falls, pressure sores, dehydration, malnourishment, isolation
- Monitor for recovery and consider specialist referral if not recovering
- *Consider follow up*

Psychosocial elements *in italics.*
SIGN, 2019

The nonpharmacologic bundles commonly used do not fully address the emotional/psychological component of delirium, although this component is one of five key domains in an influential model (Maldonaldo, 2017; see Figure 16.2). The new SIGN delirium guideline alludes to psychological interventions such as (1) assessment of causes of and treatment of agitation and/or distress, using nonpharmacologic means only, if possible, and (2) promotion of cognitive engagement and other rehabilitation strategies. However, no details regarding these psychological interventions are given (see Box 16.3).

To our knowledge, in the critical care setting, no focused research has been completed to develop or support specific psychological interventions for management of delirium by psychologists or psychiatrists. However, certain techniques have been advocated in other settings. These include psychology-led consultations to reduce delirium incidence after surgery; coordination of environmental, emotional, behavioral, and cognitive interventions for delirium; and gentle reality testing of hallucinations and delusions for patients who are ready to participate (Basten & McGuire, 2011). Research evaluating interventions for delirium, hallucinations, and delusions that occur in other settings or conditions such as geriatrics, psychosis, or disorders such as dementia or Parkinson's disease could inform interventions for critical care delirium.

Literature from geriatric medicine shows that side effects of antipsychotic medications are particularly problematic in older adults and emphasizes the need for staff to look for reasons for agitation as the first step in managing the behavior (Pritchard & Brighty, 2015). Possible reasons include the patient's inability to communicate normally about unmet needs such as pain, hunger, thirst, or loneliness. Staff should aim to assess the root cause of the patient's distress and attempt to meet their needs before patients become so agitated that they are a threat to their own or others' safety. Another possible cause is environments that are either under-stimulating or over-stimulating (and CCUs can often, paradoxically, be both of these things at different times). A third common cause is patients' perceiving (rightly or not) that they are receiving inadequate staff attention or where staff behavior is not person-centered. A comprehensive, systematic review of more than 160 studies of nonpharmacologic interventions to reduce agitation and aggression in patients with dementia found that teaching staff person-centered care and communication skills was the most successful intervention, along with sensory interventions such as massage and protocolized music therapy (Livingston et al., 2014).

Originally conceived by Carl Rogers (2004), person-centered care means that caregivers treat patients with warmth, genuineness, unconditional positive regard (acceptance), and empathic understanding, striving to be nonjudgmental. This approach is also a cornerstone of modern care for patients with psychotic disorders

TABLE 16.2.

Communication tips for critical care staff working with patients with delirium and distress

Setting the scene

Be person-centered (i.e., warm, genuine, accepting, understanding, nonjudgmental).

Build rapport: be open, honest, listening to gain trust.

Acknowledge ICU is distressing, and discussing worries is difficult.

Discuss emotions with sensitivity

Aim to assess root causes of agitation, address unmet needs (e.g., pain, thirst).

What to do

Have open, visible body language; give hallucinating patients lots of personal space.

Use caring tone of voice and manner when discussing worries and fears.

Use slow speech, simple vocabulary, and short sentences.

If a verbal patient is speaking rapidly, slow down the pace of conversation.

Talk to patients with hallucinations and delusions as rational people with unusual experiences.

If challenged by patients to confirm a delusion, say it seems unlikely to you, but you are open to learning otherwise.

Acknowledge the stress the unusual experiences are causing patients and emphasize your priority is helping them feel calm and safe.

What not to do

Make gestures that look like ordering/criticizing (e.g., pointing, arm-folding, finger-wagging).

Allow your voice to sound frustrated or irritable.

Laugh at hallucinations and delusions.

Contradict, dismiss, or minimize delusions.

Encourage paranoia.

Use phrases that sound patronizing or sarcastic.

such as schizophrenia. The research on caring for individuals with psychosis has much to offer critical care practitioners, particularly research on therapeutic communication with people having unusual experiences such as hallucinations and delusions. For example, a large qualitative review summarized evidence and advice from nurses who are expert in caring for and communicating with this population (Bowers et al., 2019). Table 16.2 gives more details about a communication style that could be helpful for critical care patients, one that is designed to calm their fears and not to increase their paranoia and sense of isolation. Further research needs to be carried out to evaluate whether training in person-centered care and enhanced communication skills could reduce delirium and agitation in critical care patients.

Few psychological studies have focused on preventing depression as a primary outcome of a critical care stay, although most studies find higher rates of depression than PTSD following a critical care stay. Physical rehabilitation and behavioral activation may offer hope for improvement, consistent with recommendations from NICE. Behavioral activation implemented by occupational therapists to address symptoms of depression and diminished physical function after acute respiratory failure is currently being evaluated by Dr. Ann Parker in the United States (ClinicalTrials.gov identifier NCT03431493).

GAPS IN RESEARCH ON POST-ICU IN-HOSPITAL REHABILITATION

The authors were unable to find any studies of psychological interventions for critical illness survivors who have been transferred to other hospital wards (although stress support sessions were frequently delivered on other units during the POPPI trial). However, further research should be carried out, as the post-critical care hospitalization period may provide patients with the space, time, and privacy needed to reflect on and process critical care experiences.

GAPS IN RESEARCH ON INTERVENTIONS IN THE POST-HOSPITAL RECOVERY PERIOD

Most critical care psychological research has focused on interventions to be delivered after hospital discharge, yet disappointingly few of these have proven to be effective. It is notable that many of the interventions described are new or innovative programs and are often nurse-led. Little has been published about individual psychological therapies offered to critical illness survivors. NICE guidance (2009) suggests psychological therapies for depression and anxiety including low-intensity interventions such as computerized CBT, guided self-help, and group-based CBT as well as high-intensity interventions such as CBT, interpersonal therapy, and short-term psychotherapy.

The revised NICE guidance (2018) for the treatment and management of PTSD also supports the effectiveness of trauma-focused psychological therapies. Ongoing studies, the results of which had not been published at the time of writing, include the PICTURE trial in Germany of three sessions of narrative therapy for post-critical care PTSD, delivered by family physicians and supervised by psychologists (ISRCTN registry 97280643) and a Cambridge case-control study of an intervention based on CBT and narrative exposure therapy (https://clinicaltrials.gov/ct2/show/NCT03315390). Another psychological therapy recommended as a second-line treatment for PTSD by NICE in the UK is eye movement desensitization and reprocessing (EMDR). A small pilot trial of EMDR in 10 post-critical care patients meeting criteria for PTSD showed reductions in PTSD and depressive symptoms after an average of five sessions, suggesting potential for treating ICU-related PTSD (Hulme, 2018). However, in the United States, EMDR has been downgraded to a "conditionally recommended" rather than "strongly recommended" treatment for PTSD (American Psychological Association, 2017). Most of the above therapies are commonly delivered to patients with PTSD resulting from a variety of traumas, not specifically critical care patients.

More and larger studies are also needed to evaluate interventions designed to reduce the incidence of persistent cognitive impairment that occurs after ICU discharge. At least one RCT, with four arms, is under way to evaluate the efficacy of physical exercise and cognitive training on cognitive function among patients aged 50 years and older who experienced delirium during a critical care admission (Wang et al., 2018).

How to conduct psychological research in a critical care-related setting

Given that there is still much to be done, how can psychologists (or other staff members interested in psychology) conduct research in the critical care area? Establishing oneself as a psychology researcher depends on the size of study the researchers plan to undertake. Psychological interventions in the critical care unit can be complex, and UK researchers who have an idea for an intervention first need to carry out an intervention development study using an accepted model such as the Medical Research Council framework for developing and evaluating complex interventions (Craig et al., 2008). An intervention development study may include some of the following essential background work: scoping reviews, systematic reviews, focus groups, Delphi processes, cohort studies, or interview studies, which are explained in Table 16.3.

TABLE 16.3.

Essential development work for psychological interventions: definitions

Examples of essential development work	Description
Scoping review	Preliminary assessment of potential, size, and scope of available research literature. Aims to identify nature and extent of research evidence. Carried out as a precursor to systematic review.
Systematic review	A review of a clearly formulated question that uses systematic, transparent, reproducible methods to identify, select, and critically appraise all relevant research, and to collect and analyze data from the studies that are included in the review
Focus group	A qualitative research method in which a trained person conducts a collective interview of typically six to eight people from similar backgrounds, with similar demographic characteristics, or similar experiences
Delphi process	A group communication method where a panel of experts arrive at a consensus over a series of questions and discussions. It is used for estimating or forecasting. A suitable facilitator is chosen and experts with relevant knowledge are selected to make sure the problem is defined well.
Cohort study	Type of longitudinal study; an approach that follows research participants who share a common characteristic or demographic similarity over a long period of time
Interview study	Qualitative research method used to collect in-depth information on people's opinions, thoughts, experiences, and feelings

This background work can be done in a library, a critical care unit where the psychology researcher works, or possibly a partnered unit if the researcher is based in a university. For example, at an early stage of the intervention development that led to the POPPI study, the first author systematically reviewed psychological risk factors and critical care outcomes; interview studies with patients experiencing flashbacks; and focus groups of nurses and patients who discussed critical care stress (Wade, 2010).

Another option is to enlist help from local research nurses if the unit has them embedded. They can share their knowledge and skills with operational issues such as screening eligible patients, patient approach, recruitment, and recording data. It is also important to develop good relationships with the multidisciplinary team of the critical care unit in order to understand the working environment and team processes. The clinical team, along with clinical researchers, can help the psychologist attend staff and team meetings to allow them to obtain a clear picture of the unit's working practices and culture. Getting to know the timing of ward rounds, bedside meetings, care plans, shift handover reports, and staff breaks allows researchers to adapt screening routines to fit the unit.

It is important for researchers to be flexible every time they arrive on a critical care unit, and to be sympathetic to the fast-changing environment. Having a regular presence on a unit helps staff become more familiar with a study and promotes teamwork between clinical staff and researchers. Two examples of a psychological researcher working with the local nurse research team are (1) a cohort study of clinical, psychological, and sociodemographic risk factors for PTSD, depression, and anxiety after critical care (Wade et al., 2012) and (2) the IPAT validation study (Wade et al., 2014) that our team carried out.

To increase awareness and support for the study, it is helpful to create attractive resources such as a study video, posters, and slide sets about studies to be used in unit meetings or training sessions. Psychology researchers should also aim to give regular updates on the progress of a study via flyers, posters, and emails, communicating with staff at their handovers to keep them engaged.

After carrying out all the essential background work to inform the development of a proposed psychological intervention, the researcher should then conduct a pilot trial to find out if the intervention is feasible to deliver in the real world and acceptable to both staff and patients involved. This would usually be conducted at a number of small sites (two to four, for example) and it would be necessary, using the same strategies as mentioned earlier, to find out about the culture and practices of the other sites, as they may include critical care units that the psychologist is not familiar with.

Once all the relevant development work has been completed, and an intervention has been piloted that is feasible and acceptable to both patients and staff, funding should be applied for, to carry out a multisite study (an RCT, for example) to evaluate the clinical effectiveness and the cost-effectiveness of the intervention. Main funding bodies need to be identified for large trials in the relevant country (e.g., the National Institute of Health in the United States and the National Institute of Health Research in the United Kingdom). An example of a rehabilitation trial with psychological elements is the Recover study (Walsh et al., 2015) conducted by a team from two Edinburgh hospitals, with support from the Chief Scientist Office, Scotland, Edinburgh University and NHS Lothian's academic health science centre. The first step in setting up the Recover study was to assemble a research team consisting of senior nurses, medical consultants, rehabilitation assistants, dietitians, physiotherapists, and speech and language therapists. A clinical trials unit consisting of trial methodologists, managers, statisticians, and health economists was commissioned to manage the running of the trial.

Guidance for creating and leading a research team

A research team, group, center, or unit can be defined as a "group of people working together in a committed way towards a common research goal" ("Vitae: Releasing the Potential of Researchers," n.d.).

A research team needs to encompass a good balance of skills and expertise, with all members working toward a shared goal. A research team leader needs to be confident that team members have, or can develop, the necessary skills and knowledge for the research in hand. Team members may have different disciplinary expertise, aspirations, and cultural backgrounds. The role of the research team leader is to provide clear goals, expectations, motivation, and inspiration for the team. If the team is involved in decision-making, it will help to build a sense of participation and commitment among members.

Evidence of this can be seen in the InS:PIRE Study (Intensive Care Syndrome: Promoting Independence and Return to Employment), a quality improvement program at Glasgow Royal Infirmary, Scotland. The 6-week rehabilitation program focused on patient education, peer support, support for family members, and self-management. The program arose from a sense among staff of a need to do something more for critical care survivors. Staff participation was voluntary, but strongly interest-based with high levels of motivation. Perceived benefits of the study included improved teamwork and enhanced quality of care (McPeake et al., 2017).

The InS:PIRE Study is an example of how innovative research methods can be used to evaluate a small project as it is scaled up over time. The Glasgow team won funding from the Health Foundation to expand their innovative rehabilitation program across five further centers in four other regions of Scotland. An independent evaluation of the scaling-up process was published (Rzewuska et al., 2019), based on ethnographic work; documentary analysis; observational activities; qualitative interviews with staff, patients, and family members; focus groups; and behavior change interviews as well as quantitative analysis of patient demographics and outcomes. This evaluation, carried out by an independent health services research unit, led to identification of the three most successful "active ingredients" of the complex intervention: (1) one-to-one time with critical care staff to discuss their critical care journey, (2) peer support, and (3) provision of patient-centered care. Less positively, they found the intervention was resource-heavy, was received by only a small proportion of patients, and had an unclear perceived mechanism of change. These findings are in contrast to the more typical intervention evaluations by RCTs that merely conclude that an intervention is effective or ineffective.

Research team leaders need to consider how to divide responsibilities, ensuring that every team member knows who is responsible for which parts of the research project. Communication is key. Everyone should know what information they can expect to receive and whom they can ask for updates. Team leaders should try to communicate clearly, early, and often to ensure the whole team has a clear vision of their goals. Communication should be a dialogue so that team members understand what is being asked of them and develop a sense of ownership over the project. The team's expectations of leadership should also be understood.

Other important issues include reporting (team members should know to whom to report, and when), milestones (team members need to be aware of all project milestones, not just the final deadline), and thinking about potential ethical dilemmas and approaches to ethical challenges. It is important for the researcher to be realistic about team members' capabilities and not give them impossible deadlines or tasks that are too complex. The lead researcher may also have to protect team members from unrealistic, distracting, or inappropriate requests made by other individuals inside and outside of the study.

Recruitment strategies and consent process

A crucial step in any research study is recruiting enough participants to ensure an adequate sample; this can be a particularly difficult challenge in a critical care setting, especially if the intervention or observation is being carried out during the acute phase of a critical care stay. Consent must be obtained for all patients taking part in research and, in order to provide an informed decision, the patient needs to understand, remember, and weigh the information being given to them. They should be given an information leaflet that tells them about the study, what it will involve, and the risks and benefits. This should be written in clear and simple language, avoiding medical jargon while still explaining the study in detail.

Patients usually need to have capacity to take part in research. However, a study of delirium or patients who require very early mobilization while still on the ventilator might involve patients without full capacity. For those patients who cannot understand and retain information due to lack of capacity and therefore cannot provide consent, a legal representative or surrogate decision-maker can consent on their behalf. The details of how this is done may differ from country to country. In the United Kingdom there are two types of legal representative:

1. A *personal* legal representative, who must have a close personal relationship with the participant and be documented as next of kin. The personal legal representative gives informed consent on behalf of the participant, and this legally represents their presumed will.

2. If no personal legal representative can be found, then a *professional* legal representative should be consulted. This can be a doctor responsible for the person's care, but they should have no connection to the research being conducted. Researchers must discuss all information with legal representatives, provide them with a study information sheet, and get their written consent.

Patients must be approached to re-consent when they regain capacity. This is intended to ensure that participants are fully informed and that they are still willing to take part. They may withdraw from the study at this point if they wish.

How to approach participants

The researcher's initial approach to presenting a study to patients, families, or legal representatives will affect their decision to participate or not. It is important to give patients a chance to ask questions and to express reservations they may have about the study so the researcher can discuss their concerns with them immediately and give reassurance where possible. The researcher should know when to defer the consent process to avoid a patient declining to participate purely because of timing or other issues that could easily be resolved. It is also valuable to spend time addressing any concerns and questions that patients and family members may have. Family members may encourage a patient to participate in a study if they believe it would be positive for the individual or for future patients. On the other hand, they might discourage participation in a study if they are worried about its potential to negatively affect the patient.

Other settings

As previously discussed, a psychological or rehabilitation study may not be designed for the critical care unit, but for settings such as other hospital wards after critical care discharge or in outpatient or community clinics (e.g., follow-up clinics or post-critical care psychology clinics) after hospital discharge. In this case, the research team will have to adapt the work to fit the relevant setting, considering the types of interventions that would be suitable in this setting and factors that might serve as enablers or barriers to a study. Preparatory work to understand settings and relevant factors will be vital to ensure the study's smooth running and success.

Another challenge for the researcher may be dealing with different staff members in a complex clinical setting where patients' conditions and needs are constantly changing. Innovative strategies may be needed to increase the number of participants in the study sample, giving careful consideration to issues such as the best times to screen patients in the sites where the researchers are working. It is important to select research sites with research capacity and capability: for example, sites where staff nurses are already familiar with research; where key leaders are likely to be supportive; where staff have good educational opportunities; and where patient throughput is large enough to support recruitment.

Conclusion

The aim of this chapter was to help potential researchers identify the main gaps that exist in the psychology and rehabilitation research related to critical care patients and to provide helpful information for psychologists or other professionals planning to set up research teams or projects in critical care psychology. Recent population studies and trials have continued to find high prevalence rates of PTSD, depression, and anxiety among critical care survivors (up to 50% depending on condition and measurement tools; e.g., Hatch et al., 2018); therefore, the development of interventions to reduce the stress and trauma endured by this vulnerable patient population remains a high priority. Critical illnesses can result in disability and reduced health-related quality of life. Although the optimal timing of components of rehabilitation is uncertain (Walsh et al., 2015), it is imperative that researchers with a passion for this area of scientific study continue to develop and define practice in future trial designs to include the whole span of the critical illness recovery trajectory.

References

Alonso-Ovies, A., & Heras, G. (2016). ICU: A branch of hell? *Intensive Care Medicine, 42*(4), 591–592.

American Psychological Association. (2017). Clinical practice guideline for the treatment of PTSD. https://www.apa.org/ptsd-guideline/ptsd.pdf

Basten, C. J., & McGuire, B. E. (2011). Delirium: The role of the psychologist in assessment and management. *Australian Psychologist, 35*(3), 201–207.

Bench, S., Day, T., Heelas, K., Hopkins, P., White, C., & Griffiths P. (2015). Evaluating the feasibility and effectiveness of a critical care discharge information pack for patients and their families: A pilot cluster randomized controlled trial. *BMJ Open, 5*(11), e006852. doi:10.1136/bmjopen-2014

Bennun, I. (2001). Intensive care unit syndrome: A consideration of psychological interventions. *British Journal of Medical Psychology, 74*(3), 369–377.

Birk, J., Sumner J., Haerizadeh M., Heyman-Kantor R., Falzon L., Gonzalez C., . . . Kronish, I. M. (2019). Early interventions to prevent post-traumatic stress disorder symptoms in survivors of life-threatening medical events: A systematic review. *Journal of Anxiety Disorders, 64*, 24–39.

Bowers, L., Brennan, G., Winship, G., & Theodoridou, C. (2019) How expert nurses communicate with acutely psychotic patients. *Mental Health Practice, 13*(7), 24–26.

Brummel, N., Girard, T., Ely, E., Pandharipande, P., Morandi, A. & Hughes, C. G. (2014). Feasibility and safety of early combined cognitive and physical therapy for critically ill medical and surgical patients: The Activity and Cognitive Therapy in ICU (ACT-ICU) trial. *Intensive Care Medicine, 40*(3), 370–379.

Carruthers, H., Gomershall, T., & Astin, F. (2018). The work undertaken by mechanically ventilated patients in intensive care: A qualitative meta-ethnography of survivors' experiences. *International Journal of Nursing Studies, 86*, 60–73.

Cohen, J., Gopal, A., Roberts, K., Anderson, E., & Siegal, A. (2019). Ventilator-dependent patients successfully weaned with cognitive behavioral therapy: A case series. *Psychosomatics, 60*(6), 612–619.

Cox, C. E., Hough, C. L., Carson, S. S., White, D. B., Kahn, J. M., Olsen, M. K., . . . Porter, L. S. (2018). Effects of a telephone- and web-based coping skills training program compared with an education program for survivors of critical illness and their family members: A randomized clinical trial. *American Journal of Respiratory and Critical Care Medicine, 197*, 66–78.

Craig, P., Dieppe, P., Macintyre, S., Michie, S., Nazareth, I., & Petticrew, M. (2008). Developing and evaluating complex interventions: The new Medical Research Council guidance. *British Medical Journal, 337*, a1655. doi:10.1136/bmj.a1655

Cuthbertson, B., Rattray, J., Campbell, M., Gager, M., Roughton, S., Smith, A., . . .Waldmann, C. (2009). The PRaCTICaL study of nurse led, intensive care follow-up programs for improving long term outcomes from critical illness: A pragmatic randomised controlled trial. *British Medical Journal, 339*, b3723.

Davydow, D., Gifford, J., Desai, S., Needham, D. M., & Bienvenu, O. J. (2008). Posttraumatic stress disorder in general intensive care survivors: A systematic review. *General Hospital Psychiatry, 30*(5), 421–434.

Ely, E., Inouye, S., Bernard, G., Gordon, S., Francis, J., & May, L. (2001). Delirium in mechanically ventilated patients: Validity and reliability of the Confusion Assessment Method for the Intensive Care Unit (CAM-ICU). *Journal of the American Medical Association, 286*(21), 2703–2710.

Fowler, D., Garety, P, & Kuipers, E. (1995). *Cognitive behaviour therapy for psychosis: Theory and practice.* John Wiley and Sons.

Garrouste-Orgeas, M., Flahault, C., Vinatier, I., Rigaud, J., Thieulot-Rolin, N., Mercier, E., . . . Timsit, J-F. (2019). Effect of an ICU diary on posttraumatic stress disorder symptoms among patients receiving mechanical ventilation: A randomized clinical trial. *Journal of the American Medical Association, 322*(3), 229–239.

Girard, T. D., Exline, M. C., Carson, S. S., Hough, C. L., Rock, P., Gong, M. N., . . . Ely, E. W. (2018). Haloperidol and ziprasidone for treatment of delirium in critical illness. *New England Journal of Medicine, 379*, 2506–2516.

Granberg, A., Bergborn Engberg, I., & Lundberg, D. (1999). Acute confusion and unreal experiences in intensive care patients in relation to the ICU syndrome. Part II. *Intensive and Critical Care Nursing, 15*(1), 19–33. doi:10.1016/s0964-3397(99)80062-7

Groves, J., Cahill, J., Sturmey, G., Peskett, M., & Wade, D., for and on behalf of the Patients and Relatives Committee of the Intensive Care Society and ICU Steps. (2020). Patient support groups: A survey of United Kingdom practice, purpose and performance. *Journal of the Intensive Care Society.* https://doi.org/10.1177/1751143720952017

Hatch, R., Young, D., Barber, V., Griffiths, J., Harrison, D., & Watkinson, P. (2018). Anxiety, depression and posttraumatic stress disorder after critical illness: A UK-wide prospective cohort study. *Critical Care, 22*, Article 310. doi:10.1186/s13054-018-2223-6

Hulme, T. (2018). Using eye movement therapy to reduce trauma after intensive care. *Nursing Times, 114*(3), 18–21.

Jackson, J., Ely, E. W., Morey, M. C., Anderson, V. M., Siebert, C. S., Denne, L. B., . . . Hoenig, H. (2012). Cognitive and physical rehabilitation of intensive care unit survivors: Results of the RETURN randomized controlled pilot investigation. *Critical Care Medicine, 40*(4), 1088–1097.

Jackson, J. C., Hart, R. P., Gordon, S. M., Hopkins, R. O., Girard, T. D., & Ely, E. W. (2007). Post-traumatic stress disorder and post-traumatic stress symptoms following critical illness in medical intensive care unit patients: Assessing the magnitude of the problem. *Critical Care, 11*, R27. https://doi.org/10.1186/cc5707

Jackson, J., Pandharipande, P., Girard, T., Brummel, N., Thompson, J., & Hughes, C. (2014). Depression, post-traumatic stress disorder, and functional disability in survivors of critical illness in the BRAIN-ICU study: A longitudinal cohort study. *Lancet Respiratory Medicine, 2*(5), 269–379.

Jackson, J. C., Santoro, M. J., Ely, T. M., Boehm, L., Keihl, A. L., Anderson, L. S., & Ely, E. W. (2014). Improving patient care through the prism of psychology: Application of Maslow's hierarchy to sedation, delirium and early mobility in the ICU. *Journal of Critical Care, 29*(3), 438–444.

Jensen, J., Egerod, I., Bestle, M., Christensen, D., Elklit, A., Hansen, R., . . . Overgaard, D. (2016). A recovery program to improve quality of life, sense of coherence and psychological health in ICU survivors: A multicenter randomized controlled trial, the RAPIT study. *Intensive Care Medicine, 42*, 1733–1743.

Jones, C., Backman, C., Capuzzo, M., Flaatten, H., Rylander, C., & Griffiths, R. (2007). Precipitants of post-traumatic stress disorder following intensive care: A hypothesis-generating study of diversity in care. *Intensive Care Medicine, 33*(6), 978–985.

Jones, C., Griffiths, R., Humphris, G., & Skirrow, P. (2001). Memory, delusions, and the development of acute posttraumatic stress disorder-related symptoms after intensive care. *Critical Care Medicine, 29*(3), 573–580. doi:10.1097/00003246-200103000-00019

Lee, H., Park, Y., Jang, E., & Lee, Y. (2019). Intensive care unit length of stay is reduced by protocolized family support intervention: A systematic review and meta-analysis. *Intensive Care Medicine, 45*(8), 1072–1081.

Livingston, G., Kelly, L., Lewis-Holmes, E., Baio, G., Morris, S., Patel, N., . . . Cooper, C. (2014). A systematic review of the clinical effectiveness and cost-effectiveness of sensory, psychological and behavioral interventions for managing agitation in older adults with dementia. *Health Technology Assessment, 18*(39), 1–226.

Maldonaldo, J. R. (2017). Acute brain failure: Pathophysiology, diagnosis, management, and sequelae of delirium. *Critical Care Clinics, 33*(3), 461–519.

McPeake, J., Hirshberg, E. L., Christie, L. M., Drumright, K., Haines, K., Hough, C. L., . . . Iwashyna, T. J. (2019). Models of peer support to remediate post-intensive care syndrome: A report developed by the society of critical care medicine thrive international peer support collaborative. *Critical Care Medicine, 47*(1), e21–e27.

McPeake, J., Shaw, M., Iwashyna, T., Daniel, M., Devine, H., Jarvie, L., . . . Quasim, T. (2017). Intensive care syndrome: Promoting independence and return to employment (InS:PIRE). Early evaluation of a complex intervention. *PLoS One, 12*(11), e0188028.

National Institute for Health and Care Excellence. (2009). Depression in adults: Recognition and management clinical guideline 90. https://www.nice.org.uk/guidance/cg90/resources/depression-in-adults-recognition-and-management-975742636741

National Institute for Health and Care Excellence. (2017). Rehabilitation after critical illness in adults: NICE Quality Standard 158. https://www.nice.org.uk/guidance/qs158/resources/rehabilitation-after-critical-illness-in-adults-pdf-75545546693317

National Institute for Health and Care Excellence. (2018). Post-traumatic stress disorder: NICE Guideline 116. https://www.nice.org.uk/guidance/ng116/chapter/Recommendations#management-of-ptsd-in-children-young-people-and-adults

Needham, D. M., Davidson, J., Cohen, H., Hopkins, R. O., Weinart, C., Wunsch, H., . . . Harvey, M. A. (2012). Improving long-term outcomes after discharge from intensive care unit: Report from a stakeholders' conference. *Critical Care Medicine, 40*(2), 502–509.

Novaes, M., Aronovich, A., Ferraz, M., & Knobel, E. (1997). Stressors in ICU: Patients' evaluation. *Intensive Care Medicine, 23*(12), 1282–1285. doi:10.1007/s001340050500

Ouimet, S., Kavanagh, B., Gottfried, S., & Skrobik, Y. (2006). Incidence, risk factors and consequences of ICU delirium. *Intensive Care Medicine, 33*(1), 66–73. doi:10.1007/s00134-006-0399-8

Pandharipande, P. P., Girard, T. D., Jackson, J. C., Morandi, A., Thompson, J. L., Pun, B. T., . . . Ely, E. W. (2013). Long-term cognitive impairment after critical illness. *New England Journal of Medicine, 369*(14), 1306–1316.

Pandharipande, P., Shintani, A., Peterson, J., Pun, B. T., Wilkinson, G. R., Dittus, R. S., . . . Ely, E. W. (2006). Lorazepam is an independent risk factor for transitioning to delirium in intensive care unit patients. *Anesthesiology, 104*(1), 21–26. doi:10.1097/00000542-200601000-00005

Peris, A., Bonizzoli, M., Iozzelli, D., Migliaccio, M., Zagli, G., Bacchereti, A., . . . Belloni, L. (2011). Early intra-intensive care unit psychological intervention promotes recovery from posttraumatic stress disorders, anxiety and depression symptoms in critically ill patients. *Critical Care, 15*(1), R41.

Pritchard, J., & Brighty, A. (2015). Caring for older people experiencing agitation. *Nursing Standard, 29*(30), 49–58.

Pun, B. T., Balas, M. C., Barnes-Daly, M. A., Thompson, J. L., Aldrich, J. M., Barr, J., . . . Ely, E. W. (2019). Caring for critically ill patients with the ABCDEF bundle. *Critical Care Medicine, 47*(1), 3–14. doi:10.1097/ccm.0000000000003482

Puntillo, K. A., Arai, S., Cohen, N. H., Gropper, M. A., Neuhaus, J., Paul, S. M., & Miaskowski, C. (2010). Symptoms experienced by intensive care unit patients at high risk of dying. *Critical Care Medicine, 38*(11), 2155–2160.

Rogers, C. (2004). *On becoming a person: A therapist's view of psychotherapy.*

Rosa, R. G., Falavigna, M., da Silva, D. B., Sganzerla, D., Martins, M., Santos, S., . . . Teixeira, C. (2019). Effect of flexible family visitation on delirium among patients in the intensive care unit. *Journal of the American Medical Association, 322*(3), 216–228.

Rzewuska, M., Morgan, H., Skea Z., Norrie, J., & Campbell, M. (2019). *InS:PIRE. Evaluation of the scaling up of a quality improvement initiative abridged report.* Health Foundation.

Scottish Intercollegiate Guidelines Network (SIGN). (2019). *Risk reduction and management of delirium.* SIGN.

Svenningsen, H., Egerod, I., Christensen, D., Tønnesen, E., Frydenberg, M., & Videbech, P. (2015). Symptoms of posttraumatic stress after intensive care delirium. *BioMed Research International, 2015,* 876947. doi:10.1155/2015/876947

Varga, K., Varga., Z, Frituz, G. (2013). Psychological support based on positive suggestions in the treatment of a critically ill ICU patient—a case report. *Interventional Medicine and Applied Science, 5*(4), 153–161.

Vitae: Releasing the Potential of Researchers. (n.d.). https://www.vitae.ac.uk/doing-research/leadership-development-for-principal-investigators-pis/building-and-managing-a-research-team

Wade, D. (2010). *Prevalence and predictors of psychological morbidity and quality of life after discharge from intensive care. Doctoral thesis,* University College London.

Wade, D., Als, N., Bell, V., Brewin, C., D'Antoni, D., Harrison, D. A., . . . Rowan, K. M. (2018). Providing psychological support to people in intensive care: Development and feasibility study of a nurse-led intervention to prevent acute stress and long-term morbidity. *BMJ Open, 8,* e021083. doi:10.1136/bmjopen-2017-021083

Wade, D., Hankins, M., Smyth, D., Rhone, E., Mythen, M., Howell, D., & Weinman, J. (2014). Detecting acute distress and risk of future psychological morbidity in critically ill patients: Validation of the intensive care psychological assessment tool. *Critical Care, 18,* Article 519. doi:10.1186/s13054-014-0519-8

Wade, D., Hardy, R., Howell, D., & Mythen, M. (2013). Identifying clinical and acute psychological risk factors for PTSD after critical care: A systematic review. *Minerva Anestesiologica, 79*(8), 944–963.

Wade, D., Howell, D., & Phillips, A. (2020). Psychological care of Covid-19 critical care patients: Staff guide 2/1. https://www.ics.ac.uk/ICS/COVID-19/COVID-19_patient_and_relative/Patient_and_Relative_Resources.aspx

Wade, D. M., Howell, D. C., Weinman, J. A., Hardy, R. J., Mythen, M. G., Brewin, C. R., & Raine, R. A. (2012). Investigating risk factors for psychological morbidity three months after intensive care: A prospective cohort study. *Critical Care, 16*(5), R192.

Wade, D., Moon, Z., Windgassen, S., Harrison, A., Morris, L., & Weinman, J. (2016). Non-pharmacological interventions to reduce ICU-related psychological distress: A systematic review. *Minerva Anestesiologica, 82*(4), 465–478.

Wade, D. M., Mouncey, P. R., Richards-Belle, A., Wulff, J., Harrison, D. A., Sadique, M. Z., . . . Rowan, K. M. (2019). Effect of a nurse-led preventive psychological intervention on symptoms of posttraumatic stress disorder among critically ill patients. *Journal of the American Medical Association, 321*(7), 665. doi:10.1001/jama.2019.0073

Walsh, T. S., Salisbury, L. G., Merriweather, J. L., Boyd, J. A., Griffith, D. M., Huby, G., . . . Ramsay, P. (2015). Increased hospital based physical rehabilitation and information provision after intensive care unit discharge: The RECOVER randomized clinical trial. *Journal of the American Medical Association, 175*(6), 901–910.

Wang, S., Hammes, J., Khan, S., Gao, S., Harrawood, A., Martinez, S., . . . Khan, B. (2018). Improving Recovery and Outcomes Every Day After the ICU (IMPROVE): Study protocol for a randomized controlled trial. *Trials, 19*(1), 19637.

Wilcox, M., Brummel, N., Archer, K., Ely, E., Jackson, J., & Hopkins, R. (2013). Cognitive dysfunction in ICU patients. *Critical Care Medicine, 41*, S81–S98. doi:10.1097/ccm.0b013e3182a16946

Wilson, J., Collar, E. M., Kiehl, A. L., Lee, H., Merzenich, M., Ely, E. W., & Jackson, J. (2018). Computerized cognitive rehabilitation in intensive care unit survivors: Returning to everyday tasks using rehabilitation networks-computerized cognitive rehabilitation pilot investigation. *Annals of the American Thoracic Society, 15*(7), 887–891.

Wolters, A. E., Peelen, L. M., Welling, M. C., Kok, L., de Lange, D. W., Cremer, O. L., . . . Veldhuijzen, D. S. (2016). Long term mental health problems after delirium in the intensive care unit. *Critical Care Medicine, 44*(10), 1808–1813.

World Health Organization. (2011). Psychological first aid: Guide for field workers. https://www.who.int/mental_health/publications/guide_field_workers/en/

17 Future Directions for Psychology in Critical Care
Dorothy Wade and Julie Highfield

The role of a practitioner psychologist in critical care

How will the emerging discipline of critical care psychology develop and increase its impact for the benefit of patients, families, and staff in future? How can the impressive body of knowledge that has been developed in the past two decades about patient experience, psychological and cognitive risk factors, outcomes, and interventions in critical care be strengthened and truly be translated from testimony and theory into practice?

For this transformation to occur, changes would be required in the philosophy and practice of medicine as well as in societal trends. Historically, critical care has primarily been a medical and nursing specialty but is gradually being extended to encompass other professionals such as physiotherapists and dietitians, and, more gradually, psychologists, speech and language therapists, and occupational therapists too. The presence of these rehabilitation experts is shifting the emphasis of critical care from acute rescue to longer-term recovery. Another shift is required to highlight the importance of psychological recovery and improved quality of life as well as physical recovery. This change has only begun. This reflects society's attitude toward mental health in comparison to physical health. In some countries, there is still stigma attached to the idea of mental illness and a lack of awareness in

Dorothy Wade and Julie Highfield, *Future Directions for Psychology in Critical Care* In: *Critical Care Psychology and Rehabilitation*. Edited by: Kirk J. Stucky and Jennifer E. Jutte, Oxford University Press. © Oxford University Press 2022.
DOI: 10.1093/oso/9780190077013.003.0017

promoting mental health, which is often a "Cinderella service," lacking funding and resources compared to physical health.

Currently, most countries have very few critical care units (CCUs) with access to a psychology service; exceptions are most notably the UK, Germany, which has a psychology section within the national critical care society, and Brazil, which has a long tradition of psychologists providing consultancy to CCU teams. We will describe each of these models in further detail in the "International Comparisons" section. While much crucial research in critical care psychology has been conducted in the United States, there is still a dearth of psychologists practicing in U.S. critical care units, perhaps due to the complications of funding such services across multiple health care tiers.

Recognition of the role of psychology in critical care may be expedited by the international experience of dealing with the COVID-19 pandemic. There has been a surge of both academic and media interest in the experiences of patients hospitalized with severe COVID-19 disease, many of whom have experienced delirium and post-hospital problems such as low mood and posttraumatic stress disorder (PTSD). Television interviews with patients and webinars with psychologists have brought the difficult psychological experiences associated with critical illness and mechanical ventilation to a much wider audience. In the United Kingdom, several national guidelines on both interdisciplinary rehabilitation and trauma-focused psychological services have prompted an increasing number of critical care departments to create roles for new or extra psychology staff. In addition, community psychology practitioners have been trained in the psychological aspects of hospital and critical care for COVID-19 patients.

Even before the pandemic, the role of the CCU psychologist had taken root more firmly in the United Kingdom than in many other countries. Perhaps this has been easier to achieve in a unitary national health system where most critical care departments are structured and funded in similar ways, with only minor variations, and are subject to the same national guidelines.

Our aims for this chapter are to look at the UK guidelines for the provision of psychological support in the critical care setting; to consider how well that guidance is carried out in reality; and to visualize a critical care psychology model where those guidelines are enacted in full. We will compare and contrast this model with guidelines or models practiced in other countries. We consider how psychology is best able to provide evidence to prove its value. Finally, we look into the crystal ball to imagine the critical care department of the future—with an environment that is psychologically informed, and where psychologists are fully integrated into the health care team.

The vision is also of a future where a well-funded international organization of critical care psychologists exists to run conferences, facilitating the exchange of ideas, research, training, and robust models of care built on shared knowledge and development. Currently, critical care psychologists attend and participate in large critical care organizations and conferences, including the Society of Critical Care Medicine (SCCM) in the United States and the European Society of Intensive Care Medicine (ESICM), to ensure that psychological issues and perspectives are heard and debated by the wider critical care community. Both authors of this chapter are involved in the Intensive Care Society of the United Kingdom (ICS-UK), promoting research and education into patient, family, and staff well-being, and have spoken at critical care conferences around the world to raise the profile of psychology.

The UK model of psychological care

The psychological impact of critical illness was first officially recognized by the National Institute of Health and Care Excellence (NICE) guideline CG83 on rehabilitation after critical illness (NICE, 2009). The emphasis was more on psychological assessment than intervention and required all UK ICUs to carry out both short and complex psychological assessments, alongside physical assessments, of patients at a number of timepoints: early in the ICU, before ICU discharge, before hospital discharge, and 2 to 3 months after critical care discharge. Short psychological assessments of patients could potentially be carried out by non-expert staff members early in an ICU admission. As no simple, clinically valid measures for the psychological impact of the ICU existed, the Intensive Care Psychological Assessment Tool (IPAT) was developed and validated in London as an easy-to-use tool for ICU staff, usually nurses; it consists of 10 items concerning stress, mood, and unusual ICU experiences (e.g., hallucinations, delusions) and is used to screen patients for acute stress (Wade et al., 2014). Complex assessments of emotional, psychological, psychiatric, or cognitive morbidity at other timepoints (before hospital discharge and at follow-up clinics) using agreed-upon tools such as the Patient Health Questionnaire–9 (depression) (PHQ-9; Kroenke et al., 2001), the General Anxiety Disorder-7 (GAD-7; Spitzer et al., 2006), the Trauma Screening Questionnaire (posttraumatic stress screen) (TSQ; Brewin et al., 2002), and the Montreal Cognitive Assessment (MoCA; Nasreddine et al., 2005) require the expertise of professional psychologists.

Later surveys found that the rehabilitation guideline (CG83) was poorly implemented across the UK National Health Service (NHS) (Connolly et al., 2014). Therefore, NICE published quality standard (QS) 158 for rehabilitation after critical illness (NICE, 2017) to strengthen and clarify the requirement for all NHS hospitals to provide a clear-cut intensive care rehabilitation pathway with assessments and interventions at key milestones. Again, the QS emphasized the need for psychological as well as physical assessments and also for each patient to have short- and medium-term rehabilitation goals set within 4 days of ICU admission as well as an individualized structured rehabilitation program in place by the time of discharge from the ICU. The rehabilitation programs should include psychological and cognitive goals and interventions as well as physical and functional ones, producing a need for psychologists in ICUs to lend their expertise in developing the programs. Goals may be set even for sedated, ventilated patients, perhaps to guide mitigation of delirium or lightening of sedation. New goals may be agreed upon when patients are more conscious, to reflect their own aims and preferences.

In response to the NICE guidance, and to the growing research evidence for psychological harm incurred during critical care admissions, the ICS-UK expanded staffing guidelines for UK critical care to include practitioner psychologists in every CCU (ICS, 2019). Currently, the requirement is for a full-time senior health or clinical psychologist (principal or consultant) to be employed by large ICUs and a part-time psychologist for smaller units, dependent on bed numbers. These psychologists should assess or oversee the psychological assessment of patients and provide evidence-based psychological interventions for patients and/or families in the critical care department, on step-down wards, or in outpatient departments following hospital discharge. They should also train staff in providing psychological care to patients and themselves provide staff well-being support as well as consultancy on psychosocial aspects of care for the interdisciplinary team.

A number of UK ICUs now support this psychological model of care, overseen by a full-time senior psychologist, particularly in large teaching hospital settings. Senior ICU psychologists have created an ICU psychology professional network known as PINC-UK (Psychologists in Intensive Care in the UK). The network has grown in just a few years from a membership of under 10 to around 100 critical care psychologists (at the time of writing) and is also a strategic partner of the ICS-UK. Through this network we know that some units have gone beyond the minimum requirement and installed a senior psychologist, supported by a small team of newly qualified psychologists, assistant psychologists, or graduate practitioners. In the majority of cases, however, psychologists have been employed for anything from a couple of hours a month to several days a week, primarily to staff a follow-up service, typically with limited input to the acute critical care setting. Many UK ICUs are not yet compliant with the staffing guideline and have not employed psychological staff. They may, however, access psychological expertise from clinical health psychology or liaison psychiatry departments serving their hospital as a whole.

The goal of PINC-UK is to have the ICS-UK staffing guidelines implemented in every hospital so that all CCUs have psychologists embedded within their team. It also aims to develop guidelines setting out clearly the role of the psychology team in working with patients, families, and staff to reduce stress levels in this high-octane environment and reduce future trauma for those groups. It is important to note that this is still a growing area for the profession, and although evidence exists to support the need for psychologists (as emphasized throughout this book), there is as yet no known cost/benefit analysis or financially driven research confirming the value of embedding psychologists within these settings.

International comparisons

A number of other countries have benefited from a strong link between intensive care and psychology teams. Brazil has a strong tradition of "hospital psychologists" (known as health, rehabilitation, and medical psychologists in other countries) since the 1950s (Azevedo & Crepaldi, 2016). Today, most Brazilian hospitals have psychologists available to provide care for patients. The hospital psychologists usually have their own department and are available for consultation to other areas, including CCUs, although some psychologists are embedded in CCUs (personal communication, Dr. Luciano Pilla, intensive care consultant and cardiologist, Hospital Universitário Onofre Lopes and Hospital Rio Grande, Natal, and Dr. Ana Claudia Meira Lima, psychologist, Hospital Rio Grande, Feb. 28, 2020). Typically, the hospital psychologists visit CCUs three times each week and provide care on a daily basis, if necessary, to anxious, depressed, or distressed patients referred by the intensivists. In other cases, an ICU may be staffed by a full-time psychologist with several trainees. They deliver brief psychotherapy focused on disease and rehabilitation, run relatives' groups on the ward, assist with palliative care, and help medical staff communicate with challenging or distressed patients or relatives (Vieira & Waischunng, 2018). In public hospitals, psychology services are fully funded by the government; in private hospitals, the patients pay. Psychiatrists are always paid by the patients themselves. There is a special psychology section within the Brazilian Critical Care Society (AMIB). The Brazilian experience may be part of a broader Latin American trend: One of the earliest academic papers on the role of psychologists in ICU was written by Colombian psychologists (Novoa & Ballesteros de Valderrama, 2006), and today the Humanization of the ICU project has been adopted by 200 Latin American and Spanish ICUs (Nin Vaeza et al., 2020).

A similar growth of interest in critical care psychology can be observed in Europe. In Germany, critical care psychologists belong to an organization within the German Interdisciplinary Society for Intensive Care Medicine and Emergency Medicine that meets twice each year to document interventions they have found useful for patients and families. They have conducted small studies—for example, one on anxiety reduction during noninvasive ventilation and another on children as visitors in ICUs. They have been invited to work on guidelines for intensive care medicine (on topics such as anxiety, communication, and risk for PTSD) and are in constant dialogue with intensive care physicians and nurses through lectures at congresses. Currently, the German group consists of about 25 to 30 members, namely researchers, interested and engaged physicians and nurses, and psychologists who are integrated within ICU teams. A few psychologists also work irregularly or on demand in the ICU. The adult group also has connections with psychologists working in pediatric ICUs.

The German Interdisciplinary Society has given its support for the psychology section to build an international network. However, similar to the UK network, they lack funding or staffing to build such a network. They recently conducted a web-based survey of 226 ICU physicians and nurses to gain an overview of the state of ICU psychology in Germany. In all care areas—psychological care of patients, relatives, and support for staff—respondents indicated a significant undersupply and expressed the need for improved care (Deffner et al., 2021):

> The relatively high rates of mental stress among critically ill patients and their relatives implies the necessity of conceptually and financially embedded psychological care in intensive care units (ICUs) . . . Task areas are care for patients and relatives as well as staff support. Goals of psychological support in the ICU are detection of mental symptoms in patients and their treatment, psychological first aid for relatives in crisis situations, and support of the staff in terms of communication with patients and relatives as well as regarding development and maintenance of an adaptive coping style for dealing with emotionally challenging situations. Psychological care in the ICU is offered by psychologists, psychotherapists, or physicians with a psychotherapeutic qualification. The psychologist is integrated into the ICU team and has a proactive, resource-oriented, and supportive orientation. Psychological support can be an enrichment and a relief, both in the interdisciplinary treatment of patients as well as in the care of relatives, and also represent a resource for the team. (Deffner et al., 2020, p. 207)

Finally, efforts are also being made in the United States to create a model for psychology in the CCU. So far, to our knowledge, there are very few psychologists with a full-time clinical role in a U.S. CCU. However, a growing number of critical care psychologists have part-time roles as well as consultancy roles in many CCUs in the United States. Moreover, the American Psychological Association's Division of Rehabilitation Psychology has a critical care special interest group (CCSIG) with 30 members (including trainees, academics, and clinicians). Rehabilitation psychologists are clinical psychologists with a further 1 to 2 years of postdoctoral training in rehabilitation psychology, sometimes in neurorehabilitation settings as well. Most CCSIG members have input with either inpatient or outpatient critical care patients and/or are involved in critical care psychology research. Barriers to spreading this service are the small numbers of psychologists with the training and experience for this job and the funding mechanisms. The "fee for service" funding model, where hospitals are billed for each patient seen by the psychologist, means that their salaries are not easily covered. One promising model in Seattle has a consulting rotation of several trainees who regularly see patients on the critical care unit, with supervision provided by the attending rehabilitation psychologist (personal communication with Dr. Megan Hosey, critical care rehabilitation psychologist, Johns Hopkins Hospital, Baltimore).

The visible psychological care model in the ICU

We have seen that there are many variations in the model for psychologists working in the CCU, largely due to limited resources and an emerging evidence base. A future model of psychology in critical care would be of a visible, integrated psychological care pathway from pre-ICU to long-term follow-up. Psychological care could be provided at four levels as it is in other well-established areas (e.g., cancer; NICE, 2004).

In such a model, all staff would be expected to have core skills in the fundamentals of psychological care at level 1, while at level 2 a select group of staff are trained to provide more guidance to patients and relatives under the clinical supervision of a qualified psychologist. Trained psychological professionals would provide level 3 and 4 direct psychological approaches: Level 3 care for more straightforward problems would typically be provided by a range of professionals trained in psychological therapies, while level 4 care involves working with problems of increased complexity, usually delivered by a professional psychologist or, on occasion, a trained psychiatrist (Table 17.1). It is worth noting that the terminology for professionals trained in psychological therapies may vary between countries.

TABLE 17.1.

Levels of psychological care

Level	Group	Typical professionals	Assessment	Support or Intervention
1	All staff working with critical care patients	All staff, including nonclinical team	• Can recognize psychological distress • Can recognize boundary of competence and make appropriate referrals	• Gives general support and information • Able to communicate honestly and compassionately
2	Professionals directly responsible for the care of critical care patients	Nurses, medical staff, and allied health professionals trained and offered clinical supervision from a level 3 or 4 practitioner	• Can assess/screen general psychological well-being at key points along journey	• Gives more detailed support and information, using psychoeducation to teach coping strategies • Uses approaches such as psychological first aid • Can skillfully elicit health beliefs, supporting decision-making, mobilizing coping, and promoting adherence
3	Professionals trained and accredited in specific psychological therapies	Counselors, psychological therapists (e.g., master's-level counselors, social workers)	• Can assess for psychopathology (e.g., anxiety, depression, relationship problems) • Refers those with complex or moderate to severe problems to level 4 staff	• Can deliver standardized psychological interventions according to an explicit theoretical framework (e.g., anxiety management using a manualized cognitive-behavioral approach)
4	Professionals registered/accredited with a mental health professional body, or professionally licensed	Professional psychologists, psychiatrists	Conducts assessment of complex and severe psychological problems	• Conducts the expert assessment and management of enduring emotional distress, delirium, or cognitive difficulty • Delivers specialist and bespoke psychotherapeutic or psychiatric interventions • Coordinates care in complex cases • Responsible for the care of people with a diagnosis of preexisting severe mental illness that has been exacerbated by critical care stay

PRE-CRITICAL CARE

Where patients are known to have risk factors during a critical care admission, a psychologist would be a valuable asset to an interdisciplinary team. Psychologists can work with patients who are frail or living with long-term conditions and are effective in helping patients make advance care plans for treatment (Hacking, 2012). They may also work alongside surgeons in decision-making for high-risk surgery, enabling the decision-making process and managing expectations of outcome, and potentially discussing with patients psychological risks such as postoperative delirium and the psychological impact of a prolonged critical care stay. It is not yet known if being prepared for an experience such as ICU delirium could reduce the associated stress, but other forms of preoperative preparation have been shown to reduce stress.

DURING CRITICAL CARE ADMISSION

During a patient's stay on the critical care unit, psychologists would provide a psychological perspective on the management of the patient. This would include screening for distress or delirium and assessing early cognitive impact and psychological trauma in the de-sedated patient. They would bring a psychological formulation (a conceptual psychological model of the patient) to the interdisciplinary team, enabling more informed treatment and rehabilitation. For example, in a patient with seemingly low mood and disengagement from treatment, the psychologist would work with the team to assess for mood, differentiate when delirium is a factor, understand the patient's premorbid personality, and determine what is likely to re-engage the patient. They would provide psychological first aid (World Health Organisation, 2012) for the early post-sedation stages.

For longer-stay patients who may be slower to wean from ventilation, the psychologist will work to manage mood, including anxiety, depression, and ongoing psychological adjustment, and will help the team to understand the patient's longer-term needs. The psychologist can also work with the family to understand both the acute anxieties early in admission and the longer-term needs for longer-stay patients. The psychologist would be involved in "treatment of best interests meetings".[1]

The psychologist also has a key role in the well-being of the critical care staff, both in providing staff with psychological well-being education and support and also in helping to understand the nature of individuals who are attracted to work in a critical care environment and how that shapes skills and understanding in working with different kinds of patients. There are boundary issues to consider when just one psychologist is employed; it would be beneficial to consider a separate service for staff, with clarity of expectations and contract. The psychologist can work to enhance team cohesion; provide psychological support and intervention to staff members dealing with work-related stress, especially in relation to critical incidents; and offer psychological case discussion and reflective practice (Highfield, 2018). They would provide staff training and enhance the psychological skills of the interdisciplinary team. They may be involved in environmental design to humanize the critical care area. This can include introducing art, perhaps using calming colors and nature imagery, and music or nature sounds, to the critical care area. It can also include enlisting hospital voluntary services to provide alternative therapies, pet therapy, and materials for patient entertainment and distraction, including radios, iPads, newspapers, puzzles, games, adult coloring books, and magazines.

WARD

In a well-functioning outreach service, the team would screen patients after critical care for evidence of early signs of postintensive care syndrome (PICS) and refer to psychologists if necessary. Psychologists would then provide further information, support, assessment, and intervention, as required. They should also provide training in psychological care and psychological first aid to outreach and ward staff.

OUTPATIENTS/COMMUNITY

Psychologists would be integrated into follow-up clinics that follow an interdisciplinary model of screening, sensemaking of the critical care experience, and onward referral to other services. One further function of the follow-up service is to return the ICU diary.[2] This is a European ICU initiative where staff and relatives complete a layman's account during the ICU stay that is then returned to the patient after discharge; the original rationale was to fill a memory gap of the ICU admission, something that many patients struggle to recall, as a preventive intervention for posttraumatic stress.

Where resources allow, the psychologist would provide evidence-based interventions for psychological sequelae of a critical care stay, from expressive writing to cognitive-behavioral therapy to trauma-informed therapies including EMDR (eye movement desensitization and reprocessing), and refer on to other psychological services (e.g., mental health services, psychiatry, neuropsychology) as appropriate. The psychologist may also help to run or facilitate a critical care support group such as an ICU Steps group (ICU Steps is a UK critical care charity that provides a framework for supporting patients and families when they have returned home from the ICU).

Sustainability of staff

Over time, psychologists can help to manage not only the psychological impact of an ICU stay for patients and relatives but also the impact of working within the ICU for staff members. They also play a critical role in understanding the interface between patient complexity and staff attitudes and experience.

Evidence suggests a propensity for critical care staff to experience burnout (Vincent et al., 2019), although this represents point prevalence data rather than providing an understanding of risk factors. It does suggest that in-house psychological support in the service of mitigating risk factors may be beneficial in preventing staff burnout. Some researchers (Colville et al., 2019) have explored the impact of the nature of the work in ICU, using concepts such as moral distress (Jameton, 1984) and emotional labor (Hochschild, 1983) to make sense of what underpins burnout and, more generally, to understand the psychological sequelae of working in critical care. The job demands/ resources theory proposes that well-being is impaired if an employee is chronically overloaded (Demerouti et al., 2001). Practice suggests that psychologists are not only helpful in providing a psychological "resource" (e.g., reflection after critical incidents, providing psychological interventions for work-related stress) through intervention for staff experiencing psychological difficulties but also in helping to mitigate "demands" by shaping the workplace to enable the sustainability of staff (Highfield, 2019). Working conditions influence employees, but employees actively influence their own working conditions (Bakker & Demerouti, 2018). Thus, for optimal workplace well-being, organizational life should be modeled at the level of individual, team, and organization with these dynamic relationships in mind, and professional psychologists are well placed to bring this psychological theory into practice (British Psychological Society, 2014). Managing the clinical nature of the work by enabling space for staff to process complex feelings that arise can be beneficial, diminishing staff stress levels and also enhancing team relationships (Maben et al., 2017).

Many veteran ICU professionals have reflected upon the changing nature of the clinical demands; as medicine has progressed, we are saving more lives, but this does mean that some patients are spending more time in the ICU, with an increasing number requiring long-term ventilation. This changes the experience of work, meaning that highly technically skilled staff also are required to have high levels of interpersonal skill and ability to communicate with family members in distress as well as awake patients on ventilators. Such patients often struggle to communicate effectively and are clouded by delirium; therefore, staff patience and tolerance are required. This extra level of skill is changing the kind of workforce an ICU requires. ICU staffing will develop over time, requiring a shift toward more rehabilitation and psychologically minded care during an ICU stay.

Aspects of critical care psychology in need of further development

COGNITIVE ASSESSMENT

Compelling research evidence suggests that one of three patients experiences cognitive impairment following critical illness affecting domains including memory, information processing, and executive function. The causes of this are not completely clear, but cognitive impairment is particularly prevalent in patients who had acute respiratory distress syndrome and is also associated with delirium in the CCU, especially prolonged delirium. While an adequate set of screening tools for psychological distress and adjustment has been developed for critical care patients, there is a need for better methods to detect cognitive problems. In the United Kingdom cognitive assessments in the CCU itself are typically confined to delirium assessment or perhaps a simple abbreviated medical test to test orientation and recall. Further assessments are scarcely practical in the setting and may be confounded by the effects of delirium, sedation, analgesia, and fatigue. Cognitive assessments may also inform a wider interdisciplinary capacity assessment, but in the United Kingdom these are often carried out by physicians, not psychologists.

In some hospitals a brief cognitive assessment such as a MoCA is conducted before hospital discharge or in a follow-up clinic. However, many follow-up clinics do not carry out cognitive assessments due to lack of time to thoroughly cover physical, psychological, functional, and cognitive issues, as well as a desire to offer therapeutic value by giving patients adequate time to discuss their critical care experience and ask questions. It is certainly a rare service that can administer a comprehensive battery of neuropsychological tests. At a minimum, clinics should ask screening questions about memory and concentration and refer a patient to neuropsychology or memory clinics for further testing if indicated. In future, a brief cognitive assessment tailored to the commonly observed deficits in CCU patients should be developed and validated for use by critical care follow-up services.

EVIDENCE-BASED PSYCHOLOGICAL AND COGNITIVE INTERVENTIONS

While health and rehabilitation psychologists are trained to deliver a range of evidence-based interventions such as cognitive-behavioral therapy (CBT) or cognitive rehabilitation protocols that are applicable to many physical and mental health populations, there is a need to develop and evaluate interventions specifically tailored to the needs of critically ill patients. Research into these interventions is still in its infancy and should be accelerated in the future. Progress is perhaps delayed by the scarcity of psychologists working in critical care. In addition, the pressure of clinical demands rarely leaves time or resources for research or intervention development.

On the other hand, academic psychology researchers with more resources may lack clinical familiarity with critically ill patients and the interventions that would be feasible in a critical care setting.

Provision of a clinical psychology service in an Italian ICU led to a large reduction in both PTSD symptoms and use of psychiatric medication at 12 months (Peris et al., 2011). However, this was a single-center study using a historical control design, and no specific interventions were used or described. A number of small studies have found promising, but mixed, results for music therapy and mind–body therapies to reduce short-term stress for critically ill patients (Wade et al., 2016). The only large multicenter trial of psychological interventions in the ICU, the Provision of Psychological Support to People in Intensive Care (POPPI) randomized clinical trial, tested a complex intervention of nurse-led CBT-inspired psychological support for critical care patients in the hospital but found that it was not associated with a reduction in PTSD, depression, or anxiety (Wade et al., 2019). The authors concluded that there might be problems with timing, staffing, and population in the POPPI trial design. An intervention that could mitigate the acutely stressful nature of critical care, particularly the experience of frightening hallucinations, delusions, and delirium, and aid in the processing of intrusive ICU memories is still warranted. The best way to deliver and evaluate such an intervention remains to be determined.

In the field of cognitive rehabilitation, evidence that interventions such as goal management training or computerized brain-training exercises could improve critical care patients' cognitive performance, while promising, rests on a small number of limited studies (e.g., Jackson et al., 2012; Wilson et al., 2018). Traditional cognitive screens are not often viable in the ICU setting, but we need to develop better systems of care to identify cognitive issues early and monitor them accurately. The short-term and long-term effects of cognitive issues on the patient and family are potentially great and would benefit from both individual support and wider support to the family also.

The availability of good-quality evidence to support psychological and cognitive interventions in critical care could do much to accelerate understanding of the role of psychology in critical care medicine.

ICU of the future: integrated psychologists and psychologically informed environments

The nature of critical care admissions and survivors is changing as intensive care medicine improves and the CCU retains more patients who stay on a ventilator for longer periods. We also write this chapter during a pandemic that has affected

CCUs in medicine, teamwork, and rehabilitation (see other chapters in this book, including Chapters 1, 3, 8, and 9). No matter what the future holds, integrated professional psychology services will play a crucial part in enabling this transition.

New CCU environments need to be ergonomically designed to allow reduced noise, increased access to light and light regulation, space for mobilization, space for family engagement, and consideration of the needs of the staff through staff rest and break facilities. The use of art, music, gardens, and audiovisual entertainment should become more commonplace in CCUs to reduce critical care stress and provide mental interest and stimulation. Finally, advances in telemedicine will likely lead to creative solutions and improved communication among the critical care team, families, and the patient during follow-up.

Conclusion

Our vision is that the ICU of the future will be patient-centered and psychologically informed, with psychologists fully integrated in the health care team. Professional psychologists will work alongside teams and be essential participants in the clinical working week. For patients and families, the key to success will entail psychologists being part of treatment planning, delirium and cognition assessment and management, rehabilitation goal planning, and working with the family. A well-rounded unit will also make use of its psychology expertise to support staff in making sense of the vicarious traumatic exposure, managing the pace of the work, and coaching leaders. We hope for a future where critical care psychologists exist across the world, building an evidence base and facilitating the exchange of ideas, research, training, and robust models of care.

Notes

1. *Best interests* is a statutory principle set out in section 4 of the UK Mental Capacity Act. It states that "Any act done, or a decision made, under this Act or on behalf of a person who lacks capacity must be done, or made, in his **best interests**." In hospital settings, this relates to ongoing medical treatments.

2. A European group has developed bringing together all of the literature (www.icu-diary.org).

References

Azevedo, A. V., & Crepaldi, M. A. (2016). Psychology within a general hospital: Hospital, conceptual, and practical aspects. Estudios de Psicologia, 33(4), 573–585. https://psycnet.apa.org/record/2016-50449-002

Bakker, A., & Demerouti, E. (2018). Multiple levels in job-demands-resources theory: Implications for employee well-being and performance. In E. Diener, S. Oishi, & L. Tay (Eds.), Handbook of wellbeing. DEF Publishers.

Brewin, C. R., Rose, S., Andrews, B., Green, J., Tata, P., McEvedy, C., . . . Foa, E. B. (2002). Brief screening instrument for post-traumatic stress disorder. British Journal of Psychiatry, 181, 158–162.

British Psychological Society. (2014). Implementing culture change within the NHS: Contributions from occupational psychology. British Psychological Society.

Colville, G. A., Dawson, D., Rabinthiran, S., Chaudry-Daley, Z., & Perkins-Porras, L. (2019). A survey of moral distress in staff working in intensive care in the UK. Journal of the Intensive Care Society, 20(3), 196–203. doi:10.1177/1751143718787753

Connolly, B., Douiri, A., Steier, J., Moxham, J., Denehy, L., & Hart, N. (2014). A UK survey of rehabilitation following critical illness: Implementation of NICE Clinical Guidance 83 (CG83) following hospital discharge. BMJ Open, 4(5), e004963. doi:10.1136/bmjopen-2014-004963

Deffner, T., Michels, G., Nojack, A., Robler, I., Stierle, D., Sydlik, M., . . . Wicklein, K. (2020). Psychological care in the intensive care unit: Task areas, responsibilities, requirements, and infrastructure. Medizinische Klinik, Intensivmedizin und Notfallmedizin, 115(3), 205–212. doi:10.1007/s00063-018-0503-1

Deffner, T., Schwarzkopf, D., & Waydhas, C. (2021). Psychological care in German intensive care units: Results of a survey among the members of the German Interdisciplinary Association for Intensive Care and Emergency Medicine. Medizinische Klinik, Intensivmedizin und Notfallmedizin, 116(2), 146–153. doi:10.1007/s00063-019-00638-2

Demerouti, E., Bakker, A. B., Machreiner, F., & Shaufeli, W. B. (2001). The job demands resources model of burnout. Journal of Applied Psychology, 86, 499–512.

Hacking, B. (2013). Testing the feasibility, acceptability and effectiveness of a "decision navigation" intervention for early stage prostate cancer patients in Scotland: A randomised controlled trial. Psycho-oncology, 22(5), 1017–1024. doi.org/10.1002/pon.3093

Highfield, J. (2019). The sustainability of the critical care workforce. Nursing Critical Care, 24(1), 6–8. https://doi.org/10.1111/nicc.12394

Hochschild, A. R. (1983). The managed heart: The commercialization of human feeling. University of California Press.

Intensive Care Society. (2019). Guidelines for the provision of intensive care services *(version 2)*. Intensive Care Society.

Jackson, J., Ely, E. W., Morey, M. C., Anderson, V. M., Siebert, C. S., Denne, L. B., . . . Hoenig, H. (2012). Cognitive and physical rehabilitation of intensive care unit survivors: Results of the RETURN randomized controlled pilot investigation. Critical Care Medicine, 40(4), 1088–1097.

Jameton, A. (1984). Nursing practice: The ethical issues. Prentice-Hall.

Kroenke, K., Spitzer, R. L., & Williams, J. B. (2001). The PHQ-9: Validity of a brief depression severity measure. Journal of General Internal Medicine, 16(9), 606–613.

Maben, J. T., Taylor, C., Dawson. J., Leamy, M., McCarthy, I., Reynolds, E., . . . Foot, C. (2017). A realist informed mixed methods evaluation of Schwartz Rounds in England. NIHR Journals Library.

Nasreddine, Z. S., Phillips, N. A., Bédirian, V., Charbonneau, S., Whitehead, V., Collin, I., . . . Chertkow, H. (2005). The Montreal Cognitive Assessment, MoCA: A brief screening tool for mild cognitive impairment. Journal of the American Geriatrics Society, 53(14), 695–699.

NICE. (2004). Cancer service guideline 4: *Improving supportive and palliative care for adults with cancer*. NICE.

NICE. (2009). *Clinical guideline 38. Rehabilitation after critical illness in adults*. NICE.

NICE. (2017). *Quality standard 158. Rehabilitation after critical illness in adults*. NICE.

Nin Vaeza, N., Martin Delgado, M., & Heras La Calle, G. (2020). Humanizing intensive care. Critical Care Medicine, 48(3), 385–390. doi: 10.1097/ccm.0000000000004191

Novoa, M., & Ballesteros de Valderamma, B. P. (2006). The role of the psychologist in an intensive care unit. Universitas Psychologica, 5(3), 599–612.

Peris, A., Bonizzoli, M., Iozzelli, D., Migliaccio, M. L., Zagli, G., Bacchereti, A., . . . Belloni, L. (2011). Early intra-intensive care unit psychological intervention promotes recovery from post traumatic stress disorders, anxiety and depression symptoms in critically ill patients. Critical Care, 15(1), R41.

Spitzer, R. L., Kroenke, K., Williams, J. B. W., & Lowe, B. (2006). A brief measure for assessing generalized anxiety disorder. Archives of Internal Medicine, 166, 1092–1097.

Vieira, A. G., & Waischunng, C. D. (2018). The practice of the hospital psychologist in intensive care units: The attention given to patients, family and staff: A review. Revista da SBPH, 21(1), 132–153.

Vincent, L., Brindley, P. G., Highfield, J., Innes, R., Greig, P., & Suntharalingam, G. (2019). Burnout syndrome in UK intensive care unit staff: Data from all three burnout syndrome domains and across professional groups, genders and ages. Journal of the Intensive Care Society, 20(4), 363–369. doi:10.1177/1751143719860391

Wade, D., Hankins, M., Smyth, D., Rhone, E., Mythen, M., Howell, D., & Weinman, J. (2014). Detecting acute distress and risk of future psychological morbidity in critically ill patients: Validation of the Intensive Care Psychological Assessment Tool. Critical Care, 18(5), Article 519. doi:10.1186/s13054-014-0519-8

Wade, D., Moon, Z., Windgassen, S., Harrison, A., Morris, L., & Weinman, J. (2016). Non-pharmacological interventions to reduce ICU-related psychological distress: A systematic review. Minerva Anestesiologica, 82(4), 465–478.

Wade, D. M., Mouncey, P. R., Richards-Belle, A., Wulff, J., Harrison, D. A., & Sadique, M. Z., . . . Rowan, K. M. (2019). Effect of a nurse-led preventive psychological intervention on symptoms of posttraumatic stress disorder among critically ill patients: A randomized controlled trial. Journal of the American Medical Association, 321(7), 665. doi:10.1001/jama.2019.0073

Wilson, J., Collar, E. M., Kiehl, A. L., Lee, H., Merzenich, M., Ely, E. W., & Jackson, J. (2018). Computerized cognitive rehabilitation in intensive care unit survivors: Returning to everyday tasks using rehabilitation networks-computerized cognitive rehabilitation pilot investigation. Annals of the American Thoracic Society, 15(7), 887–891.

World Health Organization. (2012). *Psychological first aid: Guide for field workers*.https://www.who.int/mental_health/publications/guide_field_workers/en/

Trauma-Informed Care Practices in the Intensive Care Unit

The processes we describe here are offered to support the humanity of patients, families, and intensive care unit (ICU) staff, in complex and emotionally stressful settings. At the time of this writing, during the height of the COVID-19 pandemic, ICUs have found themselves at capacity and safety precautions prevent family visits, so providers have reduced latitude for improving the patient experience. When options for choice diminish for frightened and often confused patients in the ICU, consistently compassionate human presence and attention to patient comfort remain essential and may become the only tools for staff to mitigate trauma. Psychologists can play an integral role in reducing traumatizing experience or traumatization of patients and staff. With their specialized knowledge of psychological principles and the intricacies of the human experience, the following practices naturally fit within a psychologist's scope. Psychologists are primed to model these practices for the rest of the team in the ICU.

Optimize hygiene, comfort, and privacy

In a setting where acute lifesaving measures need to be prioritized, daily habits and routines may be forgone. As soon as possible following medical stabilization, attention should be turned to personal hygiene and other daily routines, including bathing, bathing alternatives (e.g., bed bath), dental hygiene, and hair care (Furr et al., 2004; Wilson et al., 2019), with patient participation, direction, or assent.

The physical space in intensive care settings is designed for optimal observation of patients, not privacy. As they regain toileting function, patients may need to use a bedside commode in rooms lacking a toilet. Staff may not be able to change the infrastructure, but they can explain the safety rationale and maximize privacy as possible.

Support the patient's identity

When patients are unable to perform basic functions such as ambulating, toileting, and eating independently, there is exquisite dependency on the people and machines assisting them. However, opportunities for independence and choice can be offered according to the patient's ability to process information at that time. For example, when a patient needs to be repositioned to support better oxygenation and avoid pressure ulcers, health care providers can explain and offer choices around positioning as possible.

In communications between health care providers, patients may be identified as their diagnosis or treatment (e.g., "the laryngectomee in Room 3"). This communication may seem more efficient when time is limited, but it fails to recognize patients as unique individuals who are not defined solely by their condition. It is important to be cognizant of shared spaces and the need to protect patient privacy. When the space allows for HIPAA compliance, patient names should be used.

Introduce self and role; explain procedures

Many who participate in hospital functions and patient care may enter patient rooms to perform tasks and attend to urgent needs. They should introduce themselves and their role in every interaction, as well as what the patient may expect from their care. It is important that they explain what they are doing so that patients hear what is happening around them or to their body; this may be comforting and may empower them to consent or object and to be part of their care.

Acknowledge patients when attending to medical equipment

The mechanical equipment in the ICU is used to maintain biologic homeostasis. Alarms sound in response to inconsistencies in critical life functions, and staff may respond quickly to the alarm with minimal acknowledgment of the patient. We recommend providing information when changing a setting on a ventilator, flushing an intravenous line, checking sequential compression devices, and so forth, even when the patient's comprehension is uncertain due to their condition or level of consciousness. Although at times the task at hand may require complete focus on the equipment, typically there is an opportunity for a simple greeting and an explanation of what is happening and of any sensations or movement the patient might experience.

Provide specific supports during mechanical ventilation, waking from sedation, and ventilator liberation

Mechanical ventilation typically involves some period of medical sedation and often is accompanied by confusion requiring physical restraint. As sedation levels are reduced, such as during spontaneous breathing trials, patients may awaken confused and frightened, with vague and disturbing memories. It is important that nurses and/or respiratory therapists quickly explain what is going on, and—depending on the patient's ability—guide and encourage modified communication (e.g., picture/letter board, consistent signaling for yes/no). Various trained team members should regularly assess for and explain delirium in basic terms, repeating the information as necessary. Giving patients information about their conditions and providing reassurance, encouragement, and compassion during the waking process may help to alleviate the stress of a new environment and constraints of movement and speech. An ICU diary allows them to review later and process what has transpired while they were unconscious or disoriented, helping to piece together their story.

Discontinuation of mechanical ventilation, when medically indicated, continues to be one of the most challenging activities in intensive care settings. For patients who have been on extended ventilatory support and are having difficulty during discontinuation, the threatening impact of withdrawal and the shortness of breath associated with anxiety can be mitigated by gaining assent for a preplanned duration of initial trials, and ending a trial as a success rather than after the patient reaches a limit of tolerance. This is also a less aversive experience for the providers.

Involve family and other social support

To counteract the isolation of the ICU patient experience, and to harness existing supports, health care teams can include family and friends in the patient's care to the extent possible, adjusting as needed to the particulars of family dynamics. For example, a procedure known to be painful or distressing can be scheduled during a time when a friend or family member can be present. As another example, prior to initiating liberation from mechanical ventilation, anticipatory guidance can be provided to the patient's family or friends so they can help the patient prepare and can advise the team about the best ways to help the patient relax (e.g., favorite music). It is important to recognize that family and friends may have their own history of trauma that will influence and impact their responses and engagement. (At the time of this writing, family visits to patients positive for COVID and in the ICU were severely restricted or prohibited.) Technology such as tablets or smartphones with video calling capability can be used to maintain family involvement in patient care when COVID or other circumstances prevents in-person visitors.

Mitigate the impact of critical incidents

Patients in the ICU often experience, or are witness to, life-threating events. Critical change in status, mechanical dysfunction, or medical complications may culminate in rapid assessment and lifesaving interventions, with alarms, commotion, and highly coordinated, rapid actions by multiple team members. When possible, explain to patients what occurred or is occurring, what they will experience, and the next steps in their care. With witnessed events, acknowledge what is occurring and the limits of what you can say about other patients. Provide presence and reassurance. For staff to do this, their own humanity and suffering must be recognized, and support and relief must be made available to them as well.

Promote team communication and transparency

Like many previously trending improvements to ICU processes, ICU team rounding, with discussion in patients' rooms, has been attenuated or not implemented during the COVID crisis. Trauma-informed practice helps to promote transparency and allows patients and their families to be active participants in care. When the pharmacist, nurse, respiratory therapist, physical therapist, physicians, and other team members are in the room with the patient, the patient can hear the team's input, concerns, and plan. This is an opportunity to participate in shared decision-making and treatment planning. Family presence during team rounding can address patient and family questions, provide updates on medical status and interventions, and discuss goals of care, resuscitation preferences, life-sustaining treatment, and the dying process when relevant. Patient and family participation in rounding yields greater transparency and understanding of care. Though it may not be possible during COVID for family to be physically present, technology can be used to continue family engagement in team rounding and care discussions.

Critical Care Resources

ARDS Foundation
https://ardsglobal.org/other-resources/

Blake, H., & Bermingham, F. (2020). *Psychological wellbeing for health and care workers: Mitigating the impact of COVID-19 on psychological wellbeing.* University of Nottingham.
https://www.nottingham.ac.uk/toolkits/play_22794

Critical Illness, Brain Dysfunction, and Survivorship (CIBS) Center. *Monitoring delirium in the ICU*
https://www.icudelirium.org/medical-professionals/delirium/monitoring-delirium-in-the-icu

Critical Illness, Brain Dysfunction, and Survivorship (CIBS) Center. *The ICU recovery center at Vanderbilt*
https://www.icudelirium.org/the-icu-recovery-center-at-vanderbilt

Faculty of Intensive Care Medicine. (2019). *Guidelines for the provision of intensive care services* (version 2)
https://www.ficm.ac.uk/standards-research-revalidation/guidelines-provision-intensive-care-services-v2#:~:text=Guidelines%20for%20the%20Provision%20of%20Intensive%20Care%20Services%20(GPICS)%20second,of%20UK%20Intensive%20Care%20Services

Johns Hopkins Medicine. *COVID-19 survivor's tools*
https://gerocentral.org/wp-content/uploads/2020/07/COVID-survivors-toolkit_Hopkins-Rush.pdf

Korupolu, R., Francisco, G. E., Levin, H., & Needham, D. M. (2020). Rehabilitation of criti-cally ill COVID-19 survivors. *Journal of the International Society of Physical and Rehabilitation Medicine, 3*(2), 45–52.
http://www.jisprm.org/preprintarticle.asp?id=286460

Psychology Tools. *Critical illness, intensive care, and post-traumatic stress disorder (PTSD)* (patient and family guide to the ICU experience and recovery)
https://www.psychologytools.com/assets/covid-19/critical_illness_intensive_care_and_ptsd_en-us.pdf

Richmond Agitation Sedation Scale
https://www.mnhospitals.org/Portals/0/Documents/ptsafety/LEAPT%20Delirium/RASS%20Sedation%20Assessment%20Tool.pdf

Scott, K. K., & Cheshire, D. (2015, June 5). Treating hidden wounds: The case for putting psy-chologists in trauma ICUs. *The Conversation* (University of Florida).
https://theconversation.com/treating-hidden-wounds-the-case-for-putting-psychologists-in-trauma-programs-42584

Society of Critical Care Medicine: THRIVE Initiative
https://www.sccm.org/MyICUCare/Home

World Health Organization. (2020, March 18). *Mental health and psychosocial considerations dur-ing the COVID-19 outbreak*
https://afri-can.org/wp-content/uploads/2020/04/mental-health-considerations.pdf

Anxiety Management and Ventilator Liberation Strategies

The goal is to assist patients in transitioning from a more dependent state (vent-dependent) to a more independent state (weaning off the vent).

To that end, you will help patients to:

- Regain the ability to relax
- Feel less distressed by scary vent-related memories and reminders
- Search for an accurate and healthy understanding of the event and what it means to them or about them
- Identify the need for psychological follow-up in an outpatient clinic

Note: Short-acting anxiolytic medications (e.g., benzodiazepines) are associated with increased risk for delirium and can reduce the patient's ability to self-manage anxiety.

Note: Learning can occur whereby an individual "learns" that certain aspects of the environment are anxiety-provoking. This can include the learning that occurs in the context of nursing care and therapeutic tasks. Verbal and nonverbal behaviors on the part of staff can trigger or exacerbate underlying vulnerability to the anxiety response.

Prior to weaning, determine if the patient has delirium. One tool that can be used for assessment is the CAM-ICU (see Appendix B: Critical Care Resources).

Anxiety management for patients without delirium

1. Assist the patient in identifying their preferred method for communication—mouthing words, using phone or iPad to text/write, writing with pad/pencil, communication board, or eye gaze equipment.

2. Seek to understand the patient's anxiety experience in the context of their medical diagnosis and background history, as well as their "typical" ways of managing stress prior to their illness or injury.

3. Provide the patient with accurate information as to the nature of sympathetic nervous system arousal, or physiologic "sensations."

4. Normalize that the panic/anxiety they describe are "sensations" that are "normal" and harmless.

5. Let the patient know that emotional feelings of terror/fear/panic can occur suddenly and repeatedly and that in the ICU they often are triggered at least initially by physiologic changes that are perceived as catastrophic (e.g., changes in respiration).

6. Let the patient know that anticipatory anxiety can occur and can be very intense.

7. Offer reassurance that you expect anxiety symptoms to decrease in frequency and intensity over time.

8. For some patients, distraction can be a useful anxiety management strategy—for example, they can listen to music, watch TV, reach out to family, or engage in other activities to distract from the sensation of breathing.

9. Consider whether the patient should do time-limited versus untimed trials. Some patients may need to start with a set amount of time and build up, as trying for an unspecified amount of time can feel too overwhelming.

10. One of the core components of relaxation is breathing, which is one of the most effective ways to reduce tension in the body. You can teach patients to become more aware of and to control their breathing, which in turn can help to control the physical and mental effects of anxiety. This will be largely dependent on the mode of mechanical ventilation. Many patients are on pressure-support modes of ventilation, in which they are able to have some control over the rate of respirations, if not the depth, and therefore you can engage them in some breathing retraining exercises. The focus here is on "calm" breathing, not "deep" breathing.

11. Patients who are mechanically ventilated also can be guided to imagine what their breathing felt like when it was "normal" and to reflect on this thought or image while engaging in calming breathing.

12. Patients can be instructed to identify an image that is pleasing, calming, or relaxing to them and then can be guided to better formulate and reflect on all the details of the image.

13. A perceived sense of dyscontrol can be a main contributor to anxiety states. One way in which patients can establish a better sense of personal control is by modifying their environment. There are several ways in which we may achieve this: (1) moving them to a room near the nurses' station; (2) moving physiologic monitors either away from or toward the patient; or (3) instructing physicians and other care providers to provide either less or more information to the patient.

14. For some patients, their anxiety states may reduce their motivation, or otherwise present a barrier, to engage in a variety of recommended health care treatments, including mechanical ventilation, early mobilization, or medication adherence. Motivational interviewing is a patient-centered counseling approach that is brief and time-limited. It works by activating the patient's own motivation for change and adherence to treatment by identifying discrepancies between their current behavior (e.g., anxiety) and goals (e.g., recovery).

Anxiety management for patients with delirium

1. Provide reassurance and reorientation.
2. Provide distraction.
3. Do not try to reason with the patient or have prolonged discussions.
4. Speak softly, using only the most important words. Use concrete rather than abstract language.
5. Keep the environment quiet and calm, to the extent possible.

Glossary

ABCDEF bundle A coordinated effort across disciplines for management of critically ill patients that comprises:

Assess, prevent, and manage pain
Both spontaneous awakening trials (SATs) and spontaneous breathing trials (SBTs)
Choice of analgesia and sedation
Delirium: assess, prevent, and manage
Early mobility and Exercise
Family engagement and empowerment.

Acceleration/deceleration injuries Diffuse brain injuries that occur following unrestricted movement of the head creating tensile, shear, and compressive strains that often follow high-speed events (e.g., motor vehicle accidents, falls).

Acute respiratory distress syndrome (ARDS) A type of acute, diffuse inflammatory lung injury characterized by respiratory failure that is not fully explained by cardiac failure or fluid overload and has the clinical features of hypoxemia and bilateral opacities identified via a chest radiograph or a computed tomography (CT) scan. ARDS is a severe and often life-threatening medical condition because the lungs are unable to supply sufficient oxygen to the arterial blood, resulting in hypoxemia. This can in turn lead to anoxic/hypoxic brain injury and many other systemic problems. Patients usually require a mechanical ventilator until their lungs adequately recover to allow for ventilator weaning trials. The severity of ARDS is further differentiated as follows:

Mild (PaO_2/FiO_2 between 200 and 300 mmHg with PEEP or CPAP $\geq$ 5 cmH_2O)

Moderate (PaO_2/FiO_2 between 100 and 200 mmHg, with PEEP ≥ 5 cmH_2O)
Severe (PaO_2/FiO_2 ≤ 100 mmHg with PEEP ≥ 5 cmH_2O).

Acute stress disorder (ASD) A psychiatric condition whose diagnostic criteria are similar to those for posttraumatic stress disorder (PTSD). The diagnosis is made only within the first month following a traumatic event. If symptoms persist longer than 30 days, the diagnosis changes to PTSD. Risk factors include prior PTSD diagnosis, premorbid psychiatric dysfunction, and exposure to prior trauma.

Advance directive Formal written instructions completed by the patient that provide the family and care team with guidance regarding medical treatment. An advance directive also names a durable power of attorney, which gives another person the power to make decisions about the patient's medical treatment if they are not capable of doing so. Laws regarding advance directives vary between states. Additionally, an advance directive does not expire unless the person who wrote it writes a new version. For this reason, it has been recommended that advance directives should be reviewed and updated periodically. (Also see *do-not-attempt-resuscitation order*.)

Air hunger The sensation of not being able to breathe sufficiently. It is typically triggered by excess unventilated carbon dioxide. The experience of air hunger can range from moderately anxiety-provoking to traumatic and can cause a great deal of distress.

Alcohol withdrawal syndrome (AWS) Clinically significant symptoms of withdrawal occur in about 50% of individuals with alcohol use disorders. Common symptoms reveal evidence of sympathetic arousal such as tremors, anxiety, tachycardia, sweating, hypertension, and insomnia. Other symptoms include nausea/vomiting, headache, irritability, confusion, and nightmares. Withdrawal symptoms can begin about 6 to 8 hours after significant decreases in blood alcohol levels, peak around 48 to 72 hours, and decline substantially by the fourth or fifth day. Treatment is often conducted via symptom-driven protocols such as the Clinical Institute Withdrawal Assessment for Alcohol (CIWA). Although only 5–10% of individuals with AWS experience delirium tremens (DTs), this term is often inaccurately used to describe milder forms of AWS.

Anabolism Reorganization of molecules in the interest of growth and building. In this process, simple molecules are assembled into larger, more complex ones. An example of anabolism is gluconeogenesis, where the liver and kidneys produce glucose from non-carbohydrate sources.

Analgesic A medication that reduces pain, fever, or swelling. In the ICU analgesics are used to decrease patient stress/distress, improve sleep, and reduce other undesirable symptoms (e.g., soreness, stiffness). An analgesic also can reduce side effects and discomfort caused by medical procedures.

Anastomosis A surgical connection between two structures. Most often this is a connection that is created between tubular structures, such as blood vessels or loops of intestine. This procedure is often used to repair injured or damaged arteries and veins. Additionally, when part of an intestine is surgically removed, the two remaining ends are sewn or stapled together (anastomosed).

Anemia A condition in which the level of hemoglobin in the blood is low due to decreased production, increased destruction, or loss of red blood cells (e.g., hemorrhage). Reduced iron stores can lead to anemia because the bone marrow needs iron to make hemoglobin.

Anesthetic A medication used to numb an area or lead to a temporary loss of feeling. Anesthetics also often cause somnolence and are used to help the patient feel more comfortable during an invasive procedure.

Antibiotics/antimicrobials Medications used to treat and prevent bacterial infections. Patients in the ICU may require prophylactic antibiotics if they are at high risk for infection.

Apoptosis Programmed cell death. Apoptosis is part of normal regulation and turnover of cells but also can be activated by a pathologic process, such as ischemia or physical trauma.

Arterial line (a-line or art line) A small tube in the artery, usually placed in the wrist. The care team uses this tube to check the patient's blood pressure and take blood samples. Some patients in the ICU need frequent blood draws to monitor their status and response to treatment. An arterial line is more efficient and more comfortable for the patient than repeated needlesticks.

Asterixis Often referred to as a hand-flapping tremor, this is marked by a noticeable wrist tremor when the hands and arms are extended. Asterixis can be observed in liver failure but has been observed in other types of delirium as well (e.g., Wilson's disease, metabolic encephalopathy).

Atelectasis Complete or partial collapse of a lung or lobe of a lung. Although typically asymptomatic, individuals can experience chest pain or hypoxemia or, in more severe cases, shortness of breath or respiratory failure. Diagnosis is made via chest x-ray, and treatment is of the underlying cause.

Athetosis Slow writhing-like movement.

Autonomic storms (aka autonomic hyperreflexia) A reaction of the autonomic nervous system to severe injury, metabolic disturbance, or overstimulation. Symptoms include high blood pressure, tachycardia, diaphoresis, and other signs of sympathetic hyperarousal. A common cause is a spinal cord injury above T5, during which stimulation perceived as normal in a healthy individual may generate an excessive autonomic response in the patient. Other causes of autonomic storms include illicit substance use, medication side effects, and severe brain injury.

Babinski sign Blunt stimulus of the sole of the foot results in fanning of the toes and upward flexion of the big toe. Also referred to as the "extensor plantar response." In adults and children over 2 years old, a positive Babinski sign is associated with structural or functional impairment of upper motor neurons in the corticospinal tract.

Bacteremia The presence of bacteria in the blood.

Ballismus Intermittent forceful flinging of the limbs. This is considered to be an extreme choreiform movement and usually affects only one side of the body (hemiballismus). It is typically caused by a focal (often vascular) lesion in the subthalamic nucleus. Similar to other movement disorders, ballismus does not occur during sleep.

Banana bag A 1-liter solution of normal saline that contains thiamine, folic acid, multivitamin, and magnesium sulfate, used in the ICU to correct acute deficiencies. For example, individuals with chronic alcohol use disorders often have thiamine and magnesium deficiencies that require correction. For critically ill patients, banana bags also are thought to be beneficial because magnesium can mitigate nerve pain and relieve muscle pain.

Blood–brain barrier A semipermeable membrane made up of endothelial cells that separates circulating blood from brain tissue. The blood–brain barrier allows passage of oxygen, certain gases, and nutrients from the circulating blood to brain tissue but blocks passage of most harmful toxins. Some toxins, such as lead and alcohol, pass through the blood–brain barrier. The blood–brain barrier is not fully developed until approximately 6 months gestation.

Blood pressure (BP) One of the primary vital signs; represents the pressure of circulating blood on blood vessel walls. Blood pressure is typically expressed in terms of the systolic pressure (the maximum recorded pressure during one heartbeat) over the diastolic pressure (the minimum pressure between two heartbeats). Cardiac output, total peripheral resistance, and arterial stiffness have an impact on BP, as can stress, emotions, activity, medications, and specific disease states. Long-term high blood pressure (hypertension) often damages blood vessels and organs while also increasing the risk for myocardial infarction and stroke.

Blown pupil A pupil that is dilated and unresponsive to changes in light. Following traumatic brain injury this is typically a sign of increased intracranial pressure and herniation resulting in compression of the third cranial nerve. However, dilation of the pupil also can be caused by certain drugs and/or diseases.

Brain death One of two kinds of death recognized by law in the United States. It represents extensive and permanent brain damage in which there is irreversible cessation of either (1) circulatory and respiratory functions or (2) all functions of the entire brain, including the brain stem. Some aspects of brain death criteria can vary between states, but characteristic features include no response to noxious stimuli, fixed pupils, and an isoelectric electroencephalogram indicating no brain activity. After brain death bodily functions can only be maintained artificially. In this situation life support is often turned off, but it is important to note that this is not the same as withdrawal of support. Life support is withdrawn when the patient is alive but they (via an advance directive), or their surrogate decision-maker, have elected to do so.

Brain herniation Life-threatening brain displacement from the cranial vault through the tentorial notch or foramen magnum. This is usually caused by brain edema or hemorrhage resulting in increasing intracranial pressure.

Brain reserve hypothesis (BRH) and cognitive reserve hypothesis (CRH) These are related but not synonymous hypotheses. The BRH (also called cerebral reserve) maintains that individuals vary with regard to resilience and susceptibility to brain injury and/or poor outcome. Individuals who have a prior history of neurologic injury or illness are at higher risk for complicated outcome following brain-related events. For example, elderly patients with a prior history of stroke may not recover as expected following a concussion. CRH is similar but emphasizes the potentially protective effects of higher premorbid intelligence and better quality of education prior to injury.

Bronchoscopy A visual or invasive examination of the breathing passages of the lungs, typically performed by a pulmonologist. A thin flexible tube (bronchoscope) with a camera on the end is passed through the nose or mouth, down the throat, and into the lungs. However, in certain situations (e.g., blood in the lungs, airway obstruction), a rigid bronchoscope may be needed. Bronchoscopy also can be used to obtain mucus or tissue samples, treat lung problems, or remove foreign bodies.

Cardiac arrest The sudden loss of all heart function. Cardiac arrest is not the same as a heart attack, which occurs when blockage of an artery causes sudden damage to the heart. A heart attack may lead to cardiac arrest, but cardiac arrest is usually caused by coronary artery disease, electrocution, and/or abrupt oxygen loss (e.g., drowning, choking). Cardiac arrest permanently damages the brain within about 4 to 6 minutes. Approximately 95% of people who sustain a cardiac arrest do not survive. Survivors are individuals who receive immediate intervention in the field (e.g., cardiopulmonary resuscitation [CPR]) and afterwards hospital-based critical care services.

Cardiac monitoring (aka heart monitor, electrocardiography) Performed via a noninvasive diagnostic machine that records electrical activity of the heart. Portable cardiac monitors are sometimes employed (e.g., Holter monitor, implantable loop recorder). When the data are transmitted to a distant monitoring station, it is referred to as telemetry or biotelemetry. In the ICU, cardiac monitoring primarily tracks, or is used to identify, arrhythmia, myocardial infarction, and the QT interval. Unusual heart rhythms can be related to chemical and/or mechanical problems.

Cardiopulmonary resuscitation (CPR) Medical treatment provided to someone whose heart has suddenly stopped. The procedure supplies oxygen to the lungs and keeps blood flowing in the body. Proper CPR involves three steps: circulation (done by compressions), airway (done by proper positioning), and breathing (by breathing into the mouth [or mouth and nose in an infant]). During CPR, the clinician may also use a machine to restart the heart.

Catabolism Involves the process of digestion of substances to produce energy. Large, complex molecules in the body are broken down into smaller, simple ones. An example of catabolism is glycolysis. When cells are starved and energy is not available, they may catabolize themselves in an effort to maintain cellular function. This can lead to irreparable damage and cell death.

Catheter A thin, flexible tube inserted into the patient's body so fluids can move into and out of their systems. There are many types of catheters, each with a different purpose. A catheter is important in critical care because it can provide the patient with (1) food (e.g., feeding tube), (2) relief/excretion (e.g., urinary catheter), and (3) medication (e.g., arteriovenous fistula for dialysis). The critical care team also may use peripherally inserted central catheters (PICCs), which go into a vein until it reaches the heart.

Central venous catheter (CVC or central line) A catheter placed in the neck, chest, or groin used to monitor blood flow. It also can be used to give the patient fluids, medications, or nutrients. Sometimes a CVC is placed into a large vein in the arm; this is known as a peripherally inserted central catheter (PICC). A CVC can stay in place for days or weeks, as long as it shows no signs of infection.

Cerebellitis Infection of brain tissue localized to the cerebellum, typically caused by a viral infection. Sudden onset of ataxia is a common presenting symptom.

Cerebral edema Swelling of the brain. Can be caused by multiple medical events (e.g., traumatic brain injury, hypoxia, or disorders that disrupt the blood–brain barrier such as infections) and can lead to vasogenic edema (excessive extracellular fluid). Cytotoxic edema refers to excessive intracellular fluid collection within the brain cells, which often results from cellular damage (as in the case of infarction).

Cerebral perfusion pressure (CPP) A measure of the amount of blood flow through the brain. CPP is calculated by subtracting the intracranial pressure (ICP) from the mean systemic arterial blood pressure. The level and duration of reduced CPP is a main determinant in the severity of cerebral damage. By regulating blood pressure, adequate CPP can be maintained even when ICP is high. However, when ICP is too high or blood pressure is too low, CPP may drop, resulting in diffuse ischemic damage. In acute care management the goal is to lower ICP and keep CCP at or around 60 to 70 mmHg to optimize the rate of blood flow to the brain.

Cerebral vasospasm Acute narrowing of a cerebral blood vessel that reduces the blood flow and therefore increases risk for stroke.

Chelation therapy The use of a chemical substance to remove excess or toxic metals (e.g., lead, iron, copper, calcium, mercury) before they can damage the body. While there are benefits, there also are risks, including delay of a possibly more effective treatment, hypocalcemia, kidney damage, and even death.

Chest tube A large tube inserted through the skin into the lungs. The chest tube removes air or blood that impairs breathing and can cause lung collapse.

Chorea A type of movement that involves involuntary, intermittent, and irregular jerky movements of various muscle groups (e.g., arms, legs, trunk, neck). Associated with movement disorders and conditions affecting the basal ganglia (e.g., Huntington's disease). Like other movement disorders, the abnormal activity subsides during sleep.

Chronic obstructive pulmonary disease (COPD) A chronic illness that includes multiple types of pulmonary disease (e.g., asthma, emphysema, chronic bronchitis, or a combination) in which there is progressive obstruction of expiration upon breathing, which can lead to shortness of breath and fatigue. COPD can produce chronic hypoxia and, depending on the severity, may result in cognitive impairment.

Circulatory death One of two kinds of death recognized by law in the United States. It represents extensive and permanent loss of heart and/or lung function. If a patient is not on a ventilator, breathing and the beating of the heart will stop. Some people with nonsurvivable injuries to the brain never meet full criteria for brain death because they retain some minor brain stem function. In these circumstances donation after circulatory death might be an option. The option of donating organs after circulatory death may be presented to families after it is clear that the patient cannot survive. Donation in such cases entails taking the patient off ventilated support. Once the patient's heart stops beating, the physician declares the patient dead and organs can be removed for transplant (aka "donation after circulatory death").

Clinical Institute Withdrawal Assessment for Alcohol (CIWA) A 10-item scale used in the assessment and management of alcohol withdrawal. The maximum score is 67. Mild alcohol withdrawal is defined as a score of 10 or less, moderate 11 to 15, and severe 16 or more. A CIWA protocol is a symptom-driven protocol in which patients receive medications when withdrawal symptoms worsen. Symptom-triggered benzodiazepine dosing has been associated with shorter duration of treatment and lower medication use compared with fixed-schedule dosing.

Clonus Rapid, repetitive, involuntary muscle contraction and relaxation. Clonus can occur in a wide variety of conditions (e.g., movement disorders, seizures, hyperactive tendon reflexes).

Comorbidity The presence of one or more additional diseases or disorders co-occurring (i.e., concurrent) with a primary disease or disorder. Patients on the ICU commonly have a number of comorbid conditions.

Concussion grading Multiple grading systems for mild traumatic brain injury (mTBI) have been proposed, but there is controversy regarding their value because they do not significantly assist in predicting outcome or necessarily modifying the treatment plan. For example, presence/absence of loss of consciousness was initially included in several grading systems but has been de-emphasized because of its inconsistent relationship with outcome.

Continuous positive airway pressure (CPAP) Delivery of air to the lungs with slight pressure in an effort to prevent the airways from narrowing or closing. CPAP can be administered through a mask and is often used for treatment of obstructive sleep apnea (OSA). This term is used interchangeably with PEEP, though there are different mechanisms for each (e.g., MV for PEEP).

Continuous renal replacement therapy (CRRT) Dialysis that runs 24 hours a day (vs. "regular" dialysis, which runs 3 to 4 hours a day). It is the preferred type of dialysis in the ICU because it is gentler on the body.

Critical care Field of medical practice focused on conditions that require close, constant care by a team of specially trained clinicians, typically in an intensive care setting.

Critical care nurse A highly skilled nurse who provides all aspects of care for very ill patients. This nurse helps all of the people involved, which can facilitate decision-making and coordination between the patient, family, and care team. A registered nurse who is certified by the American Association of Critical-Care Nurses in critical care is known as a CCRN.

Critical illness A condition in which life cannot be sustained without invasive therapeutic intervention. It is characterized by acute loss of physiologic reserve and can last hours to months depending on the underlying pathophysiology and response to treatment. Critical illnesses often affect multiple organ systems, including pulmonary, cardiovascular, renal, gastrointestinal, neurologic, and endocrine. Underlying contributory factors include but are not limited to infection, major trauma, burns, inhalation injury, embolism, poisoning, radiation, and cancers. Although high morbidity and mortality rates are associated with critical illnesses, more and more people are surviving, and this, in turn, can lead to a host of long-term physical, cognitive, and emotional complications (see *postintensive care syndrome [PICS]*).

Critical illness myopathy (aka ICU-acquired weakness) Diffuse, symmetric, generalized muscle weakness detected by physical examination and meeting specific strength-related criteria (namely, inability to overcome resistance on manual muscle strength testing) that develops after critical illness onset without other identifiable cause.

Decannulation The process of removing a tracheostomy once the patient no longer needs it. This is typically considered once the patient:

1. Is alert and responds to commands (preferably oriented but not always necessary)
2. No longer depends on a ventilator for assisted breathing
3. Requires infrequent tracheal suctioning (typically less than once a day) and is able to manage their oral secretions without risk of aspiration
4. Can tolerate a downsized tube and capping without respiratory difficulty or suctioning.

Deep tendon reflexes Muscular contractions that occur in response to the stretching of a muscle.

Defibrillator A machine that sends an electrical charge through the chest to the heart in order to restart the heart or stop an abnormal rhythm. *Defibrillation* is the act of electrically shocking the heart

Delayed post-hypoxic leukoencephalopathy (DPHL) An uncommon condition following anoxic/hypoxic brain injury in which there is initially good recovery and return to near or full independence, followed days or weeks later by abrupt onset of marked neurologic and cognitive decline.

Delirium A reversible, acute-onset syndrome that typically develops suddenly over a short period of time and results in transient global cognitive dysfunction that represents a change from baseline. (See Chapter 6 for more detail.)

Delirium tremens (DTs; aka severe Wernicke's encephalopathy) An extreme form of alcohol withdrawal characterized by global confusion, autonomic hyperactivity, hallucinations, agitation, and/or seizures. DTs are always a medical emergency because if not addressed they can result in death, myocardial infarction, stroke, seizures, and other serious complications. The cause is chronic alcohol use with marked thiamine deficiency. Despite overuse in the literature and medical records, DTs occur in only 5% to 10% of patients with alcohol withdrawal syndrome. In rare cases, DTs can last up to 2 weeks, but they usually subside within 5 days. Some patients who survive DTs experience a persistent major neurocognitive disorder, Wernicke–Korsakoff syndrome.

Dialysis A way to clean a patient's blood when their kidneys are no longer able to do so. It involves removing waste from the blood with special medical equipment. There are two general types of dialysis: hemodialysis and peritoneal dialysis. In hemodialysis, the blood is pumped out of the body and into an external machine and then returned to the body via tubes. In peritoneal dialysis, the inside lining of the patient's own belly acts as a natural filtration system.

Dialysis catheter A tube placed in the groin or neck that connects to a machine. The tube and machine work together to clean the patient's blood when their kidneys are not able to do so.

Diffuse axonal injury (DAI) or traumatic axonal injury Caused by the stretching of myelinated axons between brain tissues of differing densities (e.g., gray–white matter junction). DAI is strongly related to the effects of secondary injury, such as deleterious biochemical and metabolic cascades, and not just the primary injury. In other words, DAI evolves over time. Advanced magnetic resonance imaging (MRI) techniques (e.g., diffusion tensor and weighted susceptibility imaging) show some promise in evaluating the extent of DAI, although they are not available in all settings and no cross-validated criteria have yet been established. DAI is not observable on conventional MRI or computed tomography (CT) scans because axons cannot be viewed with neuroimaging. Technically speaking, DAI is a neuropathologic diagnosis confirmed via microscopic analysis on autopsy.

Donation after cardiac death (DCD) A process that occurs when the patient meets the criteria for circulatory death and the family has elected to donate their organs after the removal of life support.

Do-not-attempt-resuscitation order (DNAR or DNR) Explicit written instructions in the medical chart written by the clinician but based on patient request. The order tells the care team not to attempt cardiopulmonary resuscitation (CPR) if the patient's heart stops. It reflects a choice to forgo CPR but agree to all other appropriate medical treatments. (Also see *advance directive*, as this term may be used depending on the state where the patient is hospitalized.)

Drip A bag of fluids, medications, or nutrients that go into the vein to help the patient get better. The bag runs constantly on a pump.

Durable power of attorney (DPOA) A legal document that gives another person the power to make decisions about the patient's medical treatment. The person is granted this power only if the patient becomes too ill to make decisions on their own. The document typically includes (1) a sworn, signed statement from the patient that confirms who will make the decisions; (2) a list of medical treatments the patient desires and under what circumstances; (3) the name and contact information of the appointed decision-maker and two other people if the original person is not able to make the decisions; and (4) the amount of time for which the person will have this duty.

Dysarthria A speech articulation disorder caused by impaired muscular control due to damage to the central or peripheral nervous system. There are several types, including spastic, hyperkinetic, hypokinetic, and ataxic dysarthria, reflecting damage to different regions of the brain. Dysarthria is distinct from verbal or oral apraxia, which is always due to central nervous system (CNS) damage and is a higher-order speech problem characterized by impaired sequencing of the muscles used in speech (tongue, lips, jaw muscles, vocal cords).

Dysdiadochokinesia Impaired ability to smoothly alternate hand movements.

Dysmetria Inaccurate range of movement during motion-based activities.

Dyspnea Shortness of breath; the patient may experience chest tightness, inability to breathe deeply, or "air hunger."

Early mobility Physical activity, range of motion, and mobility that occurs within 24 to 48 hours after ICU admission. Mobilizing patients who are critically ill, and often mechanically ventilated, in the ICU has been shown to reduce complications such as neuromuscular weakness and delirium. However, this has not yet become common practice in ICUs across the United States.

Emergency department (ED) A place where clinicians evaluate and attempt to stabilize the patient, often before transport to the ICU or another hospital unit for further treatment.

Encephalomyelitis Inflammation of the brain and spinal cord.

Encephalopathy A disorder or disease of the brain characterized by significant global cognitive dysfunction. The term can be used to describe both reversible/acute and chronic/permanent conditions. Consequently, in the medical literature, it has been used to describe a wide variety of brain disorders with very different etiologies, prognoses, and implications.

End-of-life care Medical care that a very ill patient receives when they will not regain health. Most ICUs have specific policies, procedures, and protocols in place for this type of care. The goal of end-of-life care is to make sure the patient experiences as much dignity and proper pain management during the transition toward death. End-of-life care can take place in the hospital, at home, or in a hospice unit (see also *palliative care*).

Endotracheal tube (ETT) A tube that is inserted through the mouth or nose and connected to a machine to help the patient breathe. Oxygen moves from the machine, through the tube, into the lungs, and throughout the body.

Epidural (extradural) hematoma (EDH) Hematoma caused by rupture of arteries between the skull and dura. Because of the high pressure in arteries, bleeding into the epidural space can result in a rapidly expanding hematoma that causes compression of brain tissue, which in turn can lead to tentorial herniation and death. Outcome from EDH has a somewhat binomial distribution, with some patients recovering similar to mild TBI if the EDH is evacuated quickly versus high morbidity and mortality if the patient does not receive timely neurosurgical management.

Extracorporeal membrane oxygenation (ECMO) A type of life support machine used during life-threatening conditions such as severe lung or cardiac injury or illness. The ECMO machine is connected to a patient through various cannulas placed in large veins and arteries in the legs, neck, or chest. The machine pumps blood into an artificial lung (i.e., oxygenator) that adds oxygen and removes carbon dioxide. It then pumps the blood back into the patient, thus replacing heart function.

Extubation Removal of an endotracheal tube following mechanical ventilation.

Facilitated sensemaking A theory proposing that clinicians can impact the period of adjustment beginning in the ICU to optimize the perceived experience, the family's ability to support the patient, and the family's ability to participate in decision-making and eventually to optimize emotional adjustment after the ICU. Clinicians can help family members to make sense of their role as caregivers while also making sense of what is happening during the period of critical illness or injury.

FiO$_2$ Fraction of inspired oxygen; the concentration of oxygen supplied by a mask or catheter during mechanical ventilation. Initial levels are higher than those supplied by "room air" and attempts are made to titrate down throughout the course of mechanical ventilation.

Fistula An abnormal connection between two hollow spaces (technically, two epithelialized surfaces), such as blood vessels, intestines, or other hollow organs. Fistulas are usually caused by injury or surgery, but they can also result from an infection or inflammation.

Foley catheter (aka urinary catheter) A tube inserted into the bladder and kept in place by a balloon. The urinary catheter drains the bladder and helps the care team measure how much urine the patient is producing. It helps them determine if that amount is normal or if the patient's kidneys are dysfunctional.

Forced expiratory volume (FEV) Measures how much air a person can exhale during a forced breath. It is measured during spirometry and is the most important measurement of lung function. It is used to diagnose disorders such as asthma and chronic obstructive pulmonary disease, to determine the effectiveness of medications, and to determine whether lung disease is worsening.

Glasgow Coma Scale (GCS) A scale that assesses responsiveness in patients who have sustained brain injury. There are three parameters: eye opening, motor response, and verbal response. The scale ranges from 3 to 15, with scores of 8 or less suggesting severe injury and scores over 13 associated with mild injuries. In severe TBI, a lower GCS score (3 to 5) is associated with increased mortality rates. GCS is not very robust in the prediction of long-term outcome following TBI because it can be affected by factors that are not related to the brain injury, such as intoxication, intubation, patient age, iatrogenic medication effects, and polytrauma.

Glutamate The most common excitatory neurotransmitter in the brain. When the brain is injured, excessive amounts of glutamate can be released into the synaptic cleft; this results in an excitotoxic state that in turn contributes to further deleterious processes in the neuron.

Hallucinations Hearing, seeing, feeling, smelling, or tasting things that are not physically present. In delirium, visual hallucinations are the most common, but auditory, tactile, olfactory, and somatosensory hallucinations have also been observed. In psychiatric illness, auditory hallucinations are more common and they are often consistent across time, without the waxing and waning commonly observed in delirium.

Health care–associated infections (HAIs) Infections that people acquire while receiving treatment for another condition in a health care setting. HAIs affect approximately one in every 20 patients in a hospital setting. They cost the U.S. health care system billions of dollars annually and are associated with increased mortality. They are considered preventable, and health care systems are increasingly being held accountable, or penalized, when they occur.

Heart monitor Machine used to monitor heart rate and rhythm. The leads—small pads on the patient's chest—are clipped onto wires connected to the monitor, which is located at the side or head of the bed.

Hepatic encephalopathy A type of delirium that occurs as the result of liver failure and/or dysfunction. When the liver begins to fail, toxic substances such as ammonia accumulate in the bloodstream. This condition is commonly treated with lactulose or other drugs that suppress the production of toxic substances in the intestine. When left untreated, it typically leads to coma and then death.

Hyperalgesia Increased sensitivity to pain.

Hypercapnia Abnormally elevated carbon dioxide (CO_2) levels in the blood. Also termed hypercarbia. Some people with lung diseases, such as chronic obstructive pulmonary disease, are unable to breathe in all the oxygen they need and expel carbon dioxide, resulting in respiratory failure.

Hypernatremia An electrolyte disturbance in which the sodium concentration in the serum is abnormally high (>145 mmol/L). Typically caused by dehydration or conditions that result in excessive water loss (e.g., diarrhea, gastroenteritis). Hypernatremia can cause cerebral dehydration, resulting in subsequent delirium.

Hyponatremia An electrolyte disturbance in which the sodium concentration in the serum falls below 135 mmol/L. It commonly occurs when water accumulates in the body at a faster rate than it can be excreted (e.g., polydipsia, congestive heart failure, syndrome of inappropriate antidiuretic hormone [SIADH]). The condition can lead to cerebral edema. Approximately 25% of cases are postoperative.

Hypothalamic–pituitary–adrenal (HPA) axis A collection of structures involved in regulating the stress response, including the periventricular nucleus of the hypothalamus, the anterior lobe of the pituitary gland, and the adrenal gland.

Hypoxemia Low oxygen concentration in the blood. It can cause mild (e.g., headaches, shortness of breath) to more severe (e.g., cardiovascular, brain-related) problems. Hypoxemia that causes low oxygen levels in the tissues is called *hypoxia*.

Ictus A sudden neurologic occurrence, such as a seizure. Ictal behaviors, or behavior changes that occur during a seizure, are often considered important lateralizing and localizing signs. *Interictal* refers to the period between seizures; for example, interictal electroencephalographic (EEG) abnormalities are changes in the EEG pattern that occur between seizures and may be helpful in localizing regions of hyperexcitability and/or seizure onset. *Postictal* refers to the period of time after a seizure occurs, as in postictal confusion or drowsiness.

Illusions (aka misperceptions) Misinterpretations of real stimuli, typically visual or auditory. Sometimes observed in the course of delirium.

Incapacitated Unable to perform a function that involves the body, thoughts, feelings, or mind (e.g., being unaware of one's surroundings).

Infarct Area of necrotic tissue resulting from obstruction of local blood supply or ischemia (e.g., by thrombus or embolus).

Informed consent A process in which patients are provided with appropriate and balanced information that allows them to make an informed choice to consent to or refuse a specific treatment. Clinicians are ethically obligated to explain the risks and benefits of treatment and must obtain informed consent before starting any treatment. For patient who do not have capacity to provide consent, a medical decision-maker must be identified.

Intensive care unit (ICU) The setting or venue where critical care is provided. There are various kinds of ICUs, including a burn or trauma unit, coronary care unit (CCU), critical care unit (CCU), medical intensive care unit (MICU), neonatal intensive care unit (NICU), neurosurgery intensive care unit (NSICU or Neuro ICU), pediatric intensive care unit (PICU), and surgical intensive care unit (SICU).

Intensivist A physician trained in critical care medicine; typically an expert in a specific specialty (e.g., surgery, internal medicine, pediatrics, anesthesiology).

Intra-aortic balloon pump A machine that helps a weak heart pump blood throughout the body. The machine has a tube that goes into the body's main artery, and the tube has a balloon that inflates and deflates to match the natural beating of the heart.

Intracranial pressure (ICP) Pressure within the skull. The intact cranium, vertebral canal, and dura are relatively inelastic, so an increase in the size of any of the contents (brain tissue, blood, or cerebrospinal fluid [CSF]) will increase ICP. ICP is measured by recording the subarachnoid fluid pressure. Increased ICP can be caused by a rise in CSF pressure due to blockage of CSF flow or by increased pressure within the brain caused by a mass lesion, edema, or bleeding. Elevated ICP can lead to brain damage as the result of reduced cerebral perfusion and brain ischemia. Common signs/symptoms of increased ICP include headache, altered mental status, nausea and vomiting, papilledema (engorgement and elevation of the optic disc), visual loss, diplopia, and Cushing's triad (hypertension, bradycardia, and irregular respiration).

Intracranial pressure catheter A small tube placed into the brain that can be used to monitor intracranial pressure and, if necessary, to drain excess cerebrospinal fluid.

Intrathecal chemotherapy Delivery of therapeutic agents directly into the cerebrospinal fluid surrounding the brain and spinal cord. This method of delivery is used to circumvent the blood–brain barrier and is administered via lumbar puncture.

Intravenous feeding (aka intravenous catheter, IV) Delivery of liquid nutrients into a vein (typically in the arm or neck) when the patient cannot eat and is not a candidate for tube feeding. This occurs when the patient's gastrointestinal system is dysfunctional or too severely damaged to digest nutrients.

Intravenous therapy Giving the patient fluids, medications, or nutrients through a tube in a vein. Some patients need this therapy once, and other patients need it nonstop.

Intubation Insertion of a tube into the body. In endotracheal intubation, a tube is inserted through the mouth down into the trachea so that air can flow freely into and out of the lungs to facilitate breathing. Intubation also permits use of a mechanical ventilator for patients who cannot breathe on their own.

Ischemia Insufficient blood supply to an organ, usually due to a blocked artery.

Ischemic-hypoxic encephalopathy The encephalopathy resulting from the combined effects of anoxia/hypoxia and ischemia. In their purest presentations, anoxia/hypoxia and ischemia may produce somewhat different neuropathology, but most cases in which the brain sustains marked disruption of oxygen supply involve both processes.

Isolation/infection control Procedures used to avoid the spread of infection. The critical care population is much more susceptible to infection for a variety of reasons, including underlying disease, invasive procedures used in their care (e.g., catheters and mechanical ventilators), frequency of contact with health care personnel, prolonged length of stay, and prolonged exposure to antimicrobial agents. Although ICUs account for a relatively small proportion of hospitalized patients, infections acquired in these units account for over 20% of all hospital-acquired infections. All providers working on the ICU should be familiar with isolation and infection control practices, including how infectious agents can be transmitted and how to protect staff and patients.

Kindling The development of an epileptogenic network by exposure to recurrent seizures. Can occur in homologous areas of the contralateral hemisphere or within the same hemisphere as seizure onset through repetitive spread of seizures to areas of the brain functionally connected to the epileptogenic cortex.

Life support The use of specialized medical equipment or treatment that maintains essential physiologic functions (e.g., breathing, circulation). Life support can fully replace or support a function. The length of time a patient is on life support varies widely based upon the underlying pathology and response to treatment.

Long-tract signs Neurologic signs related to upper motor neuron lesions, including hyperactive deep tendon reflexes, clonus, and spasticity.

Lower motor neuron (LMN) Motor neurons that originate in the anterior horn of the spinal cord. The motor cranial nerve nuclei are also classified as LMNs.

Mass effect Distortion of brain anatomy due to a mass lesion such as an epidural hematoma, subdural hematoma, abscess, or tumor. Mass effect often involves compression of a lateral ventricle, and if neurosurgical intervention does not happen promptly, brain herniation and death may occur.

Mechanical ventilation (MV) A lifesaving procedure used to address respiratory failure. The mechanical ventilator is a machine that makes it easier for patients to breathe until they are able to breathe on their own. MV addresses several critical respiratory functions: (1) improvement of pulmonary gas exchange during acute hypoxemic or hypercapnic respiratory failure with respiratory acidosis and (2) redistribution of blood flow from working respiratory muscles to other vital organs, thus aiding in the management of shock from any cause. Although lifesaving, MV also can lead to complications and thus should be removed as early as it is feasible.

Medical safety device (aka restraints) Patients in the ICU, especially those with delirium, are at risk for hurting themselves by pulling at lines and tubes, falling out of bed, scratching or picking at wounds and or dressings, and so forth. In these situations, the least restrictive medical safety device and/or other option (e.g., medication) should be used and the need for, and effectiveness of, a restraint should be reassessed throughout the day. When restraints are used as the last option, they can include hand mitts, Posey vest, enclosure bed, or wrist restraints. Restraints can agitate and even unintentionally harm patients. State laws require close monitoring and provide specific guidelines regarding use.

Minimally responsive state (aka minimally conscious state) State that occurs after the patient emerges from coma and regains lower levels of consciousness but remains unaware of their surroundings. The patient cannot follow motor commands but may spontaneously open their eyes, display facial expressions, moan, or the like. These are non-purposeful, automatic functions. As coma and minimally conscious states evolve, the patient may move into what some refer to as an unresponsive wakefulness syndrome in which they display some arousal but with no evidence of environmental awareness. Patients may open their eyes, yawn, and regain fairly normal-appearing sleep–wake cycles, which may give the false impression that the patient has regained some level of conscious awareness. This is commonly referred to as coma vigil.

Multiple organ dysfunction syndrome (MODS) (aka multiple organ failure [MOF], total organ failure [TOF], or multisystem organ failure [MSOF]) A serious medical situation in which multiple organs in the body begin to fail. The condition can be caused by factors such as sepsis, polytrauma, hypoxia/hypoperfusion, and hypermetabolism. Patients typically require life support or, if the condition is not reversible, palliative care.

Myocardial infarction (MI) (aka heart attack) A medical event that occurs when arterial blood flow to part of the heart stops or substantially decreases, causing ischemia and damage. An MI is typically caused by the blockage of an artery.

Nasogastric tube (NG tube) A tube placed into the nose, down the throat, and into the stomach that is used to feed the patient or remove acid, fluids, or blood from the stomach. NG tubes are also sometimes used to treat drug overdoses and poisonings.

Necrosis Death of tissue, typically due to insufficient blood supply or trauma.

Neuroleptic malignant syndrome (NMS) A rare complication following neuroleptic use (i.e., antipsychotic medication) marked by muscle rigidity, pallor, dyskinesia, hyperthermia, incontinence, unstable blood pressure, tachycardia, and pulmonary congestion. Treatment requires discontinuation of neuroleptics, intravenous hydration, and close monitoring of vital signs and mental status.

Neurometabolic cascade Following brain injury, a process of ionic shifts, impaired neuronal function and connectivity, altered brain metabolism, disruption of normal brain function/signal transmission, and indiscriminate neurotransmitter release can occur. In mild brain injury a gradual reversal to normal function typically occurs within days or weeks following injury. In moderate to severe brain injury, this cascade often leads to secondary injury and additional cell loss.

Nonbeneficial care or intervention (aka medical futility) Interventions that are unlikely to produce any significant benefit for the patient. Two kinds of nonbeneficial care are often distinguished: (1) quantitative futility, where the likelihood that an intervention will benefit the patient is exceedingly poor, and (2) qualitative futility, where the quality of benefit an intervention will produce is exceedingly poor. Both types refer to the prospect that a specific treatment will meaningfully benefit the patient and not simply have a physiologic effect. It is important to recognize that nonbeneficial care does not broadly refer to all treatments; instead, it should be used to describe or refer to a particular intervention at a specific time and for a specific reason. For example, "Continuation of that medication would not be beneficial for this patient at this time."

Noninvasive mechanical ventilation (NIV) Assisted ventilation delivered through a mask rather than an endotracheal tube. Patients with hypercapnic forms of respiratory failure are more likely to benefit, though those with hypoxic respiratory failure might also benefit. NIV allows patients to take deeper breaths with less effort.

Nonpenetrating traumatic brain injury A brain injury in which the dura and skull remain intact (also see *acceleration/deceleration injuries*). In the past the term "closed-head injury" was used, but this has steadily fallen out of favor for the more precise term because not all head injuries result in brain injury.

Pacemaker A machine that electrically stimulates the heart in order to maintain a normal or healthy rhythm. The pacemaker may be surgically placed under the skin for a short amount of time or for the rest of the patient's life.

Palliative care End-of-life care is a form of palliative care, but they are not the same thing. Patients can receive palliative care at any time during their illness, but end-of-life care is comfort for the dying patient. (See the World Health Organization's definition of adult and pediatric palliative care.)

Paralytic agent A drug used to prevent movement, often during the placement of lifesaving lines and tubes or to prevent patients from accidentally hurting themselves. Additional medications are typically given with the paralytic to relax patients when they are not able to move. The effect of this drug can be reversed.

Paraneoplastic syndrome (aka paraneoplastic neurologic disorder) Neurologic complications of systemic cancer caused by an immune reaction to antigens expressed by tumors and common to the nervous system; associated with several different antineural antibodies.

Partial pressure of arterial oxygen (PaO$_2$) The pressure exerted independently by a specific gas within a larger mix of gases. The PaO$_2$ in healthy adults at sea level is typically 95 to 100 mmHg. When this level rapidly drops, complex cognitive processes, memory, and judgment become impaired.

Penetrating traumatic brain injury An injury in which there is a breach of the dura mater. Examples include depressed skull fracture or gunshot wound to the head. Patients who sustain penetrating injuries are often at higher risk for certain complications, such as seizures and infection, due to blood–brain barrier compromise. In the past the term "open-head injury" was used, but this has steadily fallen out of favor for the more precise term.

Peripherally inserted central catheter (PICC) A catheter placed into a large vein in the arm. A PICC can stay in for days or weeks, as long as it shows no signs of infection.

Personal protective equipment (PPE) Specialized clothing and/or equipment worn by a hospital employee to protect against infection. In the ICU setting PPE includes gloves, gowns, masks, and the like.

Phrenic nerve A nerve that originates in the cervical region (C3–C5) and passes through the lungs and heart to reach the diaphragm. It is important for breathing function. Damage to the phrenic nerve has been associated with prolonged hospitalization and need for mechanical ventilation.

Positive end expiratory pressure (PEEP) Pressure that is applied during MV at the end of expiration to maintain alveolar recruitment; used interchangeably with continuous positive airway pressure (CPAP).

Postintensive care syndrome (PICS) New or worsening impairments in physical, cognitive, or mental health status arising after critical illness and persisting beyond acute care hospitalization. Given the high frequency with which patients experience multiple issues across domains following critical illness, the Society for Critical Care Medicine coined this term in 2010.

Posttraumatic amnesia (PTA) (aka posttraumatic confusion) PTA has been defined differently by various researchers. According to the original definition, PTA is the amount of time following brain injury that an individual remains confused and is not able to demonstrate continuous memory, including any time spent in coma. Newer definitions include the period of confusion following brain injury but do not count any period of unconsciousness or coma. This second iteration has been frequently called posttraumatic confusion (PTC). Either definition can be used. PTA is best tracked prospectively via serial testing with instruments like the Orientation Log or Children's Orientation and Amnesia Test. Relative to other outcome predictors in traumatic brain injury, such as the Glasgow Coma Scale score or time to follow commands, length of PTA is considered to be the most robust. Even so, there is no consensus regarding injury severity classification based on PTA alone. For example, some early methods classified 1 to 7 days of PTA as severe, but more recent studies have revealed that adult patients with less than 14 days of PTA often experience good functional outcomes within 1 year after the injury.

Posttraumatic seizures (PTS) Seizures following nonpenetrating brain injury are relatively uncommon (5%) but are more frequent in children than adults. There are three types: *immediate* (within 24 hours), *early* (within 1–7 days), and *late* (>1 week following injury). Regardless, seizures in the first week following nonpenetrating brain injury are not predictive of long-term risk for epilepsy, and thus continued anticonvulsant prophylaxis is not typically recommended. Alternatively, penetrating brain injury and direct injury to the cortex is a significant risk factor for seizure (30–50%).

Posttraumatic stress disorder (PTSD) Disorder in which individuals who have survived a traumatic event (e.g., physical trauma, war exposures, sexual violence, critical illness) experience intrusive symptoms (e.g., nightmares, flashbacks) related to the trauma, avoidance, negative alterations in cognition and mood, and alterations in arousal and reactivity (e.g., heightened startle response). ICU-related risk factors for PTSD include longer duration of sedation, memories of adverse ICU experiences, and delirium. PTSD is not diagnosed until the symptoms have been present for at least 1 month.

Psychological first aid (PFA) Specific practices used during or after traumatic events in critical care settings with patients as well as staff. PFA is designed to be flexible and responsive to the specific needs of an individual at a particular time. The five principles of PFA are to create a sense of safety, calm, connectedness, confidence/control, and hope after a traumatic event. Key features that are relevant to ICU patients and families include contact and engagement, safety and comfort, stabilization, information gathering, practical assistance, connection with social supports, information on coping, and linkage with collaborative services. (See Chapters 4 and 16 for more detail.)

Pulse oximeter A small machine attached to the patient's finger, nose, or ear that detects the pulse and the oxygen levels in the blood.

Quadriparesis (aka tetraparesis) Weakness in all four limbs.

QT interval The time from the start of the Q wave to the end of the T wave, which represent the time it takes for ventricular depolarization and repolarization to occur. It is inversely associated with heart rate.

Renal failure (aka kidney failure) Failure of the kidneys to work properly. This typically leads to the buildup of fluids, resulting in edema and breathing problems. Because the kidneys are no longer filtering the blood, toxic material can build up as well, resulting in uremia. There are two types of renal failure: acute (sudden cessation of kidney function) and chronic (develops slowly over time).

Reperfusion injury A complex process following restoration of cerebral circulation that results in further damage to neurons. Reperfusion injury involves multiple processes such as edema and microhemorrhages, free radical formation and nitric oxide toxicity, further glutamate release, and others.

Respiratory acidosis Condition in which body fluids, especially blood, are too acidic because the lungs cannot remove all the carbon dioxide the body produces.

Respiratory alkalosis Condition in which levels of carbon dioxide in the blood are low due to excessive breathing.

Respiratory failure A syndrome of inadequate gas exchange due to dysfunction of one or more essential components of the respiratory system. This can lead to ICU admission or occur while on the ICU. Respiratory failure may be acute, chronic, or acute on chronic. There are two main types: (1) hypoxemic, which involves failure of oxygen exchange, and (2) hypercapnic, which involves failure to exchange or remove carbon dioxide.

Sarcopenia Loss of muscle tissue as a normal part of the aging process.

Sepsis A broad term used to describe a serious infection in the bloodstream or body tissues. It can be caused by numerous types of microscopic disease-causing organisms (e.g., bacteria, viruses, fungi). Sepsis is sometimes referred to as bacteremia and/or septic syndrome (septicemia is a rarely used term as well). Severe sepsis refers to a systemic infection coupled with organ dysfunction and has been most commonly associated with white matter and blood–brain barrier compromise. Ischemic and hemorrhagic lesions are observable on magnetic resonance imaging (MRI) in approximately 10% of patients, whereas postmortem studies have revealed ischemic lesions in the majority of cases.

Septic shock A life-threatening condition that happens when a systemic infection (i.e., sepsis) leads to dangerously low blood pressure, which can then cause respiratory or heart failure, stroke, and other organ failure. Septic shock is a common cause of death in critical care settings.

Serotonin syndrome Disorder typically caused by the conjoint use of multiple serotonergic agents. In the early stages, it can be marked by mental status changes, agitation, myoclonus, hyperreflexia, diaphoresis, tremor, diarrhea, incoordination, and fever. If left untreated and intake of the medications continues, death can occur. Treatment requires the discontinuation of all serotonergic drugs and close monitoring, with improvement expected within 24 hours.

Shock Body state when the organs do not get enough oxygen and then blood pressure drops. Some causes of shock include severe blood loss, myocardial infarction, sepsis, and massive trauma. If the critical care team is unable to reverse shock quickly, the patient's organs start to shut down. Symptoms of shock include confusion, cool and clammy skin, bluish lips, dizziness, sweating, and diaphoresis.

Spasticity Increased muscle tone or increased resistance to stretching, usually caused by damage to the portion of the brain or spinal cord that controls voluntary movement.

Spirometry Test that measures the amount of air a person's lungs can move in and out, and at what rate. The test is performed with a spirometer, a recording device attached to a mouthpiece.

Spontaneous awakening trial (SAT) Procedure conducted in patients receiving mechanical ventilation (MV) to determine whether they are ready for MV withdrawal. Reducing the length of time that a patient is on MV has been shown to reduce the risk of ventilator-associated pneumonia and other complications, and a protocol of coordinated SAT and spontaneous breathing trial (SBT) has been shown to significantly reduce the number of days of MV. First the patient must pass a safety screen that determines that it is safe to begin the SAT. Then all sedating medications are stopped. To be considered a successful trial, the patient must be able to do three out of four of the following tasks: open eyes, look at caregiver, squeeze a hand, and put out their tongue; or the patient can go at least 4 hours without sedation and experience all of the following: no sustained anxiety, agitation, or pain; respiratory rate of 35 breaths/minute or more for 5 minutes; oxygen saturation of more than 88% for at least 5 minutes; normal heart rhythm; and limited or no signs of respiratory distress. If a patient does not pass the SAT, then sedating medications are reinitiated at half the prior dose and titrated up as needed.

Spontaneous breathing trial (SBT) Procedure conducted in patients receiving mechanical ventilation (MV) to determine whether they are ready for MV withdrawal. The SBT is begun after the patient has passed a spontaneous awakening trial (SAT) and begins with a safety screen, which the patient must pass. If the patient does not pass the safety screen, then sedating medications are begun at half the prior dose and titrated up if needed. Then the patient is evaluated for another SAT on the following day. If the patient does pass the SBT, then the provider is notified and extubation is considered.

Subarachnoid hemorrhage (SAH) Hemorrhage that can arise from multiple sources, including brain injury, cerebral aneurysm, arteriovenous malformation, and high blood pressure. SAH is often associated with a poorer long-term outcome in patients with moderate to severe traumatic brain injury. Generally speaking, when blood directly contacts brain tissue, there are higher risks for complications and worsening secondary injury effects.

Subdural hematoma (SDH) Hematoma caused by rupture of bridging veins between sulci on the upper surface of the brain. In high-speed injuries, hematomas are commonly found in the frontal and anterior temporal lobes due to the skull and brain's anatomic arrangement. Older adults and pediatric patients are often at higher risk for SDH, but for different reasons (i.e., widening of the sulci in the elderly vs. unique anatomic features of the head, brain, and neck in young children).

Substance use disorder According to the National Institutes of Health, "a chronic, relapsing brain disorder characterized by compulsive drug seeking and use despite negative consequences." Patients with comorbid substance use disorders are commonly seen in the ICU. Some patients may experience a substance withdrawal syndrome, which further complicates recovery.

Surrogate decision-maker Someone who makes medical decisions on the patient's behalf, usually a family member or close friend. The surrogate must be trustworthy, responsible, and ready; must know the patient's personal values; and must consider the pros and cons of each treatment. If the patient has not chosen a surrogate before becoming ill, the choice is based on hospital policy and/or applicable laws.

Swan-Ganz catheter (aka pulmonary artery catheter) A large tube in the neck or upper chest that goes into the heart and is used to measure fluid levels in the heart and consequently aspects of heart function. Commonly placed after open heart surgery.

Symptom-driven protocols Brief protocols designed to be administered at the bedside to assess symptoms. An example is the Clinical Institute Withdrawal Assessment for Alcohol (CIWA), which is used to determine best treatment approaches for patients withdrawing from alcohol.

Systemic inflammatory response syndrome (SIRS) A sepsis-like disorder that occurs in the absence of infection. Both SIRS and sepsis can ultimately progress to multiple organ dysfunction syndrome.

Tachypnea Elevated respiratory rate (i.e., breathing more rapidly than "normal").

Tidal volume The volume of gas inhaled and exhaled during one respiratory cycle.

Time to follow commands (TFC) The amount of time following acquired brain injury in which the patient is unable to follow simple motor commands and is unable to maintain arousal or awareness. It is also referred to as length of coma, although this is problematic because after several days or weeks surviving in coma, individuals typically progress to a different level of consciousness (e.g., sleep–wake cycles reemerge, may open eyes but remain minimally responsive, electroencephalographic [EEG] patterns change or evolve). Clinicians are now using other terms to describe this state, such as minimally responsive, minimally conscious, and unresponsive wakefulness syndrome. The assessment of TFC can be challenging because it must take into account the impact of sedation and paralytics. Emergence from a minimally responsive state corresponds to a score of 6 on the Motor subscale of the Glasgow Coma Scale.

Tissue plasminogen activator (tPA) The only acute anticoagulant treatment recommended by the U.S. Food and Drug Administration (FDA) for adult ischemic stroke if the patient (1) can be treated within 3 to 4.5 hours of symptom onset, (2) has significant deficits on the NIH Stroke Scale, and (3) has no evidence of hemorrhage on neuroimaging. Although clinicians typically use the 3- to 4.5-hour timeframe, FDA guidelines endorse the 3-hour time window.

Tracheostomy (aka tracheotomy) A surgical procedure performed to create an opening through the neck into the trachea for patients who are unable to breathe on their own. A temporary or permanent tube is then placed in the neck opening. This procedure is usually employed in patients who are expected to be on a mechanical ventilator for an extended time. Endotracheal tubes can cause injury over time, and after placement, a tracheostomy is less distressing and can be more easily maintained long term.

Tube feeding Giving food in the form of liquid through a tube, either from the nose to the stomach or through the skin directly into the stomach or intestines. Patients need tube feedings when they are not able to eat or obtain nutrients in another way. Tube feeding is safer and less expensive than intravenous feeding, but the patient must have a functional gastrointestinal system.

Upper motor neuron (UMN) Neurons that originate from the brain's primary motor cortex (i.e., the precentral gyrus) or from certain brain stem nuclei (e.g., the rubrospinal tract from the red nucleus).

Uremia A clinical syndrome marked by elevated concentrations of urea in the blood; most commonly develops in the context of chronic kidney disease (CKD).

Vasculitis Inflammation of blood vessels, which can lead to narrowing of the vessel, blood clot formation, or aneurysm formation due to weakening of the vessel wall, all of which increase the probability of stroke.

Vasculopathy General term used to describe any disease affecting the blood vessels; includes vascular abnormalities caused by a number of conditions and disorders (e.g., degenerative, metabolic, and inflammatory conditions; embolic diseases; coagulative disorders).

Vasopressor (aka pressor) A powerful drug that causes blood vessels to become smaller, consequently raising the patient's blood pressure.

Ventriculostomy A medical procedure in which a tube is placed through the skull, through the brain, and into the lateral ventricle. This allows intracranial pressure to be measured and extra fluid or blood to be removed if necessary.

Viral fatigue The persistent symptoms of exhaustion, low endurance, headache, and other generalized symptoms that can persist for days, weeks, or even months following resolution of a viral infection.

Vital signs (aka vitals) Assessment of the four life-sustaining functions: body temperature, blood pressure, pulse (heart rate), respiratory rate. These measurements can help determine the patient's general physical health, assist with differential diagnosis, or reveal responses to treatment. Vital signs may vary with age, weight, gender, and health status.

Watershed region Overlapping border zones in the brain between the distal supplies of two arteries that are particularly vulnerable to the effects of hypoxia/ischemia. For example, the region supplied by the distal branches of the middle and anterior cerebral arteries is a watershed region.

Weaning Process of slowly reducing the amount of breathing assistance provided by the ventilator. Weaning is done slowly so that if problems occur, ventilator settings can be quickly adjusted.

Wound therapy Medical treatment used to address large ulcers or injuries, typically involving the skin. Specialists clean and apply medication to the wound. In some cases physicians order negative-pressure wound therapy, also known as a vacuum dressing. This technique uses a sealed dressing with a suction that removes excess exudate and promotes healing. This is often used in large or chronic wounds that are not expected to respond favorably to traditional wound therapy (e.g., diabetic ulcers, open abdomen after laparotomy).

Index

For the benefit of digital users, indexed terms that span two pages (e.g., 52–53) may, on occasion, appear on only one of those pages.

Notes: Figures and tables are indicated by *f* and *t* following the page numbers. Numbers followed by n. indicate footnotes.

CPSIA information can be obtained
at www.ICGtesting.com
Printed in the USA
BVHW090929180922
646932BV00003B/4